Nutrition For Dummies®
2nd Edition

W9-BWB-009

Measurements Used in Nutrition

Abbreviation	Measurement	Equivalent
g	gram	1,000 milligrams
		1,000,000 micrograms
mg	milligram	$^{1}/_{1,000}$ gram
mcg	microgram	$^{1}/_{1,000,000}$ gram
kg	kilogram	1,000 grams
		2.2 pounds
lb	pound	45 kilograms
		16 ounces
l	liter	1,000 milliliters
		10 deciliters
dl	deciliter	$^{1}/_{10}$ liter
ml	milliliter	$^{1}/_{1,000}$ liter

Key Elements Used in Nutrition Words

Element	Meaning
Amyl-	starch
An-	without
Anti-	against
-ase	an enzyme
Di-	two
-emia	found in the blood
gastro-	referring to the stomach
Gly-	referring to sugars
Hydr-, hydro-	water (also: hydrogen)
Hyper-	above normal
Hypo-	below normal
Lact-, lacti-, lacto-	milk
Lip-, lipo-	fat
Macro-	large
Micro-	very small
Mono-	one
-ose	sugar
Tri-	three

Easy ways to cut calories

- ✔ Use lowfat or no-fat dairy products
- ✔ Use sugar substitutes instead of sugar
- ✔ Skim the fat off all soups and stews
- ✔ Choose lowfat desserts
- ✔ Serve poultry without skin
- ✔ Avoid high-fat, oily salad dressings
- ✔ Make open-face sandwiches, with just one slice of bread
- ✔ Eliminate high-fat ingredients in any dish
- ✔ Don't butter the veggies
- ✔ Rinse the fat off chopped meat with hot water

Nutrition For Dummies, 2nd Edition

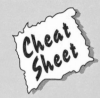

Cheat Sheet

When you may need extra nutrients

- ✔ When you are pregnant, you need extra amounts of some vitamins, minerals, and protein to meet the needs of the growing fetus.

  Ditto for when you are nursing your baby.

- ✔ Some medicines reduce your body's ability to absorb and use certain vitamins and minerals. When your doctor writes a prescription, ask her if you need supplements.

- ✔ Do you smoke? Then you use up more vitamin C than non-smokers.

- ✔ Are you a woman approaching menopause? Time for extra calcium to maintain healthy bones.

  Older men also need extra calcium.

- ✔ Is your diet strictly vegetarian — meaning no food of animal origin, not even milk and eggs? You need extra vitamin B12. You may also need extra calcium and iron.

How to keep food safe as well as nutritious

- ✔ Wash your hands before (and after) touching food.

- ✔ Wash all fruits and vegetables before you use them.

- ✔ Follow the directions on the food package for storing and preparing food safely.

- ✔ Handle all raw meat, fish, and poultry as though it were contaminated (often, it is!).

- ✔ Cook foods thoroughly.

- ✔ Keep hot foods hot, cold foods cold.

- ✔ Never eat or drink anything containing raw eggs.

- ✔ Keep your sponge dry. Better yet, microwave it.

- ✔ Use a separate cutting board for raw meat, fish, and poultry.

- ✔ Never taste any questionable food "just to be sure it's all right." When in doubt, throw it out.

The 18 essential vitamins and minerals

- ✔ Vitamin A
- ✔ Vitamin D
- ✔ Vitamin E
- ✔ Vitamin K
- ✔ Vitamin C
- ✔ Thiamin (vitamin B1)
- ✔ Riboflavin (vitamin B2)
- ✔ Niacin
- ✔ Vitamin B6

- ✔ Folate
- ✔ Vitamin B12
- ✔ Calcium
- ✔ Phosphorous
- ✔ Magnesium
- ✔ Iron
- ✔ Zinc
- ✔ Iodine
- ✔ Selenium

For Dummies™: Bestselling Book Series for Beginners

Praise for Nutrition For Dummies

"Carol Rinzler is an important women's health writer. Everything she writes is worth reading."

> — Cindy Pearson, Executive Director, National Women's Health Network

"Whether you're a fast food junkie or a health-conscious vegetarian, *Nutrition For Dummies* will show you how to get the most out of your food. It contains clear, concise information about this tricky subject and gives you practical, easy-to-follow advice for improving your diet. Before you eat your next meal, read this book."

> — Dr. Manfred Kroger, Professor of Food Science, Pennsylvania State University

"Very simply, Carol Ann Rinzler is one of the most trustworthy — and lucid — reporters on food and nutrition in the world. Rinzler will show you how to put together a healthy diet that is simple — and fun."

> — Barbara Seaman, author, Contributing Editor, *MS Magazine,* co-founder National Women's Health Network

Praise for Carol Rinzler's Estrogen and Breast Cancer

"Rinzler assumes little and explains much . . . . Her balanced and informative look at an ongoing problem may not solve it, but Rinzler offers new thoughts and a comprehensive knowledge."

> — *Publishers Weekly*

"Carol Rinzler has carefully documented the history of estrogen and breast cancer. Every woman considering post-menopausal hormonal therapy should read this book first and remember there is no free lunch."

> — Susan M. Love, M.D., author of *Dr. Susan Love's Breast Book*

"*Estrogen and Breast Cancer* should be read by any woman considering the birth control pill or hormone replacement therapy, and by prescribing physicians."

> — National Council on Women's Health

Praise for Carol Rinzler's The Complete Book of Food

" . . . makes healthy eating easier . . . a valuable compendium of culinary, nutritional and medical facts about our foods . . . . It's an asset to every food-lover's library."

— *Food & Wine* magazine

Praise for Carol Rinzler's Feed a Cold, Starve a Fever

"Ms. Rinzler tracks down the sources of these ideas and gives clear explanations for why they do not hold water. And she does this in an often whimsical way that makes the book a pleasure to read."

— Wendy Warren Keebler, Knight-Ridder News Service

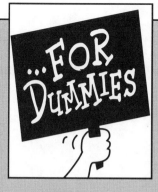 ™

References for the Rest of Us!™

BESTSELLING BOOK SERIES

Do you find that traditional reference books are overloaded with technical details and advice you'll never use? Do you postpone important life decisions because you just don't want to deal with them? Then our *...For Dummies*® business and general reference book series is for you.

...For Dummies business and general reference books are written for those frustrated and hard-working souls who know they aren't dumb, but find that the myriad of personal and business issues and the accompanying horror stories make them feel helpless. *...For Dummies* books use a lighthearted approach, a down-to-earth style, and even cartoons and humorous icons to dispel fears and build confidence. Lighthearted but not lightweight, these books are perfect survival guides to solve your everyday personal and business problems.

> *"More than a publishing phenomenon, 'Dummies' is a sign of the times."*
>
> — *The New York Times*

> *"...you won't go wrong buying them."*
>
> — *Walter Mossberg, Wall Street Journal, on IDG Books' ...For Dummies books*

> *"A world of detailed and authoritative information is packed into them..."*
>
> — *U.S. News and World Report*

Already, millions of satisfied readers agree. They have made *...For Dummies* the #1 introductory level computer book series and a best-selling business book series. They have written asking for more. So, if you're looking for the best and easiest way to learn about business and other general reference topics, look to *...For Dummies* to give you a helping hand.

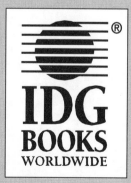

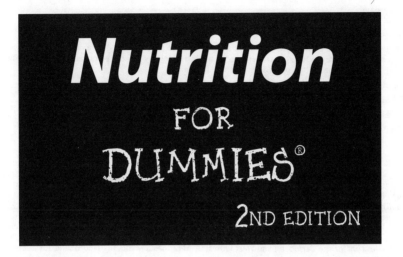

Nutrition

FOR
DUMMIES®

2ND EDITION

by Carol Ann Rinzler

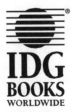

IDG BOOKS WORLDWIDE

IDG Books Worldwide, Inc.
An International Data Group Company

Foster City, CA ◆ Chicago, IL ◆ Indianapolis, IN ◆ New York, NY

Nutrition For Dummies® 2nd Edition

Published by
IDG Books Worldwide, Inc.
An International Data Group Company
919 E. Hillsdale Blvd.
Suite 400
Foster City, CA 94404
www.idgbooks.com (IDG Books Worldwide Web site)
www.dummies.com (Dummies Press Web site)

Library of Congress Catalog Card No.: 99-63210

ISBN: 0-7645-5180-9

Printed in the United States of America

10 9 8 7 6 5 4 3

2O/TQ/RS/ZZ/IN

Distributed in the United States by IDG Books Worldwide, Inc.

Distributed by CDG Books Canada Inc. for Canada; by Transworld Publishers Limited in the United Kingdom; by IDG Norge Books for Norway; by IDG Sweden Books for Sweden; by IDG Books Australia Publishing Corporation Pty. Ltd. for Australia and New Zealand; by TransQuest Publishers Pte Ltd. for Singapore, Malaysia, Thailand, Indonesia, and Hong Kong; by Gotop Information Inc. for Taiwan; by ICG Muse, Inc. for Japan; by Intersoft for South Africa; by Eyrolles for France; by International Thomson Publishing for Germany, Austria and Switzerland; by Distribuidora Cuspide for Argentina; by LR International for Brazil; by Galileo Libros for Chile; by Ediciones ZETA S.C.R. Ltda. for Peru; by WS Computer Publishing Corporation, Inc., for the Philippines; by Contemporanea de Ediciones for Venezuela; by Express Computer Distributors for the Caribbean and West Indies; by Micronesia Media Distributor, Inc. for Micronesia; by Chips Computadoras S.A. de C.V. for Mexico; by Editorial Norma de Panama S.A. for Panama; by American Bookshops for Finland.

For general information on IDG Books Worldwide's books in the U.S., please call our Consumer Customer Service department at 800-762-2974. For reseller information, including discounts and premium sales, please call our Reseller Customer Service department at 800-434-3422.

For information on where to purchase IDG Books Worldwide's books outside the U.S., please contact our International Sales department at 317-596-5530 or fax 317-596-5692.

For consumer information on foreign language translations, please contact our Customer Service department at 1-800-434-3422, fax 317-596-5692, or e-mail rights@idgbooks.com.

For information on licensing foreign or domestic rights, please phone +1-650-655-3109.

For sales inquiries and special prices for bulk quantities, please contact our Sales department at 650-655-3200 or write to the address above.

For information on using IDG Books Worldwide's books in the classroom or for ordering examination copies, please contact our Educational Sales department at 800-434-2086 or fax 317-596-5499.

For press review copies, author interviews, or other publicity information, please contact our Public Relations department at 650-655-3000 or fax 650-655-3299.

For authorization to photocopy items for corporate, personal, or educational use, please contact Copyright Clearance Center, 222 Rosewood Drive, Danvers, MA 01923, or fax 978-750-4470.

is a registered trademark under exclusive license
to IDG Books Worldwide, Inc. from International Data Group, Inc.

About the Author

Carol Ann Rinzler is a noted authority on health and nutrition and holds an M.A. from Columbia University. She is a member of the National Association of Science Writers and the National Women's Health Network. Her informative articles have appeared in numerous publications, including *The New York Times, The New York Daily News, American Health, Family Circle, Glamour, Health, Ladies' Home Journal,* and *Redbook.* Rinzler is the author of a number of health-related books, including the widely praised *The New Complete Book of Food.*

ABOUT IDG BOOKS WORLDWIDE

Welcome to the world of IDG Books Worldwide.

IDG Books Worldwide, Inc., is a subsidiary of International Data Group, the world's largest publisher of computer-related information and the leading global provider of information services on information technology. IDG was founded more than 30 years ago by Patrick J. McGovern and now employs more than 9,000 people worldwide. IDG publishes more than 290 computer publications in over 75 countries. More than 90 million people read one or more IDG publications each month.

Launched in 1990, IDG Books Worldwide is today the #1 publisher of best-selling computer books in the United States. We are proud to have received eight awards from the Computer Press Association in recognition of editorial excellence and three from Computer Currents' First Annual Readers' Choice Awards. Our best-selling ...*For Dummies*® series has more than 50 million copies in print with translations in 31 languages. IDG Books Worldwide, through a joint venture with IDG's Hi-Tech Beijing, became the first U.S. publisher to publish a computer book in the People's Republic of China. In record time, IDG Books Worldwide has become the first choice for millions of readers around the world who want to learn how to better manage their businesses.

Our mission is simple: Every one of our books is designed to bring extra value and skill-building instructions to the reader. Our books are written by experts who understand and care about our readers. The knowledge base of our editorial staff comes from years of experience in publishing, education, and journalism — experience we use to produce books to carry us into the new millennium. In short, we care about books, so we attract the best people. We devote special attention to details such as audience, interior design, use of icons, and illustrations. And because we use an efficient process of authoring, editing, and desktop publishing our books electronically, we can spend more time ensuring superior content and less time on the technicalities of making books.

You can count on our commitment to deliver high-quality books at competitive prices on topics you want to read about. At IDG Books Worldwide, we continue in the IDG tradition of delivering quality for more than 30 years. You'll find no better book on a subject than one from IDG Books Worldwide.

IDG BOOKS WORLDWIDE

John Kilcullen
Chairman and CEO
IDG Books Worldwide, Inc.

Steven Berkowitz
President and Publisher
IDG Books Worldwide, Inc.

WINNER

*Eighth Annual
Computer Press
Awards 1992*

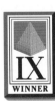

WINNER

*Ninth Annual
Computer Press
Awards 1993*

WINNER

*Tenth Annual
Computer Press
Awards 1994*

WINNER

*Eleventh Annual
Computer Press
Awards 1995*

IDG is the world's leading IT media, research and exposition company. Founded in 1964, IDG had 1997 revenues of $2.05 billion and has more than 9,000 employees worldwide. IDG offers the widest range of media options that reach IT buyers in 75 countries representing 95% of worldwide IT spending. IDG's diverse product and services portfolio spans six key areas including print publishing, online publishing, expositions and conferences, market research, education and training, and global marketing services. More than 90 million people read one or more of IDG's 290 magazines and newspapers, including IDG's leading global brands — Computerworld, PC World, Network World, Macworld and the Channel World family of publications. IDG Books Worldwide is one of the fastest-growing computer book publishers in the world, with more than 700 titles in 36 languages. The "...For Dummies®" series alone has more than 50 million copies in print. IDG offers online users the largest network of technology-specific Web sites around the world through IDG.net (http://www.idg.net), which comprises more than 225 targeted Web sites in 55 countries worldwide. International Data Corporation (IDC) is the world's largest provider of information technology data, analysis and consulting, with research centers in over 41 countries and more than 400 research analysts worldwide. IDG World Expo is a leading producer of more than 168 globally branded conferences and expositions in 35 countries including E3 (Electronic Entertainment Expo), Macworld Expo, ComNet, Windows World Expo, ICE (Internet Commerce Expo), Agenda, DEMO, and Spotlight. IDG's training subsidiary, ExecuTrain, is the world's largest computer training company, with more than 230 locations worldwide and 785 training courses. IDG Marketing Services helps industry-leading IT companies build international brand recognition by developing global integrated marketing programs via IDG's print, online and exposition products worldwide. Further information about the company can be found at www.idg.com. 1/24/99

Dedication

This book is dedicated to my husband, Perry Luntz, a fellow writer who, as always, stayed patient as a saint and even-tempered beyond belief while I was racing pell-mell (and not always pleasantly) to deadline.

Author's Acknowledgments

This new edition of *Nutrition For Dummies* has given me the opportunity to work with yet another group of thoroughly pleasant professionals at IDG. Acquisitions Editor Tami Booth moved the entire project forward. Associate Project Editor Wendy Hatch ran herd on dozens of wayward revisions — paragraphs, sentences, words, even a single letter here and there. I appreciate the clear-eyed copyediting from Darren Meiss, and I am grateful to Alfred Bushway, Ph.D., for once again reading and commenting on the manuscript.

Publisher's Acknowledgments

We're proud of this book; please register your comments through our IDG Books Worldwide Online Registration Form located at http://my2cents.dummies.com.

Some of the people who helped bring this book to market include the following:

Acquisitions, Editorial, and Media Development

Associate Project Editor: Wendy Hatch

Acquisitions Editor: Tami Booth

Copy Editor: Darren Meiss

Technical Editor: Alfred Bushway, Ph.D., Professor of Food Science, University of Maine

Editorial Coordinator: Maureen Kelly

Associate Permissions Editor: Carmen Krikorian

Editorial Manager: Rev Mengle

Editorial Assistants: Jamila Pree; Alison Walthall

Production

Project Coordinator: Maridee Ennis

Layout and Graphics: Thomas R. Emrick, Angela F. Hunckler, Brent Savage, Jacque Schneider, Janet Seib, Michael A. Sullivan, Brian Torwelle, Mary Jo Weis

Special Art: Elizabeth Kurtzman

Proofreaders: Christine Pingleton, Nancy Price, Marianne Santy

Indexer: David Heiret

General and Administrative

IDG Books Worldwide, Inc.: John Kilcullen, CEO; Steven Berkowitz, President and Publisher

IDG Books Technology Publishing Group: Richard Swadley, Senior Vice President and Publisher; Walter Bruce III, Vice President and Associate Publisher; Joseph Wikert, Associate Publisher; Mary Bednarek, Branded Product Development Director; Mary Corder, Editorial Director; Barry Pruett, Publishing Manager; Michelle Baxter, Publishing Manager

IDG Books Consumer Publishing Group: Roland Elgey, Senior Vice President and Publisher; Kathleen A. Welton, Vice President and Publisher; Kevin Thornton, Acquisitions Manager; Kristin A. Cocks, Editorial Director

IDG Books Internet Publishing Group: Brenda McLaughlin, Senior Vice President and Publisher; Diane Graves Steele, Vice President and Associate Publisher; Sofia Marchant, Online Marketing Manager

IDG Books Production for Dummies Press: Debbie Stailey, Associate Director of Production; Cindy L. Phipps, Manager of Project Coordination, Production Proofreading, and Indexing; Tony Augsburger, Manager of Prepress, Reprints, and Systems; Laura Carpenter, Production Control Manager; Shelley Lea, Supervisor of Graphics and Design; Debbie J. Gates, Production Systems Specialist; Robert Springer, Supervisor of Proofreading; Kathie Schutte, Production Supervisor

Dummies Packaging and Book Design: Patty Page, Manager, Promotions Marketing

◆

The publisher would like to give special thanks to Patrick J. McGovern, without whom this book would not have been possible.

◆

Contents at a Glance

Cartoons at a Glance

By Rich Tennant

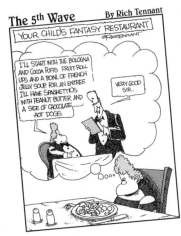

page 177

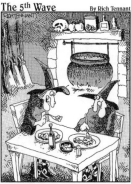

"I substitute tofu for eye of newt in all my recipes now. It has twice the protein and doesn't wriggle around the cauldron."

page 65

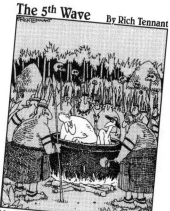

"Gee, Mark - this is an iron pot. A few bites of this stew should help you shake that anemia."

page 245

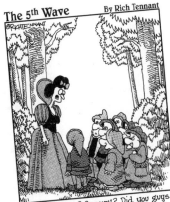

"Dopey? Sleepy? Grumpy? Did you guys forget to take your supplements again?"

page 5

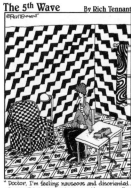

"Doctor, I'm feeling nauseous and disoriented. Do you think I'm having a reaction to something I ate?"

page 295

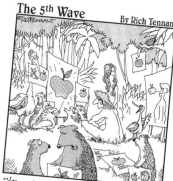

"Yes, we told them about the pectin and flavonoids, but they seem a little slow to catch on. Maybe if we just left them alone with the snake a while..."

page 331

Fax: 978-546-7747 • E-mail: the5wave@tiac.net

Table of Contents

THE INFORMATION IN THIS REFERENCE IS NOT INTENDED TO SUBSTITUTE FOR EXPERT MEDICAL ADVICE OR TREATMENT; IT IS DESIGNED TO HELP YOU MAKE INFORMED CHOICES. BECAUSE EACH INDIVIDUAL IS UNIQUE, A PHYSICIAN MUST DIAGNOSE CONDITIONS AND SUPERVISE TREATMENTS FOR EACH INDIVIDUAL HEALTH PROBLEM. IF AN INDIVIDUAL IS UNDER A DOCTOR'S CARE AND RECEIVES ADVICE CONTRARY TO INFORMATION PROVIDED IN THIS REFERENCE, THE DOCTOR'S ADVICE SHOULD BE FOLLOWED, AS IT IS BASED ON THE UNIQUE CHARACTERISTICS OF THAT INDIVIDUAL.

Introduction

● ●

*O*nce upon a time people simply sat down to dinner, eating to fill up an empty stomach or just for the pleasure of it. Nobody said, "Wow, that cream soup is loaded with calories," or asked whether the bread was a high-fiber loaf or fretted about the chicken being served with the skin still on. No longer. Today, the dinner table can be a battleground between health and pleasure. You plan your meals with the precision of a major general moving his troops into the front lines, and for most people, the fight to eat what's good for you rather than what tastes good has become a lifelong struggle.

This book is designed to end the war between your need for good nutrition and your equally compelling need for tasty meals. In fact (listen up, here!), what's good for you can also be good to eat — and vice versa.

What This Book Is About

Nutrition For Dummies, 2nd Edition, doesn't aim to send you back to the classroom, sit you down, and make you take notes about what to put on the table every day from now until you are 104 years old. Instead, this book means to give you the information you need to make wise food choices — which always means choices that please the palate and soul, as well as the body. Some of what you will read here is really, r-e-a-l-l-y basic: definitions of vitamins, minerals, proteins, fats, carbohydrates, and — can you believe this? — plain water. You'll also read tips on how to put together a nutritious shopping list and how to use food to make meals so good you can't wait to eat them.

For those who know absolutely nothing about nutrition except that it deals with food, this is a starting point. For those who know more than a little about nutrition, this is a refresher course to bring you up to speed on what has happened since the last time you checked out a calorie chart (which, by the way, you find in the Appendix).

As a bonus for you World Wide Web surfers, I've listed here and there some great Web sites that deal with our topics. Be sure to check these sites for even more information.

How This Book Is Organized

The following is a brief summary of each of the 26 "regular" chapters, four Part of Tens chapters, and the Appendix in *Nutrition For Dummies,* 2nd Edition. You can use this guide as a fast way to check out what you want to read first. One really nice thing about this book is that you don't have to start with Chapter 1 and read straight through to the end. "Au contraire," as the French like to say when they mean "on the contrary." You can dive in absolutely anywhere and still come up with tons of tasty information on how food helps your body work.

Part I: The Basic Facts about Nutrition

Chapter 1 defines nutrition and its effects on your body. This chapter also tells you how to read a nutrition study and how to judge the value of nutrition information in newspapers, magazines, and on TV. Chapter 2 is a really clear guide to how your digestive system works to transform food and beverages into the nutrients you need to sustain a healthy body. Chapter 3 concentrates on calories, the energy factor in food and beverages. Chapter 4 tells you how much of each nutrient you need to stay in tip-top form. Chapter 5 details some of the rules on dietary supplements — the pills, powders, and potions that add nutritional punch to your regular diet.

Part II: What You Get from Food

Chapter 6 gives you the facts about protein: where you get it and what it does in your body. Chapter 7 does the same job for dietary fat, while Chapter 8 explains carbohydrates: sugars, starches, and that indigestible but totally vital substance in carbohydrate foods — ta-da! — dietary fiber. Chapter 9 outlines the risks and, yes, some newly proven benefits of alcohol beverages.

Chapter 10 is about vitamins, the substances in food that trigger so many vital chemical reactions in your body. Chapter 11 is about minerals, substances that often work in tandem with vitamins. Chapter 12 explains phytochemicals, newly-important substances in food. Chapter 13 is about water, the essential liquid that comprises as much as 70 percent of your body weight. This chapter also describes the functions of electrolytes, special minerals that maintain your fluid balance (the correct amount of water inside and outside your body cells).

Part III: Healthy Eating

Chapter 14 is about *hunger* (the need for food) and *appetite* (the desire for food). Balancing these two makes it possible for you to maintain a healthful weight. Chapter 15, on the other hand, is about food preference: why you like some foods and really, really hate others. (Broccoli, anyone?) Chapter 16 tells you how to assemble a healthful diet. It's based on the Dietary Guidelines for Americans created by the U.S. Departments of Agriculture and Health and Human Services, so you know it's good for you. Chapter 17 explains how to use nutritional guidelines to plan nutritious, appetizing meals at home. Chapter 18 shows you how to take the guidelines out to dinner so that you can judge the value of foods in all kinds of restaurants, from the posh white-tablecloth ones to fast-food heaven.

Part IV: Food Processing

Chapter 19 asks and answers this simple question: What is food processing? Chapter 20 shows you how cooking affects the way food looks and tastes, as well as its nutritional value. Chapter 21 does the same for freezing, canning, drying, and irradiating techniques. Chapter 22 gives you the lowdown on chemicals used to keep food fresh.

Part V: Food and Medicine

Chapter 23 explains why some food gives some people hives and presents some strategies for identifying and avoiding the food to which you may be allergic. Chapter 24 is about how eating or drinking certain foods and beverages may affect your mood — a hot topic these days with nutrition researchers. Chapter 25 tells you how foods may "interact" with medical drugs, an important subject for anyone who ever has taken, now takes, or ever plans to take medicine. Chapter 26 tells you how some foods may actually act as preventive medicine or relieve the symptoms of certain illnesses ranging from the horrible-but-not-really-serious common cold to the Big Two: heart disease and cancer.

Part VI: The Part of Tens

Could there even be a *...For Dummies* book without The Part of Tens? Not a chance. This part provides ten great nutritional Web site addresses, lists ten common foods with nearly "magical" status, gives simple rules for keeping food safe, and last — but definitely not least — provides ten easy ways to cut calories from food.

Appendix

The Appendix is for chart wonks. It's a list of nutritional values for real-life servings of hundreds of common foods.

Icons Used in This Book

This little guy looks smart because he's marking the place where you find definitions of the words used by nutrition experts.

The same smart fella, this time pointing to clear, concise explanations of technical terms and processes.

The Official Word icon says, "Look here for scientific studies, statistics, definitions, and recommendations used to create standard nutrition policy."

Bull's-eye! This is information that you can use to improve your diet and health.

This is a watch-out-for-the-curves icon, alerting you to nutrition pitfalls such as (oops!) leaving the skin on the chicken — turning a lowfat food into one that is high in fat and cholesterol.

Nutrition is full of stuff that "everybody knows." This masked marvel clues you in to the real facts when (as often happens) "everybody's" wrong!

Part I

The Basic Facts about Nutrition

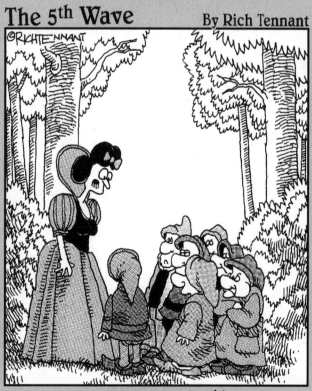

The 5th Wave   By Rich Tennant

"Dopey? Sleepy? Grumpy? Did you guys forget to take your supplements again?"

In this part . . .

To use food wisely, you need a firm grasp of the basics. In this part I define nutrition and give you a detailed explanation of digestion (how your body turns food into nutrients). I also explain why calories are useful and give you a no-nonsense guide to your daily requirements of vitamins, minerals, and other good stuff.

Chapter 1

What's Nutrition, Anyway?

• •

In This Chapter

▶ Why nutrition matters

▶ The value of food

▶ Sources for nutrition information

▶ How to read a nutrition study

• •

*W*elcome aboard! You are about to begin your very own *Fantastic Voyage.* (You know. That's the 1966 movie in which Raquel Welch and a couple of guys were shrunk down to molecule size to sail through the body of a politician shot by an assassin who had . . . hey, maybe you should just check out the next showing on The Movie Channel.)

In any event, as you read, chapter by chapter, you will follow a route that carries food (meaning food *and* beverages) from your plate to your mouth to your digestive tract and into every tissue and cell. Along the way, you will have an opportunity to see how your organs and systems work. You will observe firsthand why some foods and beverages are essential to your health. And you will learn how to manage your diet so as to get the biggest bang (nutrients) for the buck (calories). Bon voyage!

Nutrition Equals Life

Technically speaking, *nutrition* is the science of how the body uses food. In fact, nutrition is life. All living things, including you, need food and water to live. Beyond that, you need good food, meaning food with the proper nutrients, to live well. If you don't eat and drink, you will die. Period. If you don't eat and drink nutritious food and beverages

✔ Your bones may bend or break (not enough calcium).

✔ Your gums may bleed (not enough vitamin C).

✔ Your blood may not carry oxygen to every cell (not enough iron).

And on, and on, and on. Understanding how good nutrition protects you against these dire consequences requires a familiarity with the language and concepts of nutrition. Knowing some basic chemistry is helpful (don't panic: Chemistry can be a cinch when you read about it in plain English). A smattering of sociology and psychology is also useful, because although nutrition is mostly about how food revs up and sustains your body, it's also about the cultural traditions and individual differences that explain how we choose our favorite foods.

To sum up: Nutrition is about why you eat what you eat and how the food you get affects your body and your health.

First principles

Nutrition's primary task is to figure out which foods and beverages (in what quantities) provide the energy and building material you need to construct and maintain every organ and system. To do this, it concentrates on food's two basic attributes: energy and nutrients.

Energy from food

Energy is the ability to do work. Virtually every bite of food gives you energy, even when it doesn't give you nutrients. The amount of energy in food is measured in *calories,* the amount of heat produced when food is burned (metabolized) in your body cells. You can read all about metabolism in Chapter 2; Chapter 3 is your source for information about calories. But right now, all you need to know is that food is the fuel on which your body runs. Without enough food, you do not have enough energy.

Nutrients in food

Nutrients are chemical substances your body uses to build, maintain, and repair tissues. They also empower cells to send messages back and forth so as to conduct essential chemical reactions such as the ones that make it possible for you to

- ✔ Breathe
- ✔ Move
- ✔ Eliminate waste
- ✔ Think
- ✔ See
- ✔ Hear
- ✔ Smell
- ✔ Taste

. . . and do everything else natural to a living body.

Food provides two different and distinct groups of nutrients:

> ✔ **Macronutrients (macro = big):** protein, fat, carbohydrates, water
>
> ✔ **Micronutrients (micro = small):** vitamins and minerals

What's the difference between these two groups? The amount you need each day. Your daily requirements for macronutrients generally exceed one gram. (For comparison's sake, 28 grams are in an ounce.) For example, a man needs about 63 grams of protein a day (slightly more than two ounces); a woman, 50 grams (slightly less than two ounces).

Your daily requirements for micronutrients are much smaller. For example, the Recommended Dietary Allowance (RDA) for vitamin C is measured in milligrams (1/1,000th of a gram), while the RDAs for vitamin D, vitamin B12, and folate are even smaller, measured in micrograms (1/1,000,000th of a gram). You can find a lot more about the RDAs, including how they vary for people of different ages, in Chapter 4.

Essential nutrients for Fido, Fluffy, and your pet petunia

Vitamin C isn't the only nutrient that's essential for one species but not for others. Many organic compounds (substances similar to vitamins) and elements (minerals) are essential for your green or furry friends but not for you, either because you can synthesize them from the food you eat, or because they are so widely available in the human diet and you require such small amounts that you can get what you need without hardly trying.

Two good examples are the organic compounds choline and myo-inositol. *Choline* is an essential nutrient for several species of animals including dogs, cats, rats, and guinea pigs. Human beings make their own or get what they need from eggs, liver, soybeans, cauliflower, and lettuce. *Myo-inositol* is an essential nutrient for gerbils and rats, but human beings synthesize it naturally and use it in many body processes, such as transmitting signals between cells.

Here's a handy list of nutrients that are essential for animals and/or plants but not for you:

Organic compounds	Elements
Carnitine	Arsenic
Myo-inositol	Cadmium
Taurine	Lead
	Nickel
	Silicon
	Tin
	Vanadium

What's an essential nutrient?

A reasonable person might assume that an essential nutrient is one you need to sustain a healthy body. But who says a reasonable person thinks like a nutritionist? In nutrition-speak, an *essential nutrient* is a very special thing:

- **An essential nutrient cannot be manufactured in the body.** You have to get essential nutrients from food or from a nutritional supplement.

- **An essential nutrient is linked to a specific deficiency disease.** For example, people who go without protein for extended periods of time develop the protein-deficiency disease kwashiorkor. People who do not get enough vitamin C develop the vitamin-C-deficiency disease scurvy. A diet rich in the essential nutrient will cure the deficiency disease, but you need the proper nutrient. In other words, you can't cure a protein deficiency with extra amounts of vitamin C.

- **Not all nutrients are essential for all species of animals.** For example, vitamin C is an essential nutrient for human beings, but not for dogs. A dog's body makes the vitamin C it needs. Check out the list of nutrients on a can or bag of dog food. See? No C. The dog already has what it requires.

Essential nutrients for human beings include many well-known vitamins and minerals, several amino acids (the "building blocks of proteins"), and at least two fatty acids. For more about these essential nutrients see Chapters 6, 7, 10, and 11.

Other interesting substances in food

The newest flash in the nutrition sky is phytochemicals, a group of fascinating compounds in plant foods. Phytochemicals get their name from *phyto* (the Greek word for plant). While the 13-letter name may be new to you, you're probably already familiar with some phytochemicals such as beta-carotene, a deep yellow pigment in fruits and vegetables that your body can convert to a form of vitamin A. The current stars on the phytochemical stage are phytoestrogens — hormone-like chemicals in plants. These compounds are in the spotlight due to the observation that a diet high in phytoestrogens, such as the isoflavones found in soybeans, may lower the risk of heart disease and reduce the incidence of reproductive cancers (cancer of the breast, ovary, uterus, and prostate). This is very, very new and far from proven, but to find out more about phytochemicals, including phytoestrogens, check out Chapter 12. Right now, just tuck the definition away in your brain so you can access it the next time the term pops up in a fast-breaking, gee-whiz, nutrition news story.

You are what you eat

Oh boy, I bet you've heard this one before. But it bears repeating because the human body really is built from the nutrients it gets from food: water, protein, fat, carbohydrates, vitamins, and minerals. On average, when you step on the scale

- ✔ About 60 percent of your weight is water.
- ✔ About 20 percent of your weight is fat.
- ✔ About 20 percent of your weight is a combination of mostly protein plus carbohydrates, minerals, and vitamins.

An easy way to remember this formula is to think of it as the "60-20-20 Rule."

Your nutritional status

Nutritional status is a phrase used to describe the state of your health related to your diet. For example, people who are starving do not get the nutrients or calories they need for optimum health. These people are said to be *malnourished* (mal = bad), which means their nutritional status is, to put it gently, definitely not good. Malnutrition may arise from

- ✔ A diet that does not provide enough food. This might occur in times of famine or through voluntary starvation due to an eating disorder or because something in your life disturbs your appetite. For example, older people may be at risk of malnutrition because of tooth loss or age-related loss of appetite or because many live alone and sometimes just forget to eat.
- ✔ A diet that, while otherwise adequate, is deficient in a specific nutrient, such as vitamin C.
- ✔ A metabolic disorder that prevents your body from absorbing specific nutrients, such as protein or carbohydrates.
- ✔ A medical condition that prevents your body from using nutrients. For example, people who abuse alcohol are often malnourished because alcohol depresses appetite and interferes with the body's ability to metabolize the nutrients it does get.

Your doctor has many tools with which to rate your nutritional status. She can

- ✔ Review your medical history to see whether you have any conditions (such as dentures) that may make it hard for you to eat certain foods or that interfere with your ability to absorb nutrients.

✔ Perform a physical examination to look for obvious signs of nutritional deficiency such as dull hair and eyes (a lack of vitamins?), poor posture (not enough calcium to protect the spinal bones?), or extreme thinness (not enough food? an underlying disease?).

✔ Order laboratory blood and urine tests that may identify early signs of malnutrition, such as the lack of red blood cells that characterizes anemia due to an iron deficiency.

At every stage of life, the aim of a good diet is to maintain a healthy nutritional status.

Finding Nutrition Facts

Getting reliable information about nutrition can be a daunting challenge. For the most part, your nutrition information is likely to come from TV and radio talk shows or news, your daily newspaper, your favorite magazine, and a variety of nutrition-oriented books. How can you tell whether what you hear or read is really right?

Nutritional people

The people who make nutrition news may be scientists, reporters, or simply someone who wandered in with a new theory (Artichokes prevent cancer! Never eat cherries and cheese at the same meal! Vitamin C gives you hives!), the more bizarre the better. But several groups of people are most likely to give you news you can use with confidence. For example:

✔ **Nutrition scientists:** These are people with a graduate degree (usually in chemistry, biology, biochemistry, or physics) engaged in research dealing primarily with the effects of food on animals and human beings.

✔ **Nutrition researchers:** These may be either nutrition scientists or professionals in another field such as medicine or sociology whose research (study or studies) concentrates on the effects of food.

✔ **Nutritionists:** These are people who concentrate on the study of nutrition. In some states, a person who uses the title "nutritionist" must have a graduate degree in basic science courses related to nutrition.

✔ **Dietitians:** These people have an undergraduate degree in food and nutrition science or the management of food programs. A person with the letters RD after his name has completed a dietetic internship and has also passed an American Dietetic Association licensing exam.

✔ **Nutrition reporters and writers:** These are people who specialize in giving you information about the medical and/or scientific aspects of food. Like reporters who concentrate on politics or sports, nutrition reporters gain their expertise through years of covering their "beat." Most have the science background required to make it possible for them to translate technical information into language nonscientists can understand; some have been trained as dietitians, nutritionists, or nutrition scientists.

Consumer alert: Regardless of the source, nutrition news should always pass what you may call "the reasonableness test." In other words, if a story or report or study sounds ridiculous, it probably is.

Want some guidelines for evaluating nutrition studies? Read on.

Can you trust this study?

You open your morning newspaper or turn on the evening news and read or hear that a group of researchers at an impeccably prestigious scientific organization has published a study showing that yet another thing you've always taken for granted is hazardous to your health. For example:

✔ Drinking coffee stresses your heart.

✔ Adding salt to food raises blood pressure.

✔ Fatty foods increase your risk of cancer.

So you throw out the offending food or drink or rearrange your daily routine to avoid the once-acceptable, now-dangerous food, beverage, or additive. And then what happens? Two weeks, two months, or two years down the road, a second, equally prestigious group of scientists publishes a second study conclusively proving that the first group got it wrong: In fact, coffee has no effect on the risk of heart disease — and may even improve athletic performance. Salt does not cause hypertension except in certain sensitive individuals. Only *some* fatty foods are risky.

Who's right? Nobody seems to know. That leaves you, a layperson, on your own to come up with the answer. Never fear — you may not be a nutritionist, but that doesn't mean you can't apply a few common sense rules to any study you read about, rules that say: Yes, this may be true, or No, this isn't.

Does this study include human beings?

True, animal studies can alert researchers to potential problems, but working with animals alone cannot give you conclusive proof.

What's a body made of?

Sugar and spice and everything nice . . . .Oops. What I meant to say was water and fat and protein and carbohydrates and vitamins and minerals.

On average, when you step on the scale, approximately 60 percent of your weight is water, 20 percent is body fat (slightly less for a man), and 20 percent is a combination of mostly protein, plus carbohydrates, minerals, vitamins, and other naturally-occurring biochemicals.

Based on these percentages, you can reasonably expect that an average 140-pound person's body weight consists of

✔ About 84 pounds of water

✔ About 28 pounds of body fat

✔ About 28 pounds of a combination of protein (up to 25 pounds), minerals (up to 7 pounds), carbohydrates (up to 1.4 pounds), and vitamins (a trace).

Yes, you're right: Those last figures do total more than 28 pounds. That's because "up to" (as in

"up to 25 pounds protein") means that the amounts may vary from person to person.

For example, a young person's body has proportionately more muscle and less fat than an older person's, while a woman's body has proportionately less muscle and more fat than a man's. As a result, more of a man's weight comes from protein and calcium, while more of hers come from fat. Protein-packed muscles and mineral-packed bones are denser tissue than fat.

Weigh a man and a woman of roughly the same height and size, and he is likely to tip the scale higher every time.

Sources: *Recommended Dietary Allowances* (Washington D.C.: National Academy Press, 1989); Eleanor Noss Whitney, Corinne Balog Cataldo, and Sharon Rady Rolfes, *Understanding Normal and Clinical Nutrition* (Minneapolis/St. Paul: West Publishing Company, 1994)

Different species react differently to various chemicals and diseases. While outright poisons such as cyanide will clearly traumatize any living body, many foods or drugs that harm a laboratory rat will not harm you. And vice versa, too. For example, mouse and rat embryos suffer no ill effects when their mothers are given thalidomide, the sedative that may cause deformed fetal limbs when given to pregnant monkeys — and human beings.

Are enough people in this study?

Hey, it's not enough for a researcher to say, "Well, I did give this to a couple of people." The study must include sufficient numbers and a variety of individuals, too. If you don't have enough people in the study — several hundred to many thousand — to establish a pattern, there's always the possibility that an effect occurred by chance. If you don't include different types of people, which generally means young and old men and women of different racial and ethnic groups, your results may not apply across the board. For example, the original studies linking high blood levels of cholesterol to an increased risk of heart disease and small doses of aspirin to a reduced risk of a second heart attack were done only with men. It was not until follow-up studies were done with women that researchers were able to say with any certainty that high cholesterol was dangerous and aspirin, protective, for women as well as men.

Is there anything in the design or method of this study that might affect the accuracy of its conclusions?

For example, a retrospective study (which asks people to tell what they did in the past) is always considered less accurate than a prospective study (one which follows people while they are actually doing what the researchers are studying) because memory is not always accurate. People tend to forget details or, without meaning to, alter them to fit the researchers' questions.

Are the study's conclusions reasonable?

If a study comes up with a conclusion that seems illogical to you, chances are the researchers feel the same way. For example, in 1990, the long-running Nurses' Study at the Harvard School of Public Health reported that a high-fat diet raised the risk of colon cancer. But the data showed a link only to diets high in beef; there was no link to diets high in dairy fat. In short, this was a study begging for a second study to confirm (or deny) the results.

Chapter 2

Digestion: The 24-Hour Food Factory

. . . .

In This Chapter

▶ The digestive organs

▶ How food moves through your body

▶ Absorbing nutrients and passing them along to your body

. . . .

*W*hen you see (or smell) something appetizing, your digestive organs leap into action. Your mouth waters. Your stomach contracts. Intestinal glands begin to secrete the chemicals that turn food into the nutrients that build new tissues and provide the energy you need to keep zipping through the days, months, and years.

The Digestive System

Your digestive system may never win a Tony, Oscar, or Emmy, but it certainly deserves your applause for its ability to turn complex food into basic nutrients. Doing this requires not a cast of thousands, but a group of digestive organs, each designed specifically to perform one role in the process. Read on.

The digestive organs

While exceedingly well organized, your digestive system is basically one long tube that starts at your mouth, continues down through your throat to your stomach, and then on to your small and large intestine and past the rectum to end at your anus.

In between, with the help of the liver, pancreas, and gallbladder, the usable (digestible) parts of everything that you eat are converted to simple compounds that your body can easily absorb to burn for energy or build new tissue. The indigestible residue is bundled off and eliminated as waste.

Figure 2-1 shows the body parts and organs that comprise your digestive system.

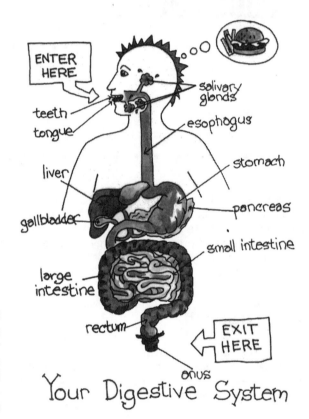

Figure 2-1:
Your
digestive
system in all
its glory.

Digestion: A two-part process

Digestion is a two-part process — half mechanical, half chemical.

 ✔ *Mechanical digestion* takes place in your mouth and your stomach. Your teeth break food into small pieces that you can swallow without choking. In your stomach, a churning action continues to break food into smaller particles.

✔ *Chemical digestion* occurs at every point in the digestive tract where enzymes and other substances such as *hydrochloric acid* (from stomach glands) and *bile* (from the gallbladder) dissolve food, releasing the nutrients inside.

How Your Body Digests Food

Each organ in the digestive system plays a specific role in the digestive drama. But the first act occurs in two places that are never listed as part of the digestive tract: your eyes and nose.

The eyes and nose

When you see appetizing food, you experience a conditioned response (for the lowdown on how your digestive system can be conditioned to respond to food, see Chapter 14; for information on your food preferences, see Chapter 15). In other words, your thoughts — Wow! That looks good! — stimulate your brain to tell your digestive organs to get ready for action.

What happens in your nose is purely physical. The tantalizing aroma of good food is transmitted by molecules that fly from the surface of the food to settle on the membrane lining of your nostrils, stimulating receptor cells on olfactory nerve fibers that stretch from your nose back to your brain. When the receptor cells communicate with your brain — hey, there's good stuff here! — your brain sends encouraging messages off to your mouth and digestive tract.

In both cases — eyes and nose — the results are the same: "Start the saliva flowing," they say. "Warm up the stomach glands. Alert the small intestine." In other words, the sight and scent of food has made your mouth water and your stomach contract in anticipatory hunger pangs.

But wait! Suppose you hate what you see or smell? For some people, even the thought of liver is enough to make them want to barf — or simply leave the room. At that point, your body takes up arms to protect you: You experience a *rejection reaction* — a reaction similar to that exhibited by babies given something that tastes bitter or sour.

Your mouth purses and your nose wrinkles as if to keep the food (and its odor) as far away as possible. Your throat tightens, and your stomach *turns* — muscles contracting not in anticipatory pangs but in movements preparatory to vomiting up the unwanted food. Not a pleasant moment.

But let's assume you like what's on your plate. Go ahead. Take a bite.

The mouth

Lift your fork to your mouth, and your teeth and salivary glands swing into action. Your teeth chew, grinding the food, breaking it into small, manageable pieces. As a result

- ✔ You can swallow without choking.
- ✔ You break down the indigestible wrapper of fibers surrounding the edible parts of some foods (fruits, vegetables, whole grains) so that your digestive enzymes can get to the nutrients inside.

At the same time, salivary glands under your tongue and in the back of your mouth secrete the watery liquid called *saliva,* which performs two important functions:

- ✔ Saliva moistens and compacts food so that your tongue can push it to the back of your mouth and you can swallow, sending the food down the slide of your *gullet* (esophagus) into your stomach.
- ✔ Saliva provides *amylases,* enzymes that start the digestion of complex carbohydrates (starches), breaking the starch molecules into simple sugars. (No protein or fat digestion occurs in your mouth.)

The stomach

If you were to lay your digestive tract out on a table, most of it would look like a simple, rather narrow tube. The exception is your stomach, a pouchy part just below your gullet (esophagus).

Like most of the digestive tube, your stomach is circled with strong muscles whose rhythmic contractions — called *peristalsis* — move food smartly along and turn your stomach into a sort of food processor that mechanically breaks pieces of food into ever smaller particles.

While this is going on, glands in the stomach wall are secreting *stomach juices* — a potent blend of enzymes, hydrochloric acid, and mucus.

One stomach enzyme — gastric alcohol dehydrogenase — digests small amounts of alcohol, an unusual nutrient that can be absorbed directly into your bloodstream even before it has been digested. For more about alcohol digestion, including why men can drink more than women without becoming tipsy, see Chapter 9.

Other enzymes, plus stomach juices, begin the digestion of proteins and fats, separating them into their basic components — amino acids and fatty acids.

Turning starches into sugars

Salivary enzymes don't lay a finger on proteins or fats, but they do begin to digest complex carbohydrates, breaking the long, chain-like molecules of starches into individual units of sugars. You can taste this for yourself with this simple experiment that allows you to experience firsthand the effects of amylases on carbohydrates.

1. **Put a small piece of plain, unsalted cracker on your tongue. No cheese, no chopped liver, just the cracker, please.**

2. **Close your mouth and let the cracker sit on your tongue for a few minutes.**

   Do you taste a sudden, slight sweetness? That's the salivary enzymes breaking a long, complex starch molecule into its component parts (sugars).

3. **Okay, you can swallow now. The rest of the digestion of the starch takes place farther down, in your small intestine.**

Stop! If the words amino acids and fatty acids are completely new to you and if you are suddenly consumed by the desire to know more about them right now this instant, stick a pencil in the book to hold your place and flip ahead to Chapter 6 and Chapter 7, where I discuss them in detail.

Stop again!! For the most part, digestion of carbohydrates comes to a screeching — though temporary — halt in the stomach because the stomach juices are so acidic that they inactivate amylases, the enzymes that break complex carbohydrates apart into simple sugars. However, stomach acid can break some carbohydrate bonds, so a bit of carb digestion does take place.

Back to the action. Eventually, your churning stomach blends its contents into a thick soupy mass called *chyme* (from *cheymos*, the Greek word for juice). When a small amount of chyme spills past the stomach into the small intestine, the digestion of carbohydrates resumes in earnest, and your body begins to extract nutrients from food.

The small intestine

Open your hand and put it flat against your belly button, with your thumb pointing up to your waist and your pinkie pointing down.

Your hand is now covering most of the relatively small space into which your 20-foot long small (20 feet? small?!?) intestine is neatly coiled. When chyme spills from your stomach into this part of the digestive tube, a whole new set of gastric juices are released. These include

✔ Pancreatic and intestinal enzymes that finish the digestion of proteins into amino acids

✔ Bile, a greenish liquid (made in the liver and stored in the gallbladder) that enables fats to mix with water

✔ Alkaline pancreatic juices that make the chyme less acidic so that amylases (the enzymes that break down carbohydrates) can go back to work separating complex carbohydrates into simple sugars

✔ Intestinal alcohol dehydrogenase that digests alcohol not previously absorbed into your bloodstream

Peephole: The first man to watch a living human gut at work

William Beaumont, M.D., was a surgeon in the United States Army in the early 19th century. His name survives in the annals of medicine because of an excellent adventure that began on June 6, 1822. Alexis St. Martin, an 18-year-old French Canadian fur trader, was wounded by a musket, which discharged accidentally, tearing through his back and out his stomach, leaving a wound that healed but did not close.

St. Martin's injury seems not to have affected what must have been a truly sunny disposition: Two years later, when all efforts to close the hole in his gut had failed, he granted Beaumont permission to use the wound as the world's first window on a working human digestive system. (To keep food and liquid from spilling out of the small opening, Beaumont kept it covered with a cotton bandage.)

Beaumont's method was simplicity itself. At noon on August 1, 1825, he tied small pieces of food (cooked meat, raw meat, cabbage, bread) to a silk string, removed the bandage, and inserted the string into the hole in St. Martin's stomach.

An hour later, he pulled the food out. The cabbage and bread were half digested; the meat, untouched. After another hour, he pulled the string out again. This time, only the raw meat remained untouched, and St. Martin, who now had a headache and a queasy stomach, called it quits for the day. But in more than 230 later trials, Beaumont — with the help of his remarkably compliant patient — discovered that while carbohydrates (cabbage and bread) were digested rather quickly, it took up to eight hours for the stomach juices to break down proteins and fats (the beef). Beaumont attributed this to the fact that the cabbage had been cut into small pieces and the bread was porous. Modern nutritionists know that carbohydrates are simply digested faster than proteins and that digesting fats (including those in beef) takes longest of all.

By withdrawing gastric fluid from St. Martin's stomach, keeping it at 100° F (the temperature recorded on a thermometer stuck into the stomach), and adding a piece of meat, Beaumont was able to clock exactly how long it took for the meat to fall apart: 10 hours.

Beaumont and St. Martin separated in 1833 when the patient, now a sergeant in the United States Army, was posted elsewhere, leaving the doctor to write "Experiments and Observations on the Gastric Juice and the Physiology of Digestion." The treatise is now considered a landmark in the understanding of the human digestive system.

While these chemicals are working, peristaltic contractions of the small intestine continue to move the food mass down through the tube so that your body can absorb sugars, amino acids, fatty acids, vitamins, and minerals into cells in the intestinal wall.

The lining of the small intestine is a series of folds covered with projections that have been described as "finger-like" or "small nipples." The technical name for these small finger/nipples is *villi* (single: villus).

Each villus is covered with smaller projections called *microvilli,* and every villus and microvillus is programmed to accept a specific nutrient — and no other.

Nutrients are absorbed not in their order of arrival in the intestine but according to how fast they are broken down into their basic parts.

- Carbohydrates — which separate quickly into single sugar units — are absorbed first.

- Proteins (as amino acids) go next.

- Fats — which take longest to break apart into their constituent fatty acids — are last. That's why a high-fat meal keeps you feeling fuller longer than a meal such as chow mein or plain tossed salad, which are mostly lowfat carbohydrates.

- Vitamins that dissolve in water are absorbed earlier than vitamins that dissolve in fat.

Once you have digested your food and absorbed its nutrients through your small intestine

- Amino acids, sugars, vitamin C, the B vitamins, iron, calcium, and magnesium are carried through the bloodstream to your liver, where they are processed and sent out to the rest of the body.

- Fatty acids, cholesterol, and vitamins A, D, E, and K go into the lymph system and then into the blood. They, too, end up in the liver, are processed, and are shipped out to other body cells.

Inside the cells, nutrients are *metabolized:* burned for heat and energy or used to build new tissues.

The metabolic process that gives you energy is called *catabolism* (from *katabole,* the Greek word for casting down). The metabolic process that uses nutrients to build new tissues is called *anabolism* (from *anabole,* the Greek word for raising up).

Chew! Chew! All aboard the Nutrient Express!

Think of your small intestine as a busy train station whose apparent chaos of arrivals and departures is actually an efficient, well-ordered system. (Please forgive the terrible pun in the title of this sidebar. My husband — who inherited a gift for this sort of thing from his mother — made me do it.)

As I was saying, the small intestine resembles a three-level, miniature Grand Central Terminal.

✔ Level 1 is the *duodenum* (at the top, right after your stomach).

✔ Level 2 is the *jejunum* (in the middle).

✔ Level 3 is the *ileum* (the last part before the colon).

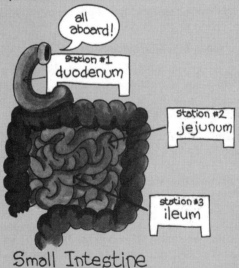

This three-station tube hums away as nutrients arrive and depart, millions of "trains" (the nutrients) running on millions of "tracks" (the microvilli) designed to accommodate only one kind of train — and no other.

The system absorbs and ships out nutrients accounting for more than 90 percent of all the protein, fat, and carbohydrates that you consume, plus smaller percentages of vitamins and minerals.

The train schedule looks something like this:

Level 1	The duodenum	Iron, calcium, magnesium
Level 2	The jejunum	Simple sugars (the end products of carbohydrate digestion) and water-soluble vitamins (vitamin C and the B vitamins — other than vitamin B12)
Level 3	The ileum	Amino acids (the end product of protein digestion), fat-soluble vitamins (vitamins A, D, E, and K), fatty acids (the end products of fat digestion), cholesterol, vitamin B12, sodium, potassium, and alcohol

How these two processes occur is, alas, a subject for another chapter. In fact, this subject is enough to fill seven different chapters, each devoted to a specific kind of nutrient. For information about metabolizing proteins, turn to Chapter 6. I discuss fats in Chapter 7, carbohydrates in Chapter 8, alcohol in Chapter 9, vitamins in Chapter 10, minerals in Chapter 11, and water in Chapter 13.

The large intestine

After every useful, digestible ingredient other than water has been wrung out of your food, the rest — indigestible waste such as fiber — moves into the top of your large intestine, the area known as your *colon.* The colon's primary job is to absorb water from this mixture and then to squeeze the remaining matter into the compact bundle known as feces.

Feces (whose brown color comes from leftover bile pigments) are made of indigestible material from food, plus cells that have sloughed off the intestinal lining and bacteria — quite a lot of bacteria. In fact, about 30 percent of the entire weight of the feces is bacteria. No, these bacteria aren't a sign you're sick. On the contrary, they prove that you're healthy and well. These bacteria are good guys, micro-organisms that live in permanent colonies in your colon where they

- Manufacture vitamin B12, which is absorbed through the colon wall
- Produce vitamin K, also absorbed through the colon wall
- Break down amino acids and produce nitrogen (which gives feces a characteristic odor)
- Feast on indigestible complex carbohydrates (fiber), excreting the gas that sometimes makes you physically uncomfortable — or a social pariah

When the bacteria have finished, the feces — the small remains of yesterday's copious feast — pass down through your rectum and out through your anus.

Digestion's done!

Chapter 3

Calories: The Energizers

· ·

In This Chapter

▶ What's a calorie?

▶ Why all calories aren't the same

▶ Why men generally need more calories than women do

▶ What happens if you get too many calories (or too few)

· ·

Automobiles burn gasoline to get the energy they need to move. Your body burns (metabolizes) food to produce energy in the form of heat. This heat warms your body and (as energy) powers every move you make.

Nutritionists measure the amount of heat produced by metabolizing food in units called *kilocalories*. A kilocalorie is the amount of energy it takes to raise the temperature of one kilogram of water one degree on the Centigrade thermometer at sea level.

In common use, nutritionists substitute the word *calorie* for *kilocalorie*. This is not scientifically accurate: Strictly speaking, a calorie is really 1/1000 of a kilocalorie. But the word calorie is easier to say and easier to remember, so that's the term you see whenever you read about the energy in food. And few nutrition-related words have caused as much confusion and concern as the lowly calorie. Read on to find out what calories mean to you and to your nutrition.

Counting the Calories in Food

When you read that a serving of food — say, one banana — has 105 calories, it means that metabolizing the banana produces 105 calories of heat that your body can use for work.

You may wonder which kinds of food have the most calories. The answer is

- ✔ One gram of protein has four calories.
- ✔ One gram of fat has nine calories.
- ✔ One gram of carbohydrates has four calories.
- ✔ One gram of alcohol has seven calories.

In other words, ounce for ounce, proteins and carbohydrates give you less than half as many calories as fat. That's why high-fat foods, such as cream cheese, are high in calories, while lowfat foods, such as bagels (minus the cream cheese) are not.

Measuring the number of calories

Nutrition scientists measure the number of calories in food by actually burning the food in a *bomb calorimeter,* a "box" with two chambers — one inside the other. They weigh a sample of the food, put the sample on a dish, and put the dish into the inner chamber of the calorimeter. They fill the chamber with oxygen and then seal it so that the oxygen cannot escape. The outer chamber is filled with a measured amount of cold water, and the oxygen in the first chamber (inside the chamber with water) is ignited with an electric spark. When the food burns, an observer records the rise in the temperature of the water in the outside chamber. If the temperature of the water goes up one degree per kilogram, the food has one calorie. Two degrees, two calories. 235 degrees, 235 calories — one eight-ounce chocolate malt!

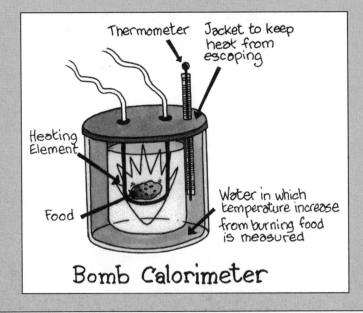

Bomb Calorimeter

But you have to watch all the angles. Sometimes foods that seem to be equally low-calorie really aren't. Here's a good example: A chicken breast and a hamburger are both high-protein foods. Both should have the same amount of calories per ounce. But if you serve the chicken without its skin, it has very little fat, while the hamburger is (sorry about this) full of it. A three-ounce serving of skinless chicken provides 140 calories; a three-ounce burger, 230 to 245 calories, depending on the cut of the meat.

Empty calories

All food provides calories. All calories provide energy. But not all calories come with a full complement of extra benefits such as amino acids, fatty acids, fiber, vitamins, and minerals.

Some foods are said to give you "empty calories." This term has nothing to do with the calorie's energy potential or with calories having a hole in the middle. It describes a "naked calorie," one with no extra benefits.

The best-known empty-calorie foods are table sugar and ethanol (the kind of alcohol found in beer, wine, and spirits). On their own, sugar and ethanol give you energy — but no nutrients. (See Chapter 8 for more about sugar and Chapter 9 for more on alcohol.)

People who abuse alcohol aren't always thin, but the fact that they often substitute alcohol for food almost always leads to nutritional deficiencies, most commonly a deficiency of thiamin (vitamin B1).

Of course, it is only fair to point out that both sugar and alcohol are often ingredients in foods that do provide other nutrients. For example, sugar is found in bread, and alcohol is found in beer — two very different foods that both have calcium, phosphorus, iron, potassium, sodium, and B vitamins.

In the United States, some people are malnourished because they cannot afford enough food to get the nutrients they need. The school lunch program — started by President Franklin Delano Roosevelt in 1935 and expanded by almost every president, Republican and Democrat, since then — has been a largely successful attempt to prevent malnutrition among poor schoolchildren.

But many Americans who can afford enough food are still malnourished because they simply do not know how to choose a diet that gives them nutrients as well as calories. For these people, eating too many foods with empty calories can cause significant health problems.

Every calorie counts

People who say that "calories don't count" or that "some calories count less than others" are usually trying to convince you to follow a diet that concentrates on one kind of food to the exclusion of most others. One common example, which seems to arise like a phoenix in every generation of dieters, is the "high-protein diet." This one says to cut back or even entirely eliminate carbohydrate foods on the assumption that, because your muscle tissue is mostly protein, the protein foods you eat will go straight from your stomach to your muscles while everything else turns to fat. In other words, this diet says that you can stuff yourself with protein foods until your eyes bug out because no matter how many calories you get, they will all be protein calories and they will all end up in your muscles, not on your hips.

Boy, wouldn't it be nice if that were true? The problem is, it isn't true.

Here's the absolute truth: All calories, no matter where they come from, give you energy. If you take in more energy (calories) than you spend each day, you'll gain weight. If you take in less than you use up, you'll lose weight. This nutrition rule is an equal opportunity, one-size-fits-all proposition that applies to everyone.

How Many Calories Do You Need?

Think of your energy requirements as a bank account. You make deposits when you consume calories. You make withdrawals when your body spends energy on work. Nutritionists divide the amount of energy you withdraw each day into two parts:

- ✔ The energy you need when your body is at rest
- ✔ The energy you need when you are actively working

To keep your energy account in balance, you need to take in enough each day to cover your withdrawals.

Resting energy expenditures

Even when you are at rest, your body is busy. Your heart beats. Your lungs expand and contract. Your intestines digest food. Your liver processes nutrients. Your glands secrete hormones. Your muscles flex, usually gently. Cells send electrical impulses back and forth among themselves, and your brain continually signals to every part of your body.

The energy your resting body uses to do all this stuff is called (surprise! surprise!) *resting energy expenditure,* abbreviated to REE. The REE, also known as the *basal metabolism,* accounts for a whopping 60 to 70 percent of all the energy you need each day.

As a general rule, infants and adolescents burn more energy per pound than adults do, because they are continually making large amounts of new tissue. An average man burns more energy than an average woman because his body is larger and has more muscle.

To find your resting energy expenditure (REE), you must first figure out your weight in kilograms (kg). One kilogram equals 2.2 pounds. So to get your weight in kilograms, divide the amount in pounds by 2.2. For example, if you weigh 150 pounds, that's equal to 68.2 kg (150 divided by 2.2). Plug that into the appropriate equation in Table 3-1 — and bingo! You have your REE.

Table 3-1 shows you how to calculate your own REE (the energy used when you are at rest) based on your age and sex.

Table 3-1 How Many Calories Do You Need When You're Resting?

Sex and Age	Use This Equation to Figure Out Your REE
Males	
0-3 years	(60.9 x weight in kg) – 54
3-10 years	(22.7 x weight in kg) + 495
10-18 years	(17.5 x weight in kg) + 651
18-30 years	(15.3 x weight in kg) + 679
30-60 years	(11.6 x weight in kg) + 879
>60 years	(13.5 x weight in kg) + 487
Females	
0-3 years	(61.0 x weight in kg) – 51
3-10 years	(22.5 x weight in kg) + 499
10-18 years	(12.2 x weight in kg) + 746
18-30 years	(14.7 x weight in kg) + 496
30-60 years	(8.7 x weight in kg) + 829
>60 years	(10.5 x weight in kg) + 596

Source: The National Research Council, *Recommended Dietary Allowances* (Washington, D.C.: National Academy Press, 1989).

Sex, glands, and chocolate cake

A *gland* is an organ that secretes *hormones,* chemical substances that can change the function — and sometimes the structure — of other body parts.

For example, your pancreas secretes *insulin,* a hormone that enables you to digest and metabolize carbohydrates. At puberty, your sex glands secrete either the female hormones estrogen and progesterone or the male hormone testosterone; these hormones trigger the development of secondary sex characteristics such as body and facial hair that make us look like either men or women.

Hormones can also affect your REE. Your pituitary gland, a small structure in the center of your brain, stimulates your thyroid gland (which sits at the front of your throat) to secrete hormones that influence the rate at which your tissues burn nutrients to produce energy.

If your thyroid gland does not secrete enough hormones (a condition known as *hypothyroidism*), you burn food more slowly and your REE drops. If your thyroid secretes excess amounts of hormones (a condition known as *hyperthyroidism*), you burn food faster and your REE is higher.

When you are frightened or excited, your adrenal glands (two small glands, one on top of each kidney) release *adrenaline,* the hormone that serves as your body's call to battle stations. Your heartbeat increases. You breathe faster. Your muscles clench. And you burn food faster, converting it as fast as possible to the energy you need for the reaction commonly known as "fight or flight." But these effects are temporary. The effects of the sex glands last as long as you live.

How your hormones affect your energy needs

If you are a woman, you know that your appetite rises and falls in tune with your menstrual cycle. In fact, this fluctuation parallels what's happening to your REE, which goes up just before or at the time of ovulation. Your appetite is highest when menstrual bleeding starts, and then falls sharply. Yes, you really are hungrier (and need more energy) just before you get your period.

Being a man (and making lots of testosterone) makes satisfying your nutritional needs on a normal American diet easier. Your male bones are naturally more dense, so you are less dependent on dietary or supplemental calcium to prevent *osteoporosis* (severe loss of bone tissue) late in life. You don't lose blood through menstruation, so you need only two-thirds as much iron. Best of all, you can eat more than a woman of the same weight without putting on the pounds.

It's no accident that teenage boys develop wide shoulders and biceps while teenage girls get hips. Testosterone, the male hormone, promotes the growth of muscle and bone. Estrogen gives you fatty tissue.

As a result, the average male body has proportionally more muscle; the average female body, proportionally more fat. Muscle is *active* tissue. It expands and contracts. It works. And in doing so, it uses more energy than fat, which insulates the body and provides a source of stored energy, but does not move an inch on its own. This means that the average man's REE is about 10 percent higher than the average woman's. In practical terms, this means that a 140-pound man can hold his weight steady while eating about 10 percent more than a 140-pound woman who is the same age and performs the same amount of physical work.

No amount of dieting will change this unfair situation. A woman who exercises strenuously may reduce her body fat so dramatically that she no longer menstruates, an occupational hazard for some professional athletes. But she will still have proportionately more body fat than an adult man of the same weight. If she eats what he does and they perform the same amount of physical work, she still requires fewer calories than he to hold her weight steady.

And here's a really rotten possibility. Muscle weighs more than fat. This is an interesting fact that many people who take up exercise to lose weight discover by accident. One month into the barbells and step-up-step-down routine, their clothes fit better, but the scale points slightly higher because they've traded fat for muscle — and you know what that means: Sometimes you can't win for losing. (Sorry, but I just couldn't resist.)

Energy for work

Your second largest chunk of energy is the energy you withdraw to spend on physical work. That's everything from brushing your teeth in the morning to hoeing a row of petunias in the garden or working out in the gym.

Your total energy requirement (the number of calories you need each day) is your REE plus enough calories to cover the amount of work you do.

Does thinking about this use up energy? Yes, but not as much as you might imagine. To solve a crossword puzzle — or write a chapter of this book — the average brain uses about one calorie every four minutes. That's only one-third the amount needed to keep a 60-watt bulb burning for the same length of time.

Table 3-2 defines the energy level of various activities ranging from the least energetic (sleep) to the most (playing football, digging ditches). Table 3-3 shows how many calories you use in an hour's worth of different kinds of work.

Table 3-2	How Active Are You When You're Active?
Activity Level	*Activity*
Resting	Sleeping, reclining
Very light	Seated and standing activities, painting, driving, laboratory work, typing, sewing, ironing, cooking, playing cards, playing a musical instrument
Light	Walking on a level surface at 2.5 to 3 mph, garage work, electrical trades, carpentry, restaurant trades, housecleaning, child care, golf, sailing, table tennis
Moderate	Walking 3.5 to 4 mph, weeding and hoeing, carrying a load, cycling, skiing, tennis, dancing
Heavy	Walking with a load uphill, tree felling, heavy manual digging, basketball, climbing, football, soccer
Exceptionally heavy	Professional athletic training

Source: The National Research Council, "Recommended Dietary Allowances" (Washington, D.C.: National Academy Press, 1989).

Table 3-3	How Many Calories Do You Need to Do the Work You Do?
Activity Level	*Calories Needed for This Work for One Hour*
Very light	80–100
Light	110–160
Moderate	170–240
Heavy	250–350
Exceptionally heavy	350+

Source: "Food and Your Weight," *House and Garden Bulletin,* No. 74 (Washington, D.C.: U.S. Department of Agriculture).

Too Much and Too Little

One pound of body fat equals 3,500 calories. So

✔ If you cut your calorie consumption from 2,000 calories a day to 1,700 and continue to do the same amount of physical work, you will lose one pound of fat in just about 12 days.

✔ If you go the other way, increasing your consumption from 1,700 to 2,000 calories a day without increasing the amount of work you do, 12 days later you will be one pound heavier.

Moderate calorie deprivation produces healthful moderate weight loss. You experience this on a sensible weight-loss diet that includes a wide variety of different foods containing sufficient amounts of essential nutrients.

Severe calorie deprivation can cause life-threatening weight loss coupled with nutritional deficiency diseases such as scurvy (the vitamin C deficiency disease) or night blindness due to a lack of vitamin A. If severe calorie deprivation continues unabated, the ultimate result is death by starvation. You may experience calorie deprivation if you have a serious eating disorder or live in an area where there is continual famine.

Some people starve themselves voluntarily because they have an eating disorder such as anorexia nervosa or because they are trying to fit their normal-size bodies into a social stereotype that is thinner than they should be. But widespread involuntary starvation, a continuing tragedy in parts of the Third World or under wartime conditions, is rare in the United States.

In fact, just the opposite is true. Statistics show that as many as 24 percent of American men and 27 percent of American women are obese, meaning that they weigh 20 percent or more than standard height-weight charts *suggest* they should.

How much should you weigh?

Over the years, a number of charts have purported to lay out "standard" or "healthy" weights for adult Americans, but some set the figures so low that you can hardly get there without severely restricting your diet — or being born again, this time with a different body, preferably with light bones and no curves.

Table 3-4 is one moderate, eminently usable set of weight recommendations that originally appeared in the 1990 edition of *Nutrition and Your Health: Dietary Guidelines for Americans,* a publication of the U.S. Department of Agriculture and the U.S. Department of Health and Human Services. The weights in this chart are listed in ranges for people (men and women) of specific heights. Naturally, you know that height is measured without shoes; weight, without clothes.

Because most people do gain some weight as they get older, Table 3-4 does a really sensible thing by dividing the ranges into two broad categories, one for men and women age 19 to 34, the other for men and women age 35 and older.

If you have a small frame and proportionately more fat tissue than muscle tissue (muscle is heavier than fat), you are likely to weigh in at the low end. If you have a large frame and proportionately more muscle than fat, you are likely to weigh in at the high end. As a general (but by no means invariable) rule, this means that women — who have smaller frames and less muscle — weigh less than men of the same height and age. People who far exceed the weights shown here are called obese (see the sidebar "What do they mean when they say that you're fat?").

I feel honor bound to tell you that later editions of the *Dietary Guidelines* leave out the higher weight allowances for older people, which means that the "healthy" weights for everyone, young or old, are the ones listed in the column for 19- to 34-year olds. I am going to go out on a limb here and say that, even though I am not fat and easily meet the later standards, I prefer the 1990 recommendations because they are

✔ Achievable without constant dieting

✔ Realistic about how your body changes as you get older

✔ Less likely to make you totally crazy about your weight

. . . which is a pretty good description of how nutritional guidelines should work, don't you think?

Table 3-4	How Much Should You Weigh?	
Height	**Weight (Pounds) for 19- to 34-Year Olds**	**Weight (Pounds) for 35+ Year Olds**
5'	97 – 128	108 – 138
5'1"	101 – 132	111 – 143
5'2"	104 – 137	115 – 148
5'3"	107 – 141	119 – 152
5'4"	111 – 146	122 – 157
5'5"	114 – 150	126 – 162
5'6"	118 – 155	130 – 167
5'7"	121 – 160	134 – 172
5'8"	125 – 164	138 – 178
5'9"	129 – 169	142 – 183
5'10"	132 – 174	146 – 188
5'11"	136 – 179	151 – 194

Height	Weight (Pounds) for 19- to 34-Year Olds	Weight (Pounds) for 35+ Year Olds
6′	140 – 184	155 – 199
6′1″	144 – 189	159 – 205
6′2″	148 – 195	164 – 210
6′3″	152 – 200	168 – 216
6′4″	156 – 205	173 – 222
6′5″	160 – 211	177 – 228
6′6″	164 – 216	182 – 234

Source: *Nutrition and Your Health: Dietary Guidelines for Americans,* 3rd ed. (Washington D.C.: U.S. Department of Agriculture, U.S. Department of Health and Human Services, 1990).

Another way to rate your weight

As you run your finger down the chart in Table 3-4, remember that the numbers are guidelines — no more, no less.

Squeezing people into neat little boxes is a reassuring exercise, but in real life, human beings constantly confound The Rules. We all know chubby people who live long and happy lives and trim and skinny ones who leave us sooner than they should. However, people who are overweight do have a higher risk of developing some illnesses, such as diabetes. So you need a way to find out if your current weight puts you at risk for this kind of illness.

One good guide is the Body Mass Index (BMI), a number that measures the relationship between your weight and your height and offers some predictive estimate of your risk of weight-related disease.

What do they mean when they say that you're fat?

Obesity is a specific medical condition in which the body accumulates an over-abundance of fatty tissue. One way nutritionists determine who's obese is by comparing a person's weight with the figures on the weight/height charts:

✔ If your weight is 20 to 40 percent higher than the chart, you're mildly obese.

✔ If your weight is 40 to 99 percent higher, you're moderately obese.

✔ If your weight is more than double the weight on the chart, you're severely obese.

To calculate your BMI, perform the following steps:

1. **Divide your weight (in pounds) by your height (in inches) squared.**
2. **Multiply the result of Step 1 by 705.**

For example, if you are 5'3" (63 inches) tall and weigh 138 pounds, the equations for your BMI looks like this:

$$BMI = \frac{138}{63 \times 63 \text{ inches}} \times 705 = 24.5$$

Current nutritional research suggests that the most healthy BMI is about 21.0. A BMI higher than 28 (168 pounds for a 5'5" woman; 195 pounds for a 5'10" man) doubles the risk of illness (especially diabetes and heart disease) and death.

How reliable are the numbers?

Weight charts and tables and numbers and stats are so plentiful that you might think they are totally reliable in predicting who's healthy and who's not. So here's a surprise: They aren't.

The problem is that real people and their differences keep sneaking into the equation. For example, the value of the BMI in predicting your risk of illness or death appears to be tied to your age. If you are in your 30s, a lower BMI is clearly linked to better health. If you are in your 70s or older, there is no convincing evidence that how much you weigh plays a significant role in determining how healthy you are or how much longer you will live. In-between, from age 30 to age 74, the relationship between your BMI and your health is, well, in-between — more important early on, less important later in life.

In other words, the simple evidence of your own eyes is true. Although Americans sometimes seem totally obsessed with the need to lose weight, the fact is that many larger people, even people who are clearly obese, do live long, happy, and healthy lives. To figure out why, many nutrition scientists are now focussing not just on weight or weight/height (the BMI), but on the importance of *confounding variables*, which is science-speak for "something else is going on here."

Here are three potential confounding variables in the obesity/health equation:

> ✔ Maybe people who are overweight are more prone to illness because they exercise less, in which case stepping up the workouts might reduce the perceived risk of being overweight.

✔ Maybe people who are overweight are more likely to be sick because they eat lots of "bad" foods (such as foods high in saturated fat), which is why they are fat, in which case the remedy may be simply a change in diet.

✔ Maybe people who are overweight have a genetic predisposition to a serious disease. If that's true, you would have to ask whether losing 20 pounds really reduces their risk of disease to the level of a person who is naturally 20 pounds lighter. Perhaps not: In a few studies, people who successfully lost weight actually had a higher rate of death.

Adding to the confusion is the fact that an obsessive attempt to lose weight may itself be hazardous to your health (see Chapter 14). Every year, Americans spend $30 to $50 billion (yes, you read that right) on diet clubs, special foods, and over-the-counter remedies aimed at weight loss. Often the diets, the pills, and the foods don't work, which may leave dieters feeling worse than they did before they started.

But that's only half the bad news. Here's the rest: Some foods that effectively lower calorie intake and some drugs that effectively reduce appetite have potentially serious side effects. For example, some fat substitutes prevent your body from absorbing important nutrients (see Chapter 19), and some prescription diet drugs, such as the combination once known as "Phen-Fen," are linked to serious, even fatal, diseases.

Right about here, you probably feel the strong need for a really big chocolate bar. Hold on, wrestle that craving to a standstill, and consider the alternative — realistic rules that allow you to control your weight safely and effectively:

✔ **Rule # 1: Not everybody starts out with the same set of genes — or fits into the same pair of jeans.** Some people are naturally larger and heavier than others. If that's you, and all your vital stats satisfy your doctor, don't waste time trying to fit someone else's idea of perfection. Relax and enjoy your own body.

✔ **Rule # 2: If you are overweight and your doctor agrees with your decision to diet, you don't have to set world records to improve your health.** Even a moderate drop in poundage can be highly beneficial. According to a recent editorial in *The New England Journal of Medicine* (www.nejm.org on the Net), losing just 10 to 15 percent of your body weight can lower high blood sugar, high cholesterol, and high blood pressure, reducing your risk of diabetes, heart disease, and stroke.

The last word on calories

Calories are not your enemy. On the contrary, they are the energy you need to live a healthy life.

The trick is to manage your calories, not let them manage you. Once you know that fats are more fattening than proteins and carbohydrates and that your body burns food to make energy, you can strategize your energy intake to match your energy expenditure, and vice versa. Here's how: Turn straight to Chapter 16 to find out about a healthful diet and Chapter 17 to find out about planning nutritious meals.

Chapter 4

How Much Nutrition Do You Need?

• •

In This Chapter

▶ What the Recommended Dietary Allowances (RDAs) are

▶ The difference between an RDA and an Estimated Safe and Adequate Daily Dietary Intake

▶ The DRI: A new way of looking at nutrition

▶ Why who you are determines the amount of nutrients you need

• •

A healthful diet provides sufficient amounts of all the nutrients your body needs. The question is, how much is enough?

Today, three sets of recommendations provide the answers, each with its own virtues and deficits. The first, and most familiar, is the RDA (short for Recommended Dietary Allowance). The second, the Estimated Safe and Adequate Daily Dietary Intakes (ESADDIs), describes recommended amounts of nutrients for which no RDAs exist. The third is the DRI (Dietary Reference Intake), a new umbrella term that includes RDAs plus several innovative categories of nutrient recommendations.

Confused? Not to worry. I spell it all out in this chapter.

RDAs: Guidelines for Good Nutrition

The Recommended Dietary Allowances (RDAs) were created in 1941 by the Food and Nutrition Board, a subsidiary of the National Research Council which is part of the National Academy of Sciences in Washington, D.C.

RDAs were originally designed to make it easy for you to plan several days' meals in advance. The "D" in RDA stands for dietary, not daily, because the RDAs are an average. You may get more one day, less the next, but the idea is to hit an average over several days.

For example, the current RDA for vitamin C is 60 mg for adults (age 18 and up), half of what you get from just one 8-ounce glass of fresh orange juice. So you could have an 8-ounce glass of orange juice on Monday, skip Tuesday, and still meet the RDA for the two days.

The amounts provided by the RDAs provide a "margin of safety" for healthy people, but they're not therapeutic. In other words, RDA servings won't cure a nutrient deficiency, but they can prevent one from occurring.

The essentials

The most recent RDAs, published in 1989, include recommendations for protein as well as 18 essential vitamins and minerals:

- ✔ Vitamin A
- ✔ Folate
- ✔ Vitamin D
- ✔ Vitamin B12
- ✔ Vitamin E
- ✔ Calcium
- ✔ Vitamin K
- ✔ Phosphorus
- ✔ Vitamin C

- ✔ Magnesium
- ✔ Thiamin (vitamin B1)
- ✔ Iron
- ✔ Riboflavin (vitamin B2)
- ✔ Zinc
- ✔ Niacin
- ✔ Iodine
- ✔ Vitamin B6
- ✔ Selenium

Recommendations for carbohydrates, fats, dietary fiber, and alcohol

What nutrients are missing from that list of essentials? Carbohydrates, fiber, fat, and alcohol. The reason is simple: If your diet provides enough protein, vitamins, and minerals, it is almost certain to provide enough carbohydrates and probably more than enough fat. Although no RDAs exist for carbohydrates and fat, recommendations definitely exist for them and for dietary fiber and alcohol.

In 1980, the U.S. Public Health Service and the U.S. Department of Agriculture joined forces to produce the first edition of Dietary Guidelines for Americans (see Chapter 16).

This report, modified in 1991 and 1995, sets parameters for what you can consider reasonable amounts of fat, saturated fat, total carbohydrates, fiber, and alcohol. According to the current guidelines:

✔ The total amount of fat in your diet should not exceed 30 percent of the calories you consume each day. In other words, if your daily diet is about 2,000 calories, no more than 600 calories should come from fat.

✔ No more than 10 percent of the calories you consume should come from saturated fat. On a 2,000-calorie diet, that's 200 for saturated fat.

✔ Carbohydrates (primarily the complex ones from fruits, vegetables, and whole grains) should account for 60 percent of your daily calories. That's 1,200 calories on a 2,000-calorie diet.

✔ You should get 11.5 grams of dietary fiber for every 1,000 calories you consume. That's 23 grams fiber in a 2,000-calorie day.

✔ Moderate drinking, which may contribute to a healthy lifestyle, means one drink a day for a woman, two for a man.

Note: For details on how to use the Dietary Guidelines, see Chapter 16.

Different people, different needs

Because different bodies require different amounts of nutrients, there are currently RDAs for 17 specific categories of human beings: boys and girls, men and women, from infancy through middle age.

For example, the RDA for protein is set in terms of grams of protein per kilogram (2.2 pounds) of body weight. Because the average man weighs more than the average woman, his RDA for protein is higher than hers. The RDA for an adult male, age 25 to 50, is 79 grams; for a woman, 63 grams.

Because women of childbearing age lose iron when they menstruate, their RDA for iron is 15 mg; for a man, 10 mg.

Just about the only category not yet covered in detail is older Americans. After 50, they are all grouped together as "51+."

But that is expected to change when the next edition of the RDAs is issued, perhaps late in 1999. In 1990, the U.S. Census counted 31,100,000 million Americans older than 65. By the year 2050, the U.S. Government expects more than 60,000,000.

As a result, the next set of RDAs, to be issued by the year 2000, will likely have separate categories for people who are middle-aged (perhaps 51 to 70), elderly (perhaps 71 to 85), and very old (85+).

ESADDI: A Second Set of Nutritional Numbers

In addition to the RDAs, the Food and Nutrition Board created Estimated Safe and Adequate Daily Dietary Intakes (sometimes abbreviated ESADDIs) for seven nutrients considered necessary for good health, even though nobody really knows exactly how much your body needs. ESADDIs are proposed for people in seven different age groups: birth to six months, six months to a year, one to three years, four to six years, seven to ten years, eleven to fourteen years, and adults (people older than 18).

The nutrients in this category are:

- ✔ Biotin
- ✔ Fluoride
- ✔ Pantothenic acid
- ✔ Chromium
- ✔ Copper
- ✔ Molybdenum
- ✔ Manganese

DRI: A New Nutrition Guide

In 1993, four years after the last RDAs were published, the Food and Nutrition Board's Dietary Reference Intake committee established panels to review the RDAs and other recommendations for major nutrients (vitamins, minerals, and other food components) in light of new research and nutrition information.

The panels' first order of business was to establish a new standard for nutrient recommendations called the Dietary Reference Intakes (DRI). The DRI is an umbrella term embracing several categories of nutritional measurements for vitamins, minerals, and other nutrients. It includes:

- ✔ **Estimated Average Requirement (EAR):** The amount that meets the nutritional needs of half the people in any one group (such as teenage girls, or people older than 70). Nutritionists use the EAR to figure out whether an entire population's normal diet provides adequate amounts of nutrients.

✔ **Recommended Dietary Allowance (RDA):** The RDA, now based on information provided by the EAR, is still a daily average for individuals, the amount of any one nutrient known to protect against deficiency.

✔ **Adequate Intake (AI):** The AI is a new measurement, the amount recommended for nutrients for which an RDA hasn't been set. It takes the place of the ESADDI.

✔ **Tolerable Upper Intake Level (UL):** The UL is the highest amount of a nutrient you can consume each day without risking an adverse effect.

The Dietary Reference Intakes Panel's first report, listing new recommendations for calcium, phosphorus, magnesium, and fluoride, appeared in 1997. Its most notable change: upping the RDA for calcium from 800 mg to 1,000 mg for adults age 31 to 50.

The second DRI Panel report appeared in 1998. The report had new recommendations for thiamin, riboflavin, niacin, vitamin B6, folate, vitamin B12, pantothenic acid, biotin and choline. The most important revision was increasing the folate recommendation to 400 mcg a day based on evidence showing that folate reduces a woman's risk of giving birth to a baby with spinal cord defects and lowers the risk of heart disease for both men and women.

As a result, the FDA ordered food manufacturers to add folates to flour, rice, and other grain products. (Multivitamin products already contain 400 mcg of folates.) In May 1999, data released by the Framingham Heart Study, which has followed heart health among residents of a Boston suburb for nearly half a century, showed a dramatic increase in blood levels of folic acid. Before the fortification of foods, 22 percent of the study participants had a folic acid deficiency; after the fortification, the number fell to 2 percent.

A third DRI report with revised recommendations for vitamin C appeared in early 1999. The reports for vitamin E, beta-carotene and other antioxidant vitamins are expected later in the year. The report for vitamin C is based on several studies, including a 1996 report from the National Institute of Diabetes, Digestive and Kidney Diseases, a division of the National Institute of Health, which states what many have long believed: The RDA (60 mg) does not provide enough vitamin C for healthy people.

In a study controlling the amount of vitamin C for seven healthy young men for four to six months, the optimum daily dose appeared to be 200 mg, the amount required to saturate the men's immune cells (create a situation where the cells held as much vitamin C as possible). Men who got less stored the vitamin until their cells were full. Men who got more simply excreted the excess in urine. *Note:* 200 mg is the amount of vitamin C in five servings of fresh fruit and/or vegetables.

The terms used to describe nutrient recommendations

RDAs for protein are listed in grams. The RDA and Estimated Safe and Effective Daily Dietary Intakes for vitamins and minerals are shown in milligrams (mg) and micrograms (mcg). A milligram is ⅟₁₀₀₀th of a gram; a microgram is ⅟₁₀₀₀th of a milligram.

Vitamin A, vitamin D, and vitamin E are special cases. One form of vitamin A is pre-formed, which means your body can use it right away. Pre-formed vitamin A, known as *retinol,* is found in food from animals — liver, milk, eggs.

Carotenoids (yellow pigments in plants) also provide vitamin A. But to get vitamin A from carotenoids, your body has to convert the pigments to chemicals similar to retinol.

Because retinol is the ready-made nutrient, the RDA for vitamin A is listed in units called retinol equivalents (RE). A retinol equivalent is equal to one microgram of pre-formed vitamin A.

Vitamin D consists of three compounds: vitamin D1, vitamin D2, and vitamin D3. Cholecalciferol, the chemical name for vitamin D3, is the most active of the three, so the RDA for vitamin D is measured in equivalents of cholecalciferol.

Your body gets vitamin E from two classes of chemicals in food: tocopherols and tocotrienols. The compound with the greatest vitamin E activity is a tocopherol: alpha-tocopherol. The RDA for vitamin E is measured in milligrams of alpha-tocopherol equivalents (mg a-TE).

Additional DRI reports, with recommendations for trace elements such as selenium and zinc, vitamin A, vitamin K, and other food components, including phytoestrogens (see Chapter 12), are expected between 2000 and 2003, by which point there will also be a completely new set of RDAs.

Table 4-1 shows the current RDAs. Table 4-2 shows the current ESADDIs. The numbers in parentheses are the RDA or AI recommendations of the Dietary Reference Intakes panel's reports from 1997 and 1998.

Table 4-1	The RDAs	
g = gram	R = retinol	
mg = milligram	a-TE = alpha-alpha-tocopherol equivalent	
mcg = microgram	NE = niacin equivalent	
Age (years)	**Protein (g)**	
Infants/children		
0.0–0.5	13	
0.5–1.0	14	
1–3	16	

Age (years)	Protein (g)
4–6	24
7–10	28
Males	
11–14	45
15–18	59
19–24	58
25–50	63
51+	63
Females	
11–14	46
15–18	44
19–24	46
25–50	50
51+	50
Pregnant	60
Nursing (1st 6 mos.)	65
Nursing (2nd 6 mos.)	62

Age (years)	Vitamin A (mcgRE)	Vitamin D (mcg/IU)	Vitamin E (mg/a-TE)	Vitamin K (mcg)	Vitamin C (mg)
Infants/children					
0.0–0.5	375	7.5/300	3	5	30
0.5–1.0	375	10/400	3	10	35
1–3	400	10/400	6	15	40
4–6	500	10/400	7	20	45
7–10	700	10/400	7	30	45
Males					
11–14	1,000	10/400	10	45	50
15–18	1,000	10/400	10	65	60
19–24	1,000	10/400	10	70	60
25–50	1,000	5/200	10	80	60
51+	1,000	5/200 (10/400)*	10	80	60

(continued)

Table 4-1 *(continued)*

g	= gram	R	= retinol
mg	= milligram	a-TE	= alpha-alpha-tocopherol equivalent
mcg	= microgram	NE	= niacin equivalent

Age (years)	Vitamin A (mcgRE)	Vitamin D (mcg/IU)	Vitamin E (mg/a-TE)	Vitamin K (mcg)	Vitamin C (mg)
Females					
11–14	800	10/400	8	45	50
15–18	800	10/400	8	55	60
19–24	800	10/400	8	60	60
25–50	800	5/200	8	65	60
51+	800	5/200 (10/400)*	8	65	60
Pregnant	800	10/400	10	65	70
Nursing (1st 6 mos.)	1,300	10/400	12	65	95
Nursing (2nd 6 mos.)	1,200	10/400	11	65	90

* The new AI for people age 71 and older is 15mcg/600 IU

Age (years)	Thiamin (Vitamin B1) (mg)	Riboflavin (Vitamin B2) (mg)	Niacin (mcg/NE)	Vitamin B6 (mg)	Folate (mcg)
Infants/Children					
0.0–0.5	0.3	0.4	5	0.3	25
0.5–1.0	0.4	0.5	6	0.6	35
1–3	0.7	0.8	9	1.0	50
4–6	0.9	1.1	12	1.1	75
7–10	1.0	1.2	13	1.4	100
Males					
11–14	1.3	1.5	17	1.7	150
15–18	1.5	1.8	20	2.0	200
19–24	1.5	1.7	19	2.0	200
25–50	1.5 (1.2)**	1.7 (1.3)*	19 (16)*	2.0 (1.3)*	200 (400)*
51+	1.2	1.4	15	2.0	200

Age (years)	Thiamin (Vitamin B1) (mg)	Riboflavin (Vitamin B2) (mg)	Niacin (mcg/NE)	Vitamin B6 (mg)	Folate (mcg)
Females					
11–14	1.1	1.3	15	1.4	150
15–18	1.1	1.3	15	1.5	180
19–24	1.1	1.3	15	1.6	180
25–50	1.1	1.3 (1.1)**	15 (14)**	1.6 (1.3)**	180 (400)**
51+	1.0	1.2	13	1.6	180
Pregnant	1.5	1.6	17	2.2	400
Nursing (1st 6 mos.)	1.6	1.8	20	2.1	280
Nursing (2nd 6 mos.)	1.6	1.7	20	2.1	260

** The numbers in parentheses are the RDA or AI recommendations of the Dietary Reference Intakes Panel's reports from 1997 and 1998.

Age (years)	Calcium (mg)	Phosphorus (mg)	Magnesium (mg)	Iron (mg)	Zinc (mg)
Infants/children					
0.0–0.5	400	300	40	6	5
0.5–1.0	600	500	60	10	5
1–3	800	800	80	10	10
4–6	800	800	120	10	10
7–10	800	800	170	10	10
Males					
11–14	1,200	1,200	270	12	15
15–18	1,200	1,200	400	12	15
19–24	1,200	1,200	350	10	15
25–50	800 (1,000)*	800 (700)*	350 (420)*	10	15
51+	800	800	350	10	15
Females					
11–14	1,200	1,200	280	15	12
15–18	1,200	1,200	300	15	12

(continued)

Table 4-1 *(continued)*

g = gram	R = retinol
mg = milligram	a-TE = alpha-alpha-tocopherol equivalent
mcg = microgram	NE = niacin equivalent

Age (years)	Calcium (mg)	Phosphorus (mg)	Magnesium (mg)	Iron (mg)	Zinc (mg)
19–24	1,200	1,200	280	15	12
25–50	800 (1,000)*	800 (700)*	280 (420)*	15	12
51+	800	800	280	10	12
Pregnant	1,200	1,200	320	30	15
Nursing (1st 6 mos.)	1,200	1,200	355	15	19
Nursing (2nd 6 mos.)	1,200	1,200	340	15	16

* The numbers in parentheses are the RDA or AI recommendations of the Dietary Reference Intakes Panel's reports from 1997 and 1998.

Age (years)	Iodine (mcg)	Selenium (mcg)
Infants/Children		
0.0–0.5	40	10
0.5–1.0	50	15
1–3	70	20
4–6	90	20
7–10	120	30
Males		
11–14	150	40
15–18	150	40
19–24	150	70
25–50	150	70
51+	150	70
Females		
11–14	150	45
15–18	150	45
19–24	150	55
25–50	150	55

Age (years)	Iodine (mcg)	Selenium (mcg)
51+	150	55
Pregnant	175	65
Nursing (1st 6 mos.)	200	75
Nursing (2nd 6 mos.)	200	75

Table 4-2 Estimated Safe and Adequate Daily Dietary Intakes

Age (years)	Biotin (mcg)	Pantothenic acid (mg)	Copper (mg)	Manganese (mg)	Fluoride (mg)
Infants/Children					
0.0–0.5	10	2	0.4–0.6	0.3–0.6	0.1–0.5
0.5–1.0	15	3	0.6–0.7	0.6–1.0	0.2–1.0
1–3	20	3	0.7–1.0	1.0–1.5	0.5–1.5
4–6	25	3–4	1.0–1.5	1.5–2.0	1.0–2.5
7–10	30	4–5	1.0–2.0	2.0–3.0	1.5–2.5
Males					
11–14	30–100	4–7	1.5–2.5	2.0–5.0	1.5–2.5
15–18	30–100	4–7	1.5–2.5	2.0–5.0	1.5–2.5
19–24	30–100	4–7	1.5–3.0	2.0–5.0	1.5–4.0
25–50	30–100 (30)*	4–7 (5)*	1.5–3.0	2.0–5.0	1.5–4.0
51+	30–100	4–7	1.5–3.0	2.0–5.0	1.5–4.0
Females					
11–14	30–100	4–7	1.5–2.5	2.0–5.0	1.5–2.5
15–18	30–100	4–7	1.5–2.5	2.0–5.0	1.5–2.5
19–24	30–100	4–7	1.5–3.0	2.0–5.0	1.5–4.0
25–50	30–100 (30)*	4–7 (5)*	1.5–3.0	2.0–5.0	1.5–4.0
51+	30–100	4–7	1.5–3.0	2.0–5.0	1.5–4.0
Pregnant	30–100	4–7	1.5–3.0	2.0–5.0	1.5–4.0
Nursing (1st 6 mos.)	30–100	4–7	1.5–3.0	2.0–5.0	1.5–4.0
Nursing (2nd 6 mos.)	30–100	4–7	1.5–3.0	2.0–5.0	1.5–4.0

* The numbers in parentheses are the RDA or AI recommendations of the Dietary Reference Intakes Panel's reports from 1997 and 1998.

(continued)

Table 4-1 (continued)

Age (years)	Chromium (mcg)	Molybdenum (mcg)	Choline (mcg)
Infants/Children			
0.0–0.5	10–40	15–30	Not determined
0.5–1.0	20–60	20–40	Not determined
1–3	20–80	25–50	Not determined
4–6	30–120	30–75	Not determined
7–10	50–200	50–150	Not determined
Males			
11–14	50–200	75–250	Not determined
15–18	50–200	75–250	Not determined
19–24	50–200	75–250	Not determined
25–50	50–200	75–250	Not determined (550)*
51+	50–200	75–250	Not determined
Females			
11–14	50–200	75–250	Not determined
15–18	50–200	75–250	Not determined
19–24	50–200	75–250	Not determined
25–50	50–200	75–250	Not determined (425)*
51+	50–200	75–250	Not determined
Pregnant	50–200	75–250	Not determined
Nursing (1st 6 mos.)	50–200	75–250	Not determined
Nursing (2nd 6 mos.)	50–200	75–250	Not determined

* The numbers in parentheses are the RDA or AI recommendations of the Dietary Reference 3Intakes Panel's reports from 1997 and 1998.

No Sale Is Ever Final

That slogan is on the sales slips at my favorite clothing store, but it also applies to nutritional numbers. Until the new RDAs are issued, consider the entire subject a work in progress. New studies yielding bunches of new information will affect the DRI panels' deliberations right up until the numbers are actually set in type and published. After that, the whole process will start all over again as new information becomes available in this ever-changing field.

Chapter 5

A Supplemental Story

*E*very year, Americans spend nearly $3 billion on dietary supplements, everything from plain old vitamin C to — yuck! — desiccated (dried) liver. You can stir up a good food fight in any group of nutrition experts simply by asking whether all these supplements are (a) necessary, (b) economical, or (c) safe. But when the argument's over, you still may not have a satisfactory official answer, so this brief chapter aims to provide the information you need to make your own sensible choices.

What a Dietary Supplement Is

The vitamin pill you may pop each morning is a dietary supplement. So are the calcium antacids many American women consider standard nutrition. Echinacea, the herb reputed to short-circuit your winter cold, is, and so is the vanilla-flavored meal-in-a-can liquid your granny chug-a-lugs each afternoon just before setting off on her daily mile power walk.

The Food and Drug Administration (FDA) classifies each of these as a dietary supplement because they meet the agency's definition: any pill, tablet, capsule, powder, or liquid you take by mouth that contains a dietary ingredient. Of course, that raises another question: What's a dietary ingredient?

Answer:

- ✔ Vitamins
- ✔ Minerals
- ✔ Herbs
- ✔ Amino acids (the "building blocks of protein" described in Chapter 6)
- ✔ Enzymes
- ✔ Organ tissue such as desiccated (dried) liver or shark cartilage
- ✔ Some hormones, such as melatonin, which is promoted as a sleep aid
- ✔ Metabolites (substances produced when nutrients are digested)
- ✔ Extracts

Dietary supplements may be single-ingredient products, such as vitamin E capsules, or they may be combination products, such as the nutrient-packed protein powders favored by some athletes.

Why People Use Dietary Supplements

In a country where food is plentiful and affordable, you have to wonder why so many people opt to scarf down pills instead of just plain food.

Many people consider vitamin and mineral supplements a quick and easy way to get nutrients without lots of shopping and kitchen time — and without all the pesky fat and sugars in food. Others take supplements as "nutritional insurance" (for more on recommended dietary allowances of vitamins and minerals, see Chapter 4). And some use supplements as substitutes for medical drugs.

In general, nutrition experts, including the American Dietetic Association, the National Academy of Sciences, and the National Research Council, prefer that you invest your time and money whipping up meals and snacks that supply the nutrients you need in a balanced, tasty diet. Nonetheless, every expert worth her vitamin C admits that in certain circumstances, supplements can be a definite plus.

When Food Is Not Enough

Illness, age, diet preferences, and some gender-related conditions may put you in a spot where you can't get all the nutrients you need from food alone.

Digestive illnesses, unfriendly drugs, injury, and chronic illness

Certain metabolic disorders and diseases of the digestive organs (liver, gall-bladder, pancreas, intestines) interfere with the normal digestion of food and the absorption of nutrients. Some medicines may also interfere with normal digestion, meaning you need supplements to make up the difference. People with certain chronic diseases, or who have suffered a major injury (such as a serious burn), or who have just been through surgery may need more nutrients than they can get from food. In these cases, a doctor may prescribe supplements to provide the hard-to-get vitamins, minerals, and other nutrients.

It's smart to check with your doctor before opting for a supplement you hope will have medical effects (make you stronger, smooth your skin, ease your anxiety). The bad old days when doctors were total ignoramuses about nutrition may not be gone forever, but they're fading fast. Besides, your doctor is the person most familiar with your health, knows what medications you are taking, and can warn you of potential side effects.

Vegetarianism

Vitamin B12 is found only in food from animals, such as meat, milk, and eggs. (Some seaweeds do have B12, but the suspicion is that the vitamin comes from micro-organisms living in the plant.) Without these foods, vegans — people who do not eat any foods of animal origin — are simply out of luck. They must get their vitamin B12 from supplements. Vegetarians who eat some animal foods may also need calcium, zinc, and iron supplements. These minerals are found in some plants, but only in a form your body does not absorb as easily as those in animal foods.

Using Supplements as Insurance

Healthy people who do eat a nutritious diet may still want to use supplements to "make sure" they're getting adequate nutrition. Their choice is supported by a lot of recent research.

Protecting against disease

After analyzing the data from a survey of 871 men and women (half diagnosed with colon cancer), epidemiologists at Seattle's Fred Hutchinson Cancer Center found that those taking a daily multivitamin for more than ten years were 50 percent less likely to develop colon cancer. In addition, sele-nium supplements seem to reduce the risk of prostate cancer, and Vitamin C seems to lower the risk of cataracts.

Supplementing aging appetites

As you grow older, your appetite may decline and your sense of taste and smell may falter. If food no longer tastes as good as it once did or if you have to eat alone all the time and don't enjoy cooking for one, or if dentures make it difficult to chew, you may not take in all the foods you need to get the nutri-ents you require. Dietary supplements to the rescue!

If you're so rushed that you literally never get to eat a full, balanced meal, you may benefit from supplements regardless of your age.

Meeting a woman's special needs

And what about women? At various stages of their reproductive lives, they, too, benefit from supplements-as-insurance:

- **Before menopause:** Women who lose iron each month through men-strual bleeding rarely get sufficient amounts of iron from a typical American diet providing fewer than 2,000 calories a day. For them, as well as women who are often on a diet to lose weight, supplements may be the only practical answer.

- **During pregnancy and lactation:** Women who are pregnant or nursing may need supplements to provide the nutrients they need to build new maternal and fetal tissue or to produce nutritious breast milk. In addi-tion, supplements of the B vitamin folate are now known to decrease a woman's risk of giving birth to a child with a neural tube defect (a defect of the spinal cord and column).

Never self-prescribe supplements while you're pregnant. Large amounts of some nutrients may actually be hazardous for your baby. For exam-ple, taking megadoses of vitamin A while you are pregnant can increase the risk of birth defects.

- **Through adulthood:** True, women older than 19 can get the calcium they require (1,000 mg/day) from four 8-ounce glasses of non-fat skim milk a day, or three 8-ounce containers of yogurt made with non-fat milk, or 22 ounces of canned salmon (with the soft edible bones; no, you should definitely not eat the hard bones in fresh salmon!) — or any com-bination of the above. But is it realistic to expect that women will do this balancing act every single day? Probably not. The simple alternative is calcium supplements.

Using Supplements in Place of Medicine

Everybody knows — achoo! — there is no medical cure for the common cold. Over the years, several supplements, such as zinc lozenges, have been touted as cold remedies. Most have now fallen by the wayside, but a new contender, the herb echinacea (pronounced e-kin-ay-sha), seems to relieve symptoms and hasten recovery.

A second herb, St. John's Wort, is widely used as an antidepressant in Europe. Eventually, well structured long-term tests will show whether the herb, now sold in the United States, really is a safe and effective substitute for commonly-prescribed antidepressant drugs.

Supplement Safety: An Iffy Proposition

The Food and Drug Administration (FDA) regulates food and drugs (no surprise there). Before the agency allows a new food or a new drug on the market, the manufacturer must submit proof that the product is safe. Drug manufacturers must meet a second test, showing that their new medicine is *efficacious,* a fancy way of saying that the drug (and the dosage in which it is sold) will cure or relieve the condition for which it is prescribed.

Nobody says the system's perfect. Reality dictates that manufacturers can only test a drug on a limited number of people for a limited period of time. So you can bet that some new drugs will trigger unexpected, serious, maybe even life-threatening side effects when used by thousands of people or taken for longer than the testing period.

For proof, look no further than Phen-Fen, the diet drug combination that appeared to control weight safely during pre-market testing, but turned lethal once it reached pharmacy shelves.

Sweet trouble

Nobody wants to choke down a yucky supplement, but pills that look or taste like candy may be hazardous to a child's health. Some nutrients are troublesome — or even deadly — in high doses (see Chapters 10 and 11), especially for kids. You're experienced enough to know not to triple your dose just because the supplement tastes like peppermint candy, but you can't count on a child to be that sophisticated. If you have youngsters in your house, protect them by buying neutral-tasting supplements and keeping them in a safe cabinet, preferably high and locked tight to resist tiny prying fingers.

But at least the FDA can require pre-market safety and/or effectiveness info on food and drugs. Unfortunately, the agency has no such power when it comes to dietary supplements.

Supplements and the Law

In 1994, Congress passed and the President signed into law the Dietary Supplement Health and Education Act limiting the FDA's control over dietary supplements. Under this law:

- ✔ The FDA can't require pre-market tests to prove that supplements are safe and effective.

- ✔ The FDA can't limit the dosage in any dietary supplement.

- ✔ The FDA can't halt or restrict sales of a dietary supplement unless there is evidence that the product has caused illness or injury *when used according to the directions on the package*. In other words, if you experience a problem after taking slightly more or less of a supplement than directed on the label, the FDA can't help you.

As a result, the FDA has found it virtually impossible to take products off drugstore shelves even after reports of illness and injury. For example, more than 600 reports of illness and at least 15 deaths are documented among people taking supplements containing *ephedra*, an herb promoted as an energy booster and mood elevator but which can cause abnormal heartbeat, heart attack, seizures, psychosis, and death. Yet ephedra supplements are still on the market, although the government is now attempting to limit their dosages.

By the way, ephedra isn't the only herbal supplement that can make you REALLY uncomfortable. Table 5-1 lists some equally problematic herbal products you should approach with caution — or avoid altogether. In many cases, even small amounts are hazardous.

Table 5-1	Some Potentially Hazardous Herbals
Herb	*Known Side Effects and Reactions*
Blue cohosh	Nausea, vomiting, dizziness, smooth muscle (such as the uterus) contractions
Chaparral	Liver damage, liver failure
Comfrey	Possible liver damage

Herb	Known Side Effects and Reactions
Kombuchu tea	Potentially fatal liver damage, intestinal upset
Lobelia (also known as Indian tobacco)	Potentially fatal convulsions, coma
Pennyroyal	Potentially fatal liver damage, convulsions, coma
Senna	Severe gastric irritation, diarrhea
Stephania (also known as magnolia)	Kidney damage (sometimes severe enough to require dialysis or transplant)
Valerian	Severe withdrawal symptoms

Sources: "Vitamin and nutritional supplements," *Mayo Clinic Health Letter* (supplement), June 1997; Nancy Beth Jackson, "Doctors' warning: Beware of herbs' side effects," *The New York Times,* November 18, 1998; Jane Brody, "Taking a gamble on herbs as medicine," *The New York Times,* February 9, 1999; Carol Ann Rinzler; *The Complete Book of Herbs, Spices, and Condiments* (New York: Facts on File, 1990)

Choosing the Most Effective Supplements

Okay, you've read about the virtues and drawbacks of supplements. You've decided which supplements you think might do you some good. Now it's crunch time, and all you really want to know is how to choose the safest, most effective products. The guidelines in this section should help.

Join the FDA's early warning system

Until Congress gives the FDA the tools it needs to ensure the safety of dietary supplements, the agency counts on you to holler when a dietary supplement causes problems.

If you experience an adverse effect after using a dietary supplement — you get a headache, you break out in hives, your stomach turns queasy — the FDA wants to hear from you through its FDA Medwatch program, which collects information about side effects caused by medical products, including drugs and supplements.

You can call the Medwatch hotline at 1-800-FDA-1088 or log onto the Medwatch Web site at www.fda.gov/medwatch/report/consumer/consumer.htm. After you're logged on, just follow the on-screen directions to pull up a complaint form or hook up with related sites.

To check out earlier reports of supplement side effects, visit the FDA's Special Nutritionals Events Monitoring System site at www.cfsan.fda.gov. (For more details on this terrific site, see Chapter 27.)

Choose a well-known brand

Even though the FDA can't require manufacturers to submit safety and effectiveness data, a respected name on the label offers some assurance of a quality product. It also promises a fresh product; well-known brands generally sell out more quickly. The initials USP (U.S. Pharmacopoeia, a reputable testing organization), are another quality statement, as are the words "release assured" or "proven release," which means the supplement is easily absorbed by your body.

Check the ingredient list

Check the supplement label. In the early 1990s, the FDA introduced the consumer-friendly nutrition food label with its mini-nutrition guide to nutrient content, complete ingredient listings, and dependable information about how eating certain foods may affect your risk of chronic illnesses, such as heart disease and cancer. (For more about the nutrition labels, see Chapter 17.) The FDA's new supplement labels must list all ingredients. The label for vitamin and mineral products must give you the quantity per nutrient per serving plus the %DV (percentage daily value), the percentage of the RDA. The listings for other dietary supplements, such as botanicals (herbs) and phytochemicals (see Chapter 12), must show the quantity per serving plus the part of the plant from which the ingredient is drawn (root, leaves, and so on). A manufacturer's own "proprietary" blend of two or more botanicals must list the weight of the total blend.

Figure 5-1 shows an example of the new supplement labels.

Look for the expiration date

Over time, all dietary supplements become less potent. Always choose the product with the longest useful shelf life. Pass on the ones that will expire before you can use up all the pills, such as the 100-pill bottle whose expiration date is 30 days from now.

Check the storage requirements

Even if you buy a product with the correct expiration date, it may be less effective if you don't keep it in the right place. Some supplements must be refrigerated; the rest you should store, like any food product, in a cool, dry place. Aviod putting dietary supplements in a cabinet over the stove or the refrigerator — true, the fridge is cold inside, but the motor pulsing away outside emits heat.

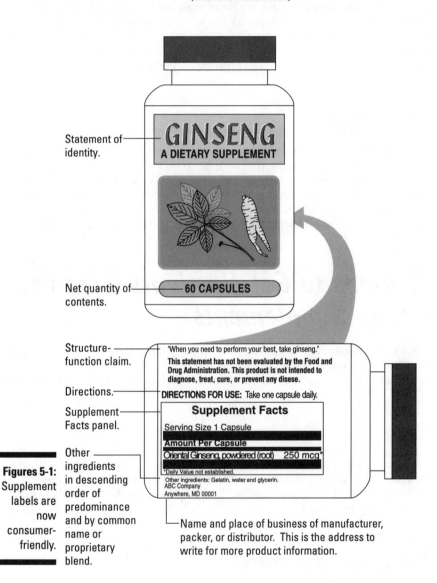

Nutrition Labeling for Dietary Supplements

(Effective March 1999)

Statement of identity.

Net quantity of contents.

Structure-function claim.

Directions.

Supplement Facts panel.

Other ingredients in descending order of predominance and by common name or proprietary blend.

Figures 5-1: Supplement labels are now consumer-friendly.

Name and place of business of manufacturer, packer, or distributor. This is the address to write for more product information.

GINSENG
A DIETARY SUPPLEMENT

60 CAPSULES

"When you need to perform your best, take ginseng."

This statement has not been evaluated by the Food and Drug Administration. This product is not intended to diagnose, treat, cure, or prevent any disese.

DIRECTIONS FOR USE: Take one capsule daily.

Supplement Facts

Serving Size 1 Capsule

Amount Per Capsule

Oriental Ginseng, powdered (root)   250 mcg*

*Daily Value not established.

Other ingredients: Gelatin, water and glycerin.
ABC Company
Anywhere, MD 00001

Choose a sensible dose

Unless your doctor prescribes a dietary supplement as medicine, you don't need products marked "therapeutic," "extra-strength," or any variation thereof. Pick one that gives you no more than the RDA for any ingredient. Luckily, you don't have to memorize the RDAs to know which products these are. Just look for the "%DV," the percentage of the Daily Value the supplement provides. For example, the DV for vitamin C is currently 60 mg for an adult. A product containing 60 mg vitamin C provides 100%DV.

Avoid hype

If the label promises something too good to be true — "Buy me! You'll live for-ever" — you know it's too good to be true. The FDA does not permit supplement marketers to claim that their products cure or prevent disease (that would make them medicines and require pre-market testing). But the agency doses allow claims that affect function such as "maintains your cho-lesterol" (the No-No medical claim would be "lowers your cholesterol").

Good Reasons to Get Nutrients from Food Rather than Supplements

Despite this chapter's focus on the wonders of supplements, I feel obligated to play Devil's Advocate and report to you the arguments in favor of healthy people getting all or most of their nutrients from food rather than supplements.

Cost

If you're willing to plan and prepare nutritious meals, you can almost always get your nutrients less expensively from fresh fruits, vegetables, whole grains, dairy products, meat, fish, and poultry. Besides, food usually tastes better than supplements.

Unexpected bonuses

Food is a package deal containing vitamins, minerals, protein, fat, carbohy-drates, and fiber, plus a cornucopia of as-yet-unidentified substances called phytochemicals (phyto = plant, chemicals = well, chemicals) that may be vital to your continuing good health. Think of lycopene, the red pigment in tomatoes recently found to reduce the risk of prostate cancer. Think of genistein and daidzein, the estrogen-like substances in soybeans that appear to reduce your risk of heart disease. Who knows what else is hiding in your apples, peaches, pears, and plums? Do you want to be the only one on your block who misses out on these goodies? Of course not. For more on the benefits of phytochemicals, see Chapter 12.

Safety

Several common nutrients may be toxic if you scarf them down in megadose servings (amounts several times larger than the RDAs). Large doses of vitamin A aren't linked just to birth defects; they may also cause symptoms similar to a brain tumor. Niacin megadoses may cause liver damage. Megadoses of vitamin B6 may cause (temporary) damage to nerves in arms and legs, fingers, and toes. All these effects are more likely to occur with supplements. Pills slip down easily, but no matter how hungry you are, you probably won't eat enough food to reach toxic levels of nutrients. (To read more about the hazards of megadoses, see Chapters 10 and 11.)

The best statement about the role of supplements in good nutrition may be a paraphrase of Abraham Lincoln's famous remark about politicians and voters: "You may fool all the people some of the time; you can even fool some of the people all the time; but you can't fool all of the people all the time."

If Honest Abe were with us now, a sensible nutritionist rather than President, he might amend his words to read: "Supplements are valuable for all of us some of the time, and some of us all of the time, but they're probably not necessary for all of us all the time."

Part II

What You Get from Food

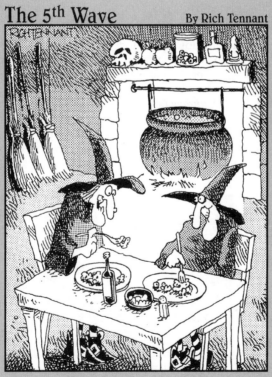

"I substitute tofu for eye of newt in all my recipes now. It has twice the protein and doesn't wriggle around the cauldron."

In this part . . .

Here's the lowdown on things you've heard about practically forever: protein, fat, carbohydrates, alcohol, vitamins, minerals, and water.

This is a *...For Dummies* book, so you don't have to read straight through protein to water to see how things work. You can skip from chapter to chapter, back and forth, side to side. Any way you take it, this part is bound to clue you in to the value of the nutrients in food.

Chapter 6

Powerful Protein

● ●

In This Chapter

▶ What's protein?

▶ Where to find the proteins in your body

▶ How to get the best quality protein from food

▶ When you need to get more (or less) protein

● ●

*P*rotein is an essential nutrient whose name comes from the Greek word *protos,* which means "first." To visualize a molecule of protein, think of a very long chain, rather like a chain of sausage links. The links in the chains are *amino acids,* commonly known as the building blocks of protein. In addition to carbon, hydrogen, and oxygen atoms, amino acids contain a nitrogen *(amino)* group. The amino group is essential for synthesizing specialized proteins in your body.

Where Your Body Puts Protein

The human body is chock-full of proteins. There are proteins in the outer and inner membranes of every living cell.

✔ Your hair, your nails, and the outer layers of your skin are made of the protein keratin. Keratin is a scleroprotein, a protein resistant to digestive enzymes. So if you bite your nails, you can't digest them.

✔ Muscle tissue contains myosin, actin, myoglobin, and a number of other proteins.

✔ Bone has lots of protein. The outer part of bone is hardened with minerals such as calcium, but the basic, rubbery inner structure is protein, and there is also protein in bone marrow, the soft material inside the bone.

✔ Red blood cells contain *hemoglobin,* a substance that carries oxygen throughout the body; globin is a protein. The clear fluid in blood (plasma) transports fat and protein particles called *lipoproteins* that ferry cholesterol around and out of the body.

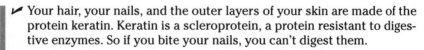

How Your Body Uses Protein

Your body uses proteins to build new cells, maintain tissues, and synthesize new proteins that make it possible for you to perform basic bodily functions.

About half the dietary protein you consume each day goes to make *enzymes,* the specialized worker proteins that do specific jobs such as digesting food and assembling or dividing molecules to make new cells and chemical substances. To perform these functions, enzymes often need specific vitamins and minerals.

Your ability to see, think, hear, move — in fact, to do just about everything that you consider part of a healthy life — requires your nerve cells to send messages back and forth to each other and to other specialized kinds of cells such as muscle cells. Sending these messages requires chemicals called *neurotransmitters.* Making neurotransmitters requires — guess what? — proteins.

Finally, proteins play an important part in the creation of every new cell and every new individual. *Nucleoproteins* are substances made of amino acids and nucleic acids. See the "DNA/RNA" sidebar later in this chapter for more information on nucleoproteins.

What Happens to the Proteins You Eat

The cells in your digestive tract can only absorb single amino acids or very small chains of two or three amino acids called *peptides.* So proteins from food are broken into their component amino acids by digestive enzymes — which are, of course, specialized proteins. Then other enzymes inside your body cells synthesize new proteins by re-assembling amino acids into specific compounds that your body needs to function. This process is called *protein synthesis.* During protein synthesis

- ✔ Amino acids hook up with fats to form *lipoproteins,* the molecules that ferry cholesterol around and out of the body. Or amino acids may join up with carbohydrates to form the *glycoproteins* found in the mucus secreted by the digestive tract.

- ✔ Proteins combine with phosphoric acid to produce phosphoproteins such as *casein,* a protein in milk.

- ✔ Nucleic acids combine with proteins to create nucleoproteins, essential components of the cell nucleus, and *protoplasm,* the living material inside each cell.

The carbon, hydrogen, and oxygen left over after protein synthesis is complete is converted to glucose and used for energy. (See Chapter 7.) The nitrogen residue (ammonia) is not used for energy. It is processed by the liver, which converts the ammonia to urea. Most of the urea produced in the liver is excreted through the kidneys in urine; very small amounts are sloughed off in skin, hair, and nails.

Every day, you *turn over* (reuse) more proteins than you get from the food you eat, so you need a continuous supply to maintain your protein status. If your diet does not contain sufficient amounts of proteins, you start to digest the proteins in your body, including the proteins in your muscles, including — in extreme cases — your heart muscle.

Not all proteins are created equal

To make all the proteins that your body needs, you require 22 different amino acids. Nine are considered *essential,* which means that you cannot synthesize them in your bodies and must obtain them from food. The rest are *nonessential* — if you do not get them in food, you can manufacture them yourself from fats, carbohydrates, and other amino acids.

TECHNICAL STUFF

DNA/RNA

Nucleoproteins are chemicals in the nucleus of every living cell. They are made of proteins linked to *nucleic acids* — complex compounds that contain phosphoric acid, a sugar molecule, and nitrogen-containing molecules made from amino acids.

Nucleic acids (molecules found in the chromosomes and other structures in the center of your cells) carry the genetic codes — genes and chromosomes that determine what you look like, your intelligence, and who you are. They contain one of two sugars, either ribose or deoxyribose. The nucleic acid containing ribose is called *ribonucleic acid* (RNA). The nucleic acid containing deoxyribose is called *deoxyribonucleic acid* (DNA).

DNA, a long molecule with two strands twisting about each other (the "double helix"), is the base of all living organisms. DNA carries and transmits your genetic inheritance in your chromosomes — genetic inheritance consists of the "instructions" that determine how your body cells are formed and how they behave. RNA, a single-strand molecule, is created in the cell according to the pattern determined by the DNA. RNA carries DNA instructions to each cell.

Knowing about DNA is important because it is the most distinctly "you" thing about your body. The chances that another person on earth will have exactly the same DNA as you is really, really small. That is why DNA analysis is used increasingly to identify criminals or exonerate the innocent. Some people are even proposing that parents should store a sample of their children's DNA so that they will have a conclusive way of identifying a missing child, even years later.

The essential amino acids are

- ✔ Histadine
- ✔ Isoleucine
- ✔ Leucine
- ✔ Lysine
- ✔ Methionine
- ✔ Phenlyalanine
- ✔ Threonine
- ✔ Tryptophan
- ✔ Valine

The nonessential amino acids are

- ✔ Alanine
- ✔ Arginine
- ✔ Aspartic acid
- ✔ Citrulline
- ✔ Cystine
- ✔ Glutamic acid
- ✔ Glycine
- ✔ Hydroxyglutamic acid
- ✔ Hydroxyproline
- ✔ Norleucine
- ✔ Proline
- ✔ Serine
- ✔ Tyrosine

High-quality and low-quality proteins

Because an animal's body is similar to ours, its proteins contain similar combinations of amino acids. That is why nutritionists call proteins from foods of animal origin — meat, fish, poultry, eggs, and dairy products — high-quality proteins. Our bodies absorb these proteins more efficiently; they can be used without much waste to synthesize other proteins. The proteins from plants — grains, fruit, vegetables, legumes (beans), nuts, and seeds — often have limited amounts of some amino acids. Our bodies do not absorb them as easily or use them as efficiently as animal proteins. Their nutritional quality is not as high.

The basic standard against which you measure the value of the proteins in food is the egg. Nutrition scientists have arbitrarily given the egg a "biological value" of 100 percent, meaning that it is the most useful to the human body. Other foods, which have proportionately more protein, may not be as valuable as the egg because their proteins are not as complete, which means they lack ample amounts of one or more essential amino acids.

For example, eggs are 11 percent protein; dry beans, 22 percent. But the proteins in beans do not provide sufficient amounts of all the essential amino acids, so they are not as valuable to human beings. The prime exception is the soybean, a *legume* (bean) that is packed with abundant amounts of all

5th-6th line

nine essential amino acids. Soybeans are an excellent source of proteins for vegetarians, especially *vegans* (vegetarians who avoid all products of animal origin, including milk and eggs). See Table 6-1 for the relative protein quality of representative foods.

Table 6-1	Scoring the Amino Acids in Food	
Food	*Protein Content (% of the calories in a serving)*	*Amino Acid Score*
Egg	33	100
Fish	61	100
Beef	29	100
Milk (cow's whole)	23	100
Soybeans	29	100
Dry beans	22	75
Rice	7	62–66
Corn	7	47
Wheat	13	50
Wheat (white flour)	12	36

Sources: *Nutritive Value of Foods* (Washington, D.C.: U.S. Department of Agriculture, 1991); George M. Briggs and Doris Howes Calloway, *Nutrition and Physical Fitness,* 11th ed. (New York: Holt, Rinehart and Winston, 1984).

Homocysteine and your heart

Homocysteine is an *intermediate,* a chemical released when you metabolize (digest) protein. Unlike other amino acids, which are vital to your health, homocysteine can be hazardous to your heart, raising your risk of heart disease by attacking cells in the lining of your arteries, by making the cells reproduce faster (the extra cells may block your coronary arteries), or by causing your blood to clot (ditto).

Years and years ago, before cholesterol moved to center stage, some smart heart researchers labeled homocysteine the major nutritional culprit in heart disease. Today, they've been vindicated. The American Heart Association has now cited high homocysteine levels as an independent risk factor for heart disease, perhaps explaining why some people with low cholesterol have heart attacks.

But wait! The good news is that information from several studies, including the Harvard/Brigham and Women's Hospital Nurses' Health Study in Boston suggest that a diet rich in the B vitamin folacin lowers blood levels of homocysteine. Most fruits and vegetables have plentiful amounts of folacin. Stocking up on them may protect your heart.

Super soy: The special protein food

Nutrition fact #1: Food from animals has complete proteins. Nutrition fact # 2: Vegetables, fruits, and grains have incomplete proteins. Nutrition fact #3: Nobody told the soybean.

Unlike other vegetables, including other beans, soybeans have complete proteins with sufficient amounts of all the amino acids essential to human health. In fact, food experts rank soy proteins on par with egg whites and casein (the protein in milk), the two proteins easiest for your body to absorb and use (see Table 6-1).

Some nutritionists think soy proteins are even better than the proteins in eggs and milk because the proteins in soy have no cholesterol and very little of the saturated fat known to clog your arteries and raise your risk of heart attack. Better yet, more than 20 recent studies suggest that adding soy foods to your diet can actually lower your cholesterol levels.

One-half cup of cooked soybeans has 14 grams protein; 4 ounces of tofu has 13. Either serving gives you approximately twice the protein you get from one large egg or one 8-ounce glass of skim milk, and two-thirds the protein in 3 ounces of lean ground beef. Eight ounces of fat-free soy milk has 7 mg protein, a mere 1 mg less than a similar serving of skim milk — and no cholesterol. Soybeans are also friendly to your digestive tract because they are jam-packed with dietary fiber that helps move food through your digestive tract.

In fact, soybeans are such a good source of food fiber that I feel obligated to add a cautionary note here. One day after I had read through a bunch of studies about soy's effect on cholesterol levels, I decided to lower my cholesterol level right away. So I had a soy burger for lunch, a half cup of soybeans and no-fat cheese for an afternoon snack, and another half cup with tomato sauce at dinner. Delicacy prohibits me from explaining in detail how irritated and upset all that fiber made my digestive track, but I'm sure you get the picture.

If you choose to use soy (or any other dry beans), take it slow — a little today, a little more tomorrow, and a little bit more on the day after that.

Complete proteins and incomplete proteins

Another way to describe the quality of proteins is to say that they are either complete or incomplete. A *complete protein* is one that contains ample amounts of the essential amino acids; an *incomplete protein* does not. A protein low in one specific amino acid is called a *limiting protein* because it can only build as much tissue as the smallest amount of the necessary amino acid. You can improve the quality in one food with incomplete proteins by eating the food along with another one that contains the missing or limited amino acids. Matching foods to create complete proteins is called *complementarity*.

For example, rice is low in the essential amino acid lysine, and beans are low in the essential amino acid methionine. By eating rice with beans, you "improve" the proteins in both. Another example is pasta and cheese. Pasta is low in the essential amino acids lysine and isoleucine; milk products have abundant amounts of these two amino acids. Shaking parmesan cheese onto pasta creates a higher-quality protein dish. In each case, the foods have complementary amino acids. Other examples of complementary protein dishes are peanut butter with bread, and milk with cereal. Many such combinations are a natural and customary part of the diet in parts of the world where animal proteins are scarce or very expensive. Table 6-2 shows categories of foods with incomplete proteins. Table 6-3 shows how to combine foods to improve the quality of their proteins.

Table 6-2	Foods with Incomplete Proteins
Category	*Examples*
Grain foods	Barley, bread, bulgar wheat, cornmeal, kasha, and pancakes
Legumes	Black beans, black-eyed peas, fava beans, kidney beans, lima beans, lentils, peanut butter, peanuts, peas, split peas, and white beans
Nuts and seeds	Almonds, Brazil nuts, cashews, pecans, walnuts, pumpkin seeds, sesame seeds (tahini), and sunflower seeds

Table 6-3	How to Combine Foods to Complement Proteins	
This Food	*Complements This Food*	*Examples*
Whole grains	Legumes (beans)	Rice & beans
Dairy Products	Whole Grains	Cheese sandwich, pasta with cheese, pancakes (wheat & milk/egg batter)
Legumes (beans)	Nuts and/or seeds	Chili (beans) with caraway seeds
Dairy products	Legumes (beans)	Chili beans with cheese
Dairy products	Nuts and seeds	Yogurt with chopped nut garnish

The lowdown on gelatin and your fingernails

Everyone "knows" that gelatin is protein that strengthens fingernails. Too bad everyone is wrong. Gelatin is produced by treating animal bones with acid, a process that destroys the essential amino acid tryptophan. Surprise: bananas are high in tryptophan. Slicing bananas onto your gelatin increases the quality of the protein. Adding milk makes it even better, but that still may not heal your splitting nails. The fastest way to a cure is a visit to the dermatologist, who can tell you whether the problem is an allergy to nail polish, too much time spent washing dishes, a medical problem such as a fungal infection, or just plain peeling nails. Then the dermatologist may prescribe a different nail polish (or none at all), protective gloves, a *fungicide* (a drug that wipes out fungi), or a lotion product that strengthens the natural "glue" that holds the layers of your nails together.

How Much Protein Do You Need?

An average healthy adult man or woman needs about 0.8 grams of high-quality protein for every kilogram (2.2 pounds) of body weight, slightly more than 0.4 grams for every pound.

For example, a 138-pound woman needs about 50 grams of protein a day; a 175-pound man, about 63 grams. This amount is easily obtained from two to three 3-ounce servings of lean meat, fish, or poultry (21 grams each). If the 138-pound woman were a vegetarian, she could get her 50 grams of proteins from 2 eggs (12–16 grams), 2 slices of prepacked fat-free cheese (10 grams), 4 slices of bread (3 grams each), and one cup of yogurt (10 grams).

As you grow older, you synthesize new proteins less efficiently, and your muscle mass (protein tissue) diminishes while your fat content stays the same or rises. This is why muscle seems to "turn to fat" in old age. But some tissues — hair, skin, and nails — never stop growing.

What happens if you don't get enough protein?

The first sign of protein deficiency is a weakening of the tissues where protein is heavily used. Children who do not get enough protein fail to grow properly. Their muscles are small and weak, their hair is thin, their skin may be covered with sores, and blood tests may show that the level of albumin in their blood is below normal. (*Albumin* is a protein that helps maintain the body's fluid balance, keeping a proper amount of liquid in and around body cells.)

The lining of the digestive tract is renewed every day and a half, and your red blood cells live for only 120 days, so people who do not get enough protein to replace these cells may have digestive problems or become *anemic* (have fewer red blood cells than they need). Protein deficiency may also show up as fluid retention (the big belly on a starving child) or hair loss and muscle wasting caused by the body's attempt to protect itself by digesting the proteins in its own muscle tissue. That is why victims of starvation are, literally, "skin and bones."

Given the high protein content of a normal American diet (which generally provides far more protein than you actually require), protein deficiency is rare in the United States except as a consequence of an eating disorder such as *anorexia nervosa* (refusal to eat) or *bulimia* (regurgitation after meals).

Who needs extra protein?

Anyone who is building new tissue quickly needs more than 0.8 grams of protein per kilogram (2.2 pounds) of body weight per day. For example:

- ✔ Infants need as much as 2.0 grams of protein for every kilogram of body weight per day.
- ✔ Adolescents need as much as 1.2 grams per kilogram per day.
- ✔ Pregnant women need an extra 10 grams a day, and women who are nursing new babies also need extra protein — 15 grams a day in the first six months, 12 grams a day in the second six months. This extra protein is used to build the fetal tissues and then to produce adequate amounts of nutritious breast milk.

Injuries also raise your protein requirements. An injured body releases above-normal amounts of protein-destroying hormones from the pituitary and adrenal glands. You need extra protein to protect existing tissues, and after severe blood loss, you need extra protein to make new hemoglobin. Cuts, burns, or surgical procedures mean that you need extra protein to make new skin and muscle cells. Fractures mean extra protein needed to make new bone. This is so important that if you have been badly injured and cannot take protein by mouth, you will be given an intravenous solution of amino acids with glucose (sugar) or emulsified fat.

Do athletes need more proteins than the rest of us? Recent research suggests that the answer may be yes, but athletes easily meet their requirements — about an additional 0.5 grams per kilogram per day — within the framework of a normal diet.

Can you ever get too much protein?

Yes. Several medical conditions make it difficult for people to digest and process proteins properly. As a result, waste products build up in different parts of the body.

People with liver disease or kidney disease either do not process protein efficiently into urea or do not excrete it efficiently through urine. The result may be uric acid kidney stones or *uremic poisoning* (an excess amount of uric acid in the blood). The pain associated with *gout* (a form of arthritis that affects nine men for every one woman) is caused by uric acid crystals collecting in the spaces around joints. Doctors usually recommend a low-protein diet in these cases.

Chapter 7

The Lowdown on Fat and Cholesterol

The chemical family name for fats and related compounds such as cholesterol is *lipids* (from *lipos,* the Greek word for fat). Liquid fats are called *oils;* solid fats are called, well, *fat.* With the exception of *cholesterol* (a fatty substance that has no calories and provides no energy), fats are high-energy nutrients. Gram for gram, fats have more than twice as much energy potential (calories) as protein and carbohydrates: nine calories per fat gram versus four calories per gram for proteins and carbs. (For more calorie facts, see Chapter 3.)

How Your Body Uses Fat

Here's a sentence that you probably never thought you'd read: A healthy body needs fat. Your body uses *dietary fat* (the fat you get from food) to make tissue and manufacture biochemicals, such as hormones. Some of the body fat made from food fat is *visible.* Even though it is covered by your skin, you can *see* the fat in the *adipose* (fatty) tissue in female breasts, hips, thighs, buttocks, and belly, or male abdomen and shoulders.

This *visible* body fat

- Provides a source of stored energy
- Gives shape to your body
- Cushions your skin (imagine sitting in a chair for a while to read this book without your buttocks to pillow your bones)
- Acts as an insulation blanket that reduces heat loss

Other body fat is *invisible.* You can't see this body fat because it is tucked away in and around your internal organs. This hidden fat

- Is part of every cell membrane (the outer "skin" that holds the cell together).
- Is a component of *myelin,* the fatty material that sheathes nerve cells and makes it possible for them to fire the electrical messages that enable you to think, see, speak, move, and perform the multitude of tasks natural to a living body. Brain tissue is also rich in fat.
- Is a shock absorber that protects your organs (as much as possible) if you fall or are injured.
- Is a constituent of hormones and other biochemicals, such as vitamin D and bile.

The Fats in Food

Food contains three kinds of fats: triglycerides, phospholipids, and sterols. *Triglycerides* are the fats you use to make adipose tissue and burn for energy.

Phospholipids are hybrids — part lipid, part *phosphate* (a molecule made with the mineral phosphorus) — that act as tiny rowboats, ferrying hormones and fat-soluble vitamins A, D, E, and K through your blood and back and forth in the watery fluid that flows across cell membranes.

Sterols are fat and alcohol compounds with no calories. Vitamin D is a sterol. So is the sex hormone testosterone. And so is cholesterol, the base on which your body builds hormones and vitamins.

The Right Amount of Fat

Getting the right amount of fat in your diet is a balancing act. Too much, and you increase your risk of obesity, diabetes, heart disease, and some forms of cancer. (The risk of colon cancer seems to be tied more clearly to a diet high in fat from meat rather than fat from dairy products.) Too little, and infants do not thrive, children do not grow, and everyone, regardless of age, is unable to absorb and use fat-soluble vitamins that smooth the skin, protect vision, bolster the immune system, and keep reproductive organs functioning.

How much fat should a healthy diet have? The Dietary Guidelines for Americans (more about that in Chapter 16) recommend that

✔ No more than 30 percent of your total daily calories come from fat

✔ No more than 10 percent of your total daily calories come from saturated fat (This means that a person who consumes 2,000 calories a day should get only 600 calories or fewer from fat and 200 calories or fewer from saturated fat.)

And regardless of calorie intake, the Guidelines recommend no more than 300 milligrams of cholesterol a day.

These recommendations are for adults. While many organizations such as the American Academy of Pediatrics, the American Heart Association, and the National Heart, Lung, and Blood Institute do recommend restricting fat intake for older children, they stress that infants and toddlers require fatty acids for proper physical growth and mental development — that's why Mother Nature made human breast milk high in essential fatty acids. Never limit the fat in your baby's diet without checking with her pediatrician.

Essential fatty acids

An *essential fatty acid* is one your body cannot assemble from other fats. You have to get it whole, from food. Linoleic acid, found in vegetable oils, is an essential fatty acid. Two others — linolenic acid and arachonidonic acid — occupy a somewhat ambiguous position. You can't make them from scratch, but you can make them if you have enough linoleic acid on hand, so food scientists can work up a good fight over whether linolenic and arachonidonic acids are actually "essential." In practical terms, who cares? Linoleic acid is so widely available in food, you are unlikely to experience a deficiency of any of the three — linoleic, linolenic, or arachonidonic acid — so long as two percent of the calories you get each day come from fat.

Which Foods Are High in Fat?

As a general rule:

- ✔ Fruits and vegetables have only traces of fat, primarily unsaturated fatty acids.

- ✔ Grains have very small amounts, up to three percent of their total weight.

- ✔ Dairy products vary. Cream is a high-fat food. "Regular" milks and cheeses are moderately high in fat. Skim milk and skim milk products are lowfat foods. Most of the fat in any dairy product is saturated fatty acids.

- ✔ Meat is moderately high in fat, and most of its fats are saturated fatty acids.

- ✔ Poultry (chicken and turkey), without the skin, is relatively low in fat.

- ✔ Fish may be high or low in fat. Its fats are composed primarily of unsaturated fatty acids that stay liquid in cold water.

- ✔ Vegetable oils, butter, and lard are high-fat foods. Most of the fatty acids in vegetable oils are unsaturated; most of the fatty acids in lard and butter are saturated.

- ✔ Processed foods, such as cakes, breads, and canned or frozen meat and vegetable dishes, are generally higher in fat than plain grains, meats, fruits, and vegetables.

Here's a simple guide to which foods are high (or low) in fat. Oils are clearly high. In fact, you just can't get any higher than 100 percent. Butter and lard are close behind, but no cigar. After that, the fat level drops, from 70 percent for some nuts down to 2 percent for most bread. Here's the rule to take away from the numbers: A diet high in grains and plants is always lower in fat than a diet higher in meat and oils.

Saturated and Unsaturated Fatty Acids

Fatty acids are the building blocks of fats. Chemically speaking, a fatty acid is a chain of carbon atoms with hydrogen atoms attached and a carbon-oxygen-oxygen-hydrogen group (the unit that makes it an "acid") at one end.

Nutritionists characterize fatty acids as saturated, monounsaturated, or polyunsaturated, depending on how many hydrogen atoms are attached to the carbon atoms in the chain. The more hydrogen atoms, the more saturated the fatty acid.

A nutritional fish story

Omega-3 fatty acids are a group of unsaturates found primarily in fatty fish such as salmon and sardines. The primary omega-3 is alpha-linolenic acid, which your body converts to hormone-like substances called eicosanoids. The eicosanoids — eicosapentaenoic acid (EPA) and docosahexaenoic acid (DHA) — reduce inflammation, perhaps by inhibiting an enzyme called COX-2 which is linked to inflammatory diseases such as rheumatoid arthritis and some cancers (including skin cancer).

You can find omega-3s in:

- anchovies
- haddock
- herring
- mackeral
- salmon
- sardines
- scallops
- tuna (albacore)
- broccoli
- kale
- purslance
- spinach
- canola oil
- walnut oil
- flaxseed oil

The Arthritis Foundation says omega-3s relieve joint inflammation, swelling, and pain in people with rheumatoid arthritis. Omega-3s may also prevent the natural breakdown of bone tissue, hold minerals in bone, and increase the formation of new bone. That's precisely what happens when Purdue University nutrition professor Bruce A. Watkins, Ph.D., feeds omega-3s to female lab rats after their ovaries are removed, cutting off their natural supply of bone-protecting estrogen (a condition related to menopause in women).

How much fatty fish must you eat to get the omega-3s you need? No rules exist yet, but Watkins says you should try to increase consumption of omega-3s while reducing consumption of omega-6 fatty acids — polyunsaturates found in beef, pork, and several vegetable oils, including corn, sunflower, cottonseed, soybean, peanut, and sesame. Although they are chemical cousins, omega-6s lack the benefits of the omega-3s.

Fish oil also helps your body create calciferol, a naturally-occurring form of vitamin D, the nutrient that enables your body to absorb bone-building calcium.

The Relationship between Fatty Acids and Dietary Fat

All the fats in food are combinations of fatty acids. Depending on which fatty acids predominate, a food fat is characterized as saturated, monounsaturated, or polyunsaturated.

> ✔ A saturated fat, such as butter, has mostly saturated fatty acids. Saturated fats are solid at room temperature and get harder when chilled.
>
> ✔ A monounsaturated fat, such as olive oil, has mostly monounsaturated fatty acids. Monounsaturated fats are liquid at room temperature; they get thicker when chilled.
>
> ✔ A polyunsaturated fat, such as corn oil, has mostly polyunsaturated fatty acids. Polyunsaturated fats are liquid at room temperature; they stay liquid when chilled.

So how come margarine — made from unsaturated fats such as corn and soybean oil — is solid? Because it has been artificially saturated by food chemists who add hydrogen atoms to its unsaturated fatty acids. This process, called *hydrogenation,* turns an oil, such as corn oil, into a fat: margarine. A fatty acid with extra hydrogens is called a *hydrogenated fatty acid.* Another name for a hydrogenated fatty acid is a trans fatty acid. Hydrogenated fatty acids are thought to act much like saturated fats, raising the blood cholesterol level.

Table 7-1 shows the kinds of fatty acids found in some common dietary fats and oils. Fats are characterized according to their predominant fatty acids. For example, as you can plainly see in the table, nearly 25 percent of the fatty acids in corn oil are monounsaturated fatty acids. Nevertheless, because corn oil has more polyunsaturated fatty acid, corn oil is considered a polyunsaturated fatty acid. Note for math majors: True, some of the totals in Table 7-1 do not add up to 100 percent, because these fats and oils also contain other kinds of fatty acids in amounts so small that they do not affect the basic character of the fat.

Table 7-1	What Fatty Acids Are in That Fat or Oil?			
Fat or Oil . . .	Saturated Fatty Acid (%)	Monoun-saturated Fatty Acid (%)	Polyun-saturated Fatty Acid (%)	Kind of Fat or Oil
Canola oil	7	53	22	Monounsaturated
Corn oil	13	24	59	Polyunsaturated
Olive oil	14	74	9	Monounsaturated
Palm oil	52	38	10	Saturated
Peanut oil	17	46	32	Monounsaturated
Safflower oil	9	12	74	Polyunsaturated
Soybean oil	15	23	51	Polyunsaturated

Fat or Oil . . .	Saturated Fatty Acid (%)	Monoun- saturated Fatty Acid (%)	Polyun- saturated Fatty Acid (%)	Kind of Fat or Oil
Soybean- cottonseed oil	18	29	48	Polyunsaturated
Butter	62	30	5	Saturated
Lard	39	45	11	Saturated*

*Because more than ⅓ of its fats are saturated, nutritionists label lard a saturated fat.
Sources: *Nutritive Value of Foods* (Washington, D.C.: U.S. Department of Agriculture, 1991); *Food and Life* (New York: American Council on Science and Health, 1990).

A diet high in saturated fats increases the amount of cholesterol circulating in your blood, which is believed to raise your risk of heart disease and stroke. A diet high in unsaturated fats reduces the amount of cholesterol circulating in your blood, which is believed to lower your risk of heart disease and stroke.

But here's a puzzle: Nature's no fool. If cholesterol is uniformly bad, why do our very own bodies make so much of it? Read on.

Cholesterol and You

I mention earlier in this chapter that your body actually *needs* fat, and here's another sentence that may blow your (nutritional) mind: Every healthy body *needs* cholesterol. Look carefully and you find cholesterol in and around your cells, in your fatty tissue, in your organs, and in your glands. What's it doing there? Lots of useful things. For example, cholesterol

✔ Protects the integrity of cell membranes

✔ Helps enable nerve cells to send messages back and forth

✔ Is a building block for vitamin D (a sterol), made when sunlight hits the fat just under your skin (for more about vitamin D, see Chapter 10)

✔ Enables your gallbladder to make *bile acids,* digestive chemicals that allow you to absorb fats and fat-soluble nutrients such as vitamin A, vitamin D, vitamin E, and vitamin K

✔ Is a base on which you build steroid hormones such as estrogen and testosterone

Cholesterol and heart disease

Doctors measure your cholesterol level by taking a sample of blood and counting the milligrams of cholesterol in one deciliter (1/10 liter) of blood. When you get your annual report from the doctor, your total cholesterol level looks something like this: 225 mg/dl. Translation: You have 225 milligrams of cholesterol in every tenth of a liter of blood. Why does this matter? Because cholesterol can make its way into blood vessels, stick to the walls, and form deposits that eventually block the flow of blood. The more cholesterol floating in your blood, the more cholesterol is likely to cross into your arteries, where it may increase your risk of heart attack or stroke.

As a general rule, an adult cholesterol level higher than 250 mg/dl is said to be a "high risk" factor for heart disease. A cholesterol level between 200–250 mg/dl is considered a "moderate risk" factor. A cholesterol level below 200 mg/dl is considered a "low risk" factor. But that's not the whole story. Many people with a high cholesterol level live to a ripe old age while others with a low total cholesterol level develop heart disease. (Worse yet, recent research indicates that low cholesterol levels may increase the risk of stroke.) The reason is that total cholesterol is only one of several risk factors for heart disease. Here are some more:

- ✔ An unfavorable ratio of lipoproteins (see the following section)
- ✔ Smoking
- ✔ Obesity
- ✔ Age (being older is riskier)
- ✔ Gender (being male is riskier)
- ✔ A family history of heart disease

Living with lipoproteins

A *lipoprotein* is a fat (lipo = fat) and protein particle that carries cholesterol through your blood. Your body makes four types of lipoproteins: chylomicrons, very low density lipoproteins (VLDLs), low-density lipoproteins (LDLs), and high density lipoproteins (HDLs). As a general rule, LDLs take cholesterol into blood vessels; HDLs carry it out of the body.

Lipoproteins are like fat people on a perpetual treadmill. They start out big and fluffy. Then, as they keep moving, traveling around your body, they lose fat to end up small and dense. A lipoprotein is born as a chylomicron, made in your intestinal cells from protein and triglycerides. Chylomicrons are very low density, a term that means they have very little protein and lots of fat and cholesterol (protein is denser, that is, heavier and more compact than fat). After 12 hours of traveling through your blood and around your body, a chylomicron has lost virtually all its fats. By the time the chylomicron makes its way to your liver, the only thing left is protein.

The liver, a veritable fat and cholesterol factory, collects fatty acid fragments from your blood and uses them to make cholesterol and new fatty acids. Then your liver packages the cholesterol and fatty acids with protein as very low density lipoproteins, which have more protein and are more dense than chylomicrons. As VLDLs travel through your blood stream, they lose triglycerides, pick up cholesterol, and turn into low density lipoproteins. LDLs supply cholesterol to your body cells, which use it to make new cell membranes and manufacture sterol compounds such as hormones. That's the good news.

The bad news is that both VLDLs and LDLs are soft and squishy enough to pass through blood vessel walls. They carry cholesterol into blood vessels where it can cling to the inside wall, forming deposits (plaques). These plaques may eventually block an artery, keep blood from flowing through, and trigger a heart attack or stroke. Whew! Got all that?

VLDLs and LDLs are sometimes called "bad" cholesterol, but this is a misnomer. They aren't cholesterol; they're just the rafts on which cholesterol sails into your arteries. Traveling through the body, LDLs continue to lose cholesterol. In the end, they become high-density lipoproteins, the particles sometimes called "good" cholesterol. Once again, this is an inaccurate label. HDLs aren't cholesterol; they are simply protein and fat particles too dense and compact to pass through blood vessel walls, so they carry cholesterol out of the body rather than into arteries.

That's why a high level of HDLs may reduce your risk of heart attack regardless of your total cholesterol levels. Conversely, a high level of LDLs may raise your risk of heart attack, even if your overall cholesterol level is low. Hey, on second thought, maybe that does qualify them as "good cholesterol" and "bad cholesterol."

Diet and cholesterol

Most of the cholesterol that you need is made right in your own liver, which churns out about 1 gram (1,000 milligrams) a day from the raw materials in the proteins, fats, and carbohydrates you consume. But you also get cholesterol from food or animal origin: meat, poultry, fish, eggs, and dairy products. Although some plant foods, such as coconuts and cocoa beans, are high in saturated fats, no plants have cholesterol. Table 7-2 lists the amount of cholesterol in normal servings of some representative foods.

Plants don't have cholesterol, so no plant foods are on this list. No grains. No fruits. No veggies. No nuts and seeds. Of course, you can juice plant food up with cholesterol if you really try: Butter in the bread dough, cheese on the macaroni, cream sauce on the peas and onions, whipped cream on poached peaches, and so on.

Table 7-2	How Much Cholesterol Is on That Plate?	
Food	*Serving*	*Cholesterol (milligrams)*
Meat		
Beef (stewed) lean & fat	3 ounces	87
Beef (stewed) lean	2.2 ounces	66
Beef (ground) lean	3 ounces	74
Beef (ground) regular	3 ounces	76
Beef steak (sirloin)	3 ounces	77
Bacon	3 strips	16
Pork chop, lean	2.5 ounces	71
Poultry		
Chicken (roast) breast	3 ounces	73
Chicken (roast) leg	1.6 ounces	41
Turkey, roast, breast	3 ounces	59
Fish		
Clams	3 ounces	43
Flounder	3 ounces	59
Oysters (raw)	1 cup	120
Salmon (canned)	3 ounces	34
Salmon (baked)	3 ounces	60
Tuna (water canned)	3 ounces	48
Tuna (oil canned)	3 ounces	55
Cheese		
American	1 ounce	27
Cheddar	1 ounce	30
Cream	1 ounce	31
Mozzarella (whole milk)	1 ounce	22
Mozzarella (part skim)	1 ounce	15
Swiss	1 ounce	26

Food	Serving	Cholesterol (milligrams)
Milk		
Whole	8 ounces	33
2%	8 ounces	18
1%	8 ounces	18
Skim	8 ounces	10
Other dairy products		
Butter	pat	11
Eggs, large	1	213
Other		
Lard	1 tbsp.	12

Source: *Nutritive Value of Foods* (Washington, D.C.: U.S. Department of Agriculture, 1991).

How much cholesterol you get from food may affect your liver's daily output: If you eat more cholesterol, your liver may make less. If you eat less cholesterol, your liver may make more.

To keep your cholesterol level low, the U.S. Department of Agriculture's Dietary Guidelines for Americans (which I discuss in detail in Chapter 16) recommend that you consume no more than 300 milligrams of cholesterol a day from food. But overall, the total amount of fat and saturated fat in your diet now seems to be more important than the amount of cholesterol in determining your cholesterol level.

A diet high in saturated fats increases the amount of fat in your blood, including the amount of low density lipoproteins — the fat and protein particles that carry cholesterol into blood vessels — while monounsaturated and polyunsaturated fatty acids appear to reduce the amount of fat circulating in your blood.

From Food to Energy

Fat has more energy (calories) per gram than proteins and carbohydrates, but your body has a more difficult time pulling the energy out of fatty foods. Imagine a chain of long balloons, the kind people twist into shapes that resemble dachshunds and flowers and other such amusements. If you drop one of these balloons into water, it will float. That's exactly what happens when you swallow fat-rich foods. The fat floats on top of the watery food and liquid mixture in your stomach, which means that *lipases* — fat-busting digestive enzymes in the mix below — cannot reach it. Because fat is digested more slowly than proteins and carbohydrates, you feel fuller (a condition called *satiety*) longer after eating high-fat food.

Into the intestines

When the fat moves down your digestive tract into your small intestine, an intestinal hormone called *cholestokinin* beeps your gallbladder, signaling for the release of bile. *Bile* is an emulsifier, a substance that enables fat to mix with water so that lipases can start breaking the fat into glycerol and fatty acids. These smaller fragments may be stored in special cells ("fat cells") in adipose tissue, or they may be absorbed into cells in the intestinal wall where

✔ They are combined with oxygen ("burned") to produce heat/energy, plus water and the waste product carbon dioxide, or

✔ They are used to make lipoproteins that haul fats, including cholesterol, through your bloodstream

Turning fat into energy

Glucose, the molecule you get by digesting carbohydrates, is the body's basic source of energy. Burning glucose is easier and more efficient than burning fat, so your body always goes for carbohydrates first. But if you have used up all your available glucose — you're stranded in a cabin in the Arctic, you haven't eaten for a week, a blizzard's howling outside, and the corner deli 500 miles down the road doesn't deliver — then it's time to start in on your body fat.

The first step is for an enzyme in your fat cells to break up stored triglycerides. The enzyme action releases glycerol and fatty acids, which travel through your blood to body cells where they combine with oxygen to produce heat/energy, plus water and the waste product carbon dioxide. Burning fat without glucose produces a second waste product called ketones. In high concentrations (a condition known as "ketosis"), ketones change the pH (acid/alkaline balance) of your blood and may trip you into a coma which, if untreated, can lead to death. The telltale sign of ketosis is urine or breath that smells like acetone (nail polish remover). Under normal circumstances, ketosis is more likely to occur among people with diabetes who lack the insulin needed to process carbohydrates effectively. But it can also occur in people who try an unbalanced high fat/high protein/low carbohydrate reducing diet.

The chemical structure of fatty acids

This sidebar explains the structure of saturated, monounsaturated, and polyunsaturated fatty acids. It was originally up at the front of the chapter, but my editors think it will bore you to death. If you agree, or if you already know how a fatty acid is put together, you can just skip this information.

But if you haven't a clue about the chemical structure of fatty acids, it may be worth your while to walk slowly with me through this explanation. The concepts are really simple, and the information you find here applies to all kinds of molecules, not just fatty acids.

Molecules are groups of atoms hooked together with chemical bonds. Different atoms form different numbers of bonds to other atoms. For example, a hydrogen atom can form one bond to one other atom; an oxygen atom can form two bonds to other atoms; and a carbon atom can form four bonds to other atoms.

To "see" how this works, visualize a carbon atom as one of those round pieces in a child's Erector set or Tinkertoy kit. Your carbon atom (C) has — figuratively speaking, of course — four holes: one on top, one on the bottom, and one on each side. If you stick a peg into each hole and attach a small piece of wood representing a hydrogen atom (H) to the peg on top, the peg on the bottom, and the peg on the left, you have a structure that looks like this:

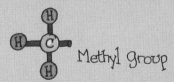

This unit, called a *methyl group*, is the first piece in any fatty acid. To build the rest of the fatty acid, you add carbon atoms and hydrogen atoms to form a chain. At the end, you tack on a group with one carbon atom, two oxygen atoms, and a hydrogen atom. This group is called an *acid group*, the part that makes the chain of carbon and hydrogen atoms a fatty acid.

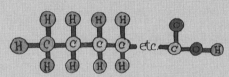

The preceding molecule is a *saturated fatty acid* because it has a hydrogen atom at every available carbon link in the chain. A monounsaturated fatty acid drops two hydrogen atoms and forms one double bond (two lines instead of one) between two carbon atoms. A polyunsaturated fatty acid drops more hydrogen atoms and forms several (poly) double bonds between several carbon atoms. Every hydrogen atom still forms one bond; every carbon atom still forms four bonds, but they do it in a slightly different way. These sketches are not pictures of real fatty acids, which have many more carbons in the chain and have their double bonds in different places, but they can give you an idea of what fatty acids "look" like:

Instead of this:

You get this:

(a saturated fatty acid)

(a monosaturated fatty acid)

or

(a polyunsaturated fatty acid)

Chapter 8

Carbohydrates: A Complex Story

● ●

In This Chapter

▶ The different kinds of carbohydrates

▶ How does your body use carbohydrates?

▶ Why athletes load up on carbohydrates before a long-distance competition

▶ The value of dietary fiber

● ●

*C*arbohydrates — the name means "carbon plus water" — are sugar compounds made by plants when the plants are exposed to light. This
process of making sugar compounds is called *photosynthesis,* from the Latin
words for "light" and "putting together."

What Are Carbohydrates?

Carbohydrates come in three varieties: simple carbohydrates, complex carbohydrates, and dietary fiber. All are composed of units of sugar. What makes
carbohydrates different from each other is how many sugar units they contain and how the units are linked together.

✔ **Simple carbohydrates:** Carbohydrates with only one or two units of
sugar.

• A carbohydrate with one unit of sugar is called a *simple sugar* or a
monosaccharide (mono = one; saccharide = sugar). Fructose ("fruit
sugar") is a monosaccharide. So are glucose ("blood sugar"), the
sugar produced when you digest carbohydrates, and galactose, the
sugar derived from digesting lactose ("milk sugar").

• A carbohydrate with two units of sugar is called a *double sugar* or a
disaccharide (di = two). Sucrose ("table sugar"), which is made of
one unit of fructose and one unit of glucose, is a disaccharide.

✔ **Complex carbohydrates:** Also known as *polysaccharides* (poly = many), these carbohydrates have more than two units of sugar linked together. Carbs with three to eight units of sugar are sometimes called *oligosaccharides.*

- Raffinose is a *trisaccharide* (tri = three) found in potatoes, beans, and beets; it has one unit each of galactose, glucose, and fructose.

- Stachyose is a *tetrasaccharide* (tetra = four) found in the same vegetables; it has one fructose unit, one glucose unit, and two galactose units.

- Starch, a complex carbohydrate in potatoes, pasta, and rice, is a definite polysaccharide, made of many units of glucose.

✔ **Dietary fiber:** A term used to distinguish the fiber in food from the natural and synthetic fibers (silk, cotton, wool, nylon) used in fabrics. Dietary fiber is a third kind of carbohydrate.

- Like the complex carbohydrates, dietary fiber (cellulose, hemicellulose, pectin, beta-glucans, gum) is a polysaccharide. Lignin, a different kind of chemical, is also called a dietary fiber.

- Some kinds of dietary fiber also contain units of *uronic acids,* chemicals derived from fructose, glucose, and galactose. (Galacturonic acid, from galactose, is an example of a uronic acid.)

Dietary fiber is not like other carbohydrates. The bonds that hold its sugar units together cannot be broken by human digestive enzymes. Although the bacteria living naturally in your intestines do convert very small amounts of dietary fiber to fatty acids, dietary fiber is not considered a source of energy. (For more about fatty acids, see Chapter 7.)

Table 8-1 shows you which sugars — and how many units of each — are in the different kinds of carbohydrates. After Table 8-1, I talk about how your body gets energy from carbohydrates. Because dietary fiber does not provide energy, I'm going to put it aside for the moment and get back to it later. If you can't wait to find out more about fiber, skip right to "Dietary Fiber: The Non-Nutrient in Carbohydrate Foods," later in this chapter.

As far as I can tell, the information in Table 8-1 has absolutely no practical value. It's strictly trivia for your own personal nutrition data bank. Of course, you could call it up for use in social situations. For example, suppose you're standing in line at the hot dog stand at Yankee Stadium, looking for a way to start up a conversation with the trim, attractive person in front of you who obviously cares about diet and health. "Wow," you may say, "did you notice the cola over there is sweetened with both fructose and sucrose — a monosaccharide and a disaccharide, both in the same drink? And given how nutrition-savvy they are here, I bet the hot dog rolls are loaded with polysaccharides." Who could resist such a high-minded, intellectual approach?

Table 8-1	Naming the Sugar Units in Carbohydrates
Carbohydrate	*Composition*
Monosaccharides (one sugar unit)	
Fructose (fruit sugar)	One unit fructose
Glucose (sugar unit used for fuel)	One unit glucose
Galactose (made from lactose [milk sugar])	One unit galactose
Disaccharides (two sugar units linked together)	
Sucrose (table sugar)	Glucose + fructose
Lactose (milk sugar)	Glucose + galactose
Maltose (malt sugar)	Glucose + glucose
Polysaccharides (many sugar units linked together)	
Raffinose	Galactose + glucose + fructose
Stachyose	Glucose + fructose + galactose + galactose
Starch	Many glucose units
Cellulose	Many glucose units
Hemicellulose	Arabinose* + galactose + mannose* + xylose** plus uronic acids
Pectin	Galactose + arabinose plus galacturonic acid
Gums	Mainly galacturonic acid

* this sugar is found in many plants
** this sugar is found in plants and wood

Carbohydrates and energy: A biochemical love story

Your body runs on glucose, the molecules your cells burn for energy. (For more information on how you get energy from food, check out Chapter 3.)

Proteins, fats, and alcohol also provide energy in the form of calories. And protein does give you glucose, but it takes a long time, relatively speaking, for your body to get it.

But all the digestible carbohydrates you get from food provide either glucose or sugar units that can be converted quickly to glucose. The glucose is then carried into your cells with the help of *insulin,* a hormone secreted by your pancreas.

How glucose becomes energy

Inside your cells, the glucose is burned to produce heat and *adenosine triphosphate,* a molecule that stores and releases energy as required by the cell. By the way, nutrition scientists, who have as much trouble pronouncing polysyllabic words as you do, usually refer to adenosine triphosphate by its initials: ATP. Smart cookies!

The transformation of glucose into energy occurs in one of two ways: with oxygen or without it. Glucose is converted to energy with oxygen in the mito-chondria — tiny bodies in the jelly-like substance inside every cell. This conversion yields energy (ATP, heat) plus water and carbon dioxide — a waste product.

Red blood cells do not have mitochondria, so they change glucose into energy without oxygen. This yields energy (ATP, heat) and lactic acid.

Glucose is also converted to energy in muscle cells. When it comes to pro-ducing energy from glucose, muscle cells are, well, double-jointed. They have mitochondria, so they can process glucose with oxygen. But if the level of oxygen in the muscle cell falls very low, the cells can just go ahead and change glucose into energy without it. This is most likely to happen when you've been exercising so strenuously that you (and your muscles) are, liter-ally, "out of breath."

Being able to turn glucose into energy without oxygen is a handy trick, but here's the down side: one by-product is lactic acid. Why is that a big deal? Too much lactic acid makes your muscles ache.

How pasta ends up on your hips when too many carbs pass your lips

Your cells budget energy very carefully. They do not store more than they need right now. Any glucose the cell does not need for its daily work is con-verted to glycogen ("animal starch") and tucked away as stored energy in your liver and muscles.

Your body can pack about 400 grams (14 ounces) of glycogen into liver and muscle cells. A gram of carbohydrates — including glucose — has four calories. If you add up all the glucose stored in glycogen to the small amount of glucose in your cells and blood, it equals about 1,800 calories of energy.

If your diet provides more carbohydrates than you need to produce this amount of stored calories in the form of glucose and glycogen in your cells, blood, muscles, and liver, the excess will be converted to fat — the ultimate energy bank. And that's how your pasta ends up on your hips.

Other ways your body uses carbohydrates

Providing energy is an important job, but it's not the only thing carbohydrates do for you.

Carbohydrates also protect your muscles. When you need energy, your body looks for carbohydrates first. If none are available — for example, because you are on a severe reducing diet or have a medical condition that prevents you from using the carbohydrates you consume — your body pragmatically begins to burn its own protein tissues (muscles). If this use of proteins for energy continues long enough, you will run out of fuel and die.

A diet that provides sufficient amounts of carbohydrates keeps your body from "eating" its own muscles. That's why a carbohydrate-rich diet is sometimes described as "protein sparing."

What else do carbohydrates do? Check out this list:

- They regulate the amount of sugar circulating in your blood so that all your cells get the energy they need.
- They provide nutrients for the friendly bacteria in your intestinal tract that help digest food.
- They assist in your body's absorption of calcium.
- They may help lower cholesterol levels and regulate blood pressure. These effects are special benefits of dietary fiber, which I discuss in the "Dietary Fiber: The Non-Nutrient in Carbohydrate Foods" section, later in this chapter.

Where to get the carbohydrates you need

The most important sources of carbohydrates are plant foods — fruits, vegetables, and grains. Milk and milk products do contain the carbohydrate lactose (milk sugar), but meat, fish, and poultry have no carbohydrates at all.

The current Dietary Guidelines for Americans, produced by the U.S. Departments of Agriculture and Health and Human Services (you can find a full discussion of these rules for healthy eating in Chapter 16) build a nutritious diet on:

- ✔ 6 to 11 servings a day of grain foods (bread, cereals, pasta, rice), plus
- ✔ 2 to 4 servings of fruit and
- ✔ 3 to 5 servings of vegetables

These foods provide simple carbohydrates, complex carbohydrates, and the natural bonus of dietary fiber. Table sugar, honey, and sweets — which provide simple carbohydrates — are recommended only on a once-in-a-while basis.

One gram of carbohydrates has four calories. To find the number of calories from the carbohydrates in a serving, multiply the number of grams of carbohydrates by 4. For example, one whole bagel has about 38 grams of carbohydrates, equal to about 152 calories (38 x 4). (You have to say "about" because the dietary fiber in the bagel provides no calories since it can't be metabolized by the body.)

Wait: That number does not account for all the calories in the serving. Remember, the foods listed here may also contain at least some protein and fat, and these two nutrients add calories. You can find the complete calorie count for hundreds of these foods in the Appendix.

Some problems with carbohydrates

Some people have a hard time handling carbohydrates.

For example, if you have diabetes, your pancreas does not produce enough insulin to carry all the glucose produced from carbohydrates into your body cells. As a result, the glucose continues to circulate in your blood until it is excreted through the kidneys; one way to tell if someone has diabetes is to test the level of sugar in the person's urine.

Other people can't digest carbohydrates because they lack the specific enzymes needed to break the bonds that hold a carbohydrate's sugar units together. For example, most Asians, Africans, Middle Easterners, South Americans, and Eastern, Central, or Southern Europeans are deficient in lactase, the enzyme that splits lactose (milk sugar) into glucose and galactose. If they drink milk or eat milk products, they will end up with a lot of undigested lactose in their intestinal tracts. This undigested lactose will make the bacteria living there happy as clams — but not the person who owns the intestines: As the bacteria feast on the undigested sugar, they excrete waste products that give their host gas and cramps.

To avoid this, many national cuisines instinctively avoid milk. (Quick! Name one native Asian dish that's made with milk. No. Coconut milk doesn't count.) Does that mean people living in these countries don't get enough calcium? No. They simply substitute high-calcium foods such as greens or soy products for milk.

A second solution for people who do not make enough lactase is to use a "predigested" milk product such as yogurt or buttermilk or sour cream, all made by adding friendly bacteria that digest the milk (that is, break the lactose apart) without spoiling it. Other solutions are lactose-free cheeses and enzyme-treated milk.

Who needs extra carbohydrates?

The small amount of glucose in your blood and cells provides the energy you need for your body's daily activities. The 400 grams of glycogen stored in your liver and muscles provides enough energy for ordinary bursts of extra activity.

But what happens if you have to work harder or longer than that? For example, what if you are a long-distance athlete, which means that you use up your available supply of glucose before you finish your competition? (That's why marathoners often run out of gas — a phenomenon called "hitting the wall" — at 20 miles, six miles short of the finish line.)

If you were stuck on an ice floe or lost in the woods for a month or so, after your body exhausted its supply of glucose, including the glucose stored in glycogen, it would start to pull energy first out of fat and then out of muscle. But extracting energy from body fat requires lots of oxygen — which is likely to be in short supply when your body has run, swum, or cycled 20 miles. So athletes have to find another way to leap the wall. Here it is: loading up on carbohydrates in advance.

Time out for the name game!

Here's an interesting bit of nutritional information. The names of all enzymes end in the letters "ase." An enzyme that digests a specific substance in food often has a name similar to the substance but with the letters "ase" at the end. For example, *proteases* are enzymes that digest protein; *lipases* are enzymes that digest fats; *galactase* is the enzyme that digests galactose.

Carbohydrate-loading is a dietary regimen designed to increase temporarily the amount of glycogen stored in your muscles. You start about a week before the event, says the University of Maine's Alfred A. Bushway, Ph.D., exercising to exhaustion in order to pull as much glycogen as possible out of your muscles. Then, for three days, you eat foods high in fat and protein and low in carbohydrates to keep your glycogen level from rising again.

Three days before the Big Day, reverse the pattern. Now you want to build and conserve glycogen stores. What you need is a diet that's about 70 percent carbohydrates, providing 6 to 10 grams of carbohydrates for every kilogram (2.2 pounds) of body weight for men as well as women. And not just any carbohydrates, mind you. What you want are the starchy ones (pasta, potatoes), rather than sugary ones (fruit, candy).

This is not a diet for every day. Nor will this diet help people competing in events lasting less than 90 minutes. It's strictly for events lasting longer than 90 minutes.

What about while you're running, swimming, or cycling? Will consuming sugar during the race give you extra short-term bursts of energy? Yes. Sugar is rapidly converted to glycogen and carried to the muscles. But you don't want "straight" sugar (candy, honey) because it's *hydrophilic* (hydro = water; philic = loving), which means that it pulls water from body tissues into your intestinal tract. That can increase dehydration and make you nauseated. So it's best to get the sugar you want from sweetened athletic drinks that provide fluids along with the energy. The label on the athletic drink tells you the liquid also contains salt (sodium chloride). Why? To replace the salt you lose when you perspire heavily. Turn to Chapter 13 to find out why this is important.

Dietary Fiber: The Non-Nutrient in Carbohydrate Foods

Dietary fiber is a group of complex carbohydrates that are not a source of energy for human beings. Because human digestive enzymes cannot break the bonds that hold fiber's sugar units together, fiber adds no calories to your diet and cannot be converted to glucose.

Ruminants (animals such as cows that "chew the cud") have a combination of digestive enzymes and digestive microbes that enables them to extract the nutrients from insoluble dietary fiber (cellulose and some hemicelluloses and pectins). But not even these creatures can pull nutrients out of lignin, an insoluble fiber in plant stems and leaves and the predominant fiber in wood. As a result, the U.S. Department of Agriculture specifically prohibits the use of wood or sawdust in animal feed.

But just because you can't digest dietary fiber doesn't mean it's not a valuable part of your diet. The opposite is true. Dietary fiber is valuable *because* you can't digest it!

The two kinds of dietary fiber

Nutritionists classify dietary fiber as either insoluble fiber or soluble fiber, depending on whether it dissolves in water. (Both kinds of fiber resist human digestive enzymes.)

✔ **Insoluble fiber,** such as cellulose, some hemicelluloses, and lignin found in whole grains and other plants. This kind of dietary fiber is a natural laxative. It absorbs water, helps you feel full after eating, and stimulates your intestinal walls to contract and relax. These natural contractions, called *peristalsis,* move solid materials through your digestive tract.

By moving food quickly through your intestines, insoluble fiber may help prevent or relieve digestive disorders such as constipation or diverticulosis (infection caused by food getting stuck in small pouches in the wall of your colon). Insoluble fiber also bulks up stool and makes it softer, reducing your risk of developing hemorrhoids and lessening the discomfort if you already have them.

✔ **Soluble fiber,** such as pectins in apples and beta-glucans in oats and barley, seems to lower the amount of cholesterol circulating in your blood (your *cholesterol level*). This may be why a diet rich in fiber appears to offer some protection against heart disease.

Here's a benefit for dieters: Soluble fiber forms gels in the presence of water, which is what happens when apples and oat bran reach your digestive tract. Like insoluble fiber, soluble fiber can make you feel full without adding calories.

Getting fiber from food

You find fiber in all plant foods — fruits, vegetables, and grains. But you find absolutely no fiber in foods from animals: meat, fish, poultry, milk, milk products, and eggs.

A balanced diet with lots of foods from plants gives you both insoluble and soluble fiber. Most foods that contain fiber have both kinds, although the balance is usually tilted toward one or the other. For example, the predominant fiber in an apple is pectin (a soluble fiber), but an apple peel also has some cellulose, hemicellulose, and lignin.

Table 8-2 shows you which foods are the best sources of what fiber. A diet rich in plant foods (fruits, vegetables, grains) gives you adequate amounts of dietary fiber. This list shows which foods are particularly good sources of specific kinds of dietary fiber.

Table 8-2	Where's the Fiber?
Fiber	*Found in . . .*
Soluble fiber	
Pectin	Fruits (apples, strawberries, citrus fruits)
Beta-glucans	Oats, barley
Gums	Beans, cereals (oats, rice, barley), seeds, seaweed
Insoluble fiber	
Cellulose	Leaves (cabbage), roots (carrots, beets), bran, whole wheat, beans
Hemicellulose	Seed coverings (bran, whole grains)
Lignin	Plant stems, leaves, and skin

How much fiber do you need?

According to the U.S. Department of Agriculture, the average American woman gets about 12 grams of fiber a day from food; the average American man, 17 grams. That's well below the current recommendations of 20 to 35 grams a day thought to confer the benefits of fiber without causing fiber-related — um — unpleasantries.

Like what unpleasantries? And how will you know?

Trust me: If you eat more than enough fiber, your body will tell you right away. In fact, it will issue an unmistakable protest in the form of intestinal gas or diarrhea. In extreme cases, if you don't drink enough liquids to carry the fiber you eat easily through your body, you can end up with an intestinal obstruction (for more on water, see Chapter 13).

Here's the lesson for you to learn: If you decide to up the amount of fiber in your diet, do it v-e-r-y gradually, a little bit more every day. That way you are less likely to experience intestinal distress.

In other words, if your current diet is heavy on no-fiber foods such as meat, fish, poultry, eggs, milk, and cheese, and low-fiber foods such as white bread and white rice, don't load up on bran cereal (35 grams dietary fiber per

3.5-ounce serving) or dried figs (9.3 grams per serving) all at once. Start by adding a serving of cornflakes (2.0 grams dietary fiber) at breakfast, maybe an apple (2.8 grams) at lunch, a pear (2.6 grams) at mid-afternoon, and a half cup of baked beans (7.7 grams) at dinner. Four simple additions, and already you're up to 15 grams dietary fiber.

Another way to painlessly add fiber is to follow the recommendations of the Food Guide Pyramid (see Chapter 17) and increase your consumption of grain products, vegetables, and fruits — all good sources of dietary fiber.

Finally, always check the nutrition label whenever you shop (for more about the wonderfully informative guides, see Chapter 17). When choosing between similar products, just take the one with the higher fiber content per serving. For example, white pita bread generally has about 1.6 grams dietary fiber per serving. Whole wheat pita bread has 7.4 grams. From a fiber standpoint, you know which works better for your body. Go for it!

By the way, dietary fiber is like a sponge. It sops up liquid, so increasing your fiber intake may deprive your cells of the water they need to perform their daily work (for more on how your body uses the water you drink, see Chapter 13). Unless you're already drinking at least six 8-ounce glasses of water every day, the American Academy of Family Physicians (among others) suggests upping your fluid intake when you consume more fiber.

Table 8-3 shows the amount of all types of dietary fiber — insoluble plus soluble — in a 100-gram (3.5-ounce) serving of specific foods. (For a more comprehensive list of foods and their fiber content, see the Appendix.) By the way, nutritionists like to measure things in terms of 100-gram portions because that makes comparing foods at a glance possible.

To find the amount of dietary fiber in your own serving, divide the gram total for the food shown in Table 8-3 (or the Appendix) by 3.5 and multiply the result by the number of ounces in your portion. For example, if you're having one ounce of cereal, the customary serving of ready-to-eat breakfast cereals, divide the gram total of dietary fiber by 3.5; then multiply by one. If your slice of bread weighs one-half ounce, divide the gram total by 3.5; then multiply the result by 0.5 (one-half).

Or — let's get real! — you can look at the nutrition label on the side of the package that gives the nutrients per portion.

Finally, the amounts on this chart are averages. Different brand-name processed products (bread, some cereals, cooked fruits, and vegetables) may have more (or less) fiber per serving.

Fiber factoid

The amount of fiber in a serving of food may depend on whether the food is raw or cooked. For example, as you can see from Table 8-3, a 3.5-ounce serving of plain dried prunes has 7.2 grams of fiber while a 3.5-ounce serving of stewed prunes has 6.6 grams of fiber.

Why? When you stew prunes, they "plump up" — which means they absorb water. The water adds weight but (obviously) no fiber. So a serving of prunes-plus-water has slightly less fiber per ounce than a same-weight serving of plain dried prunes.

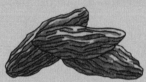

dried prunes

VS.

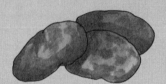

stewed prunes

Table 8-3	Getting Fiber from Food
Food	*Grams of Fiber in a 100-Gram (3.5-Ounce) Serving*
Bread	
Bagel	2.1
Bran bread	8.5
Pita bread (white)	1.6
Pita bread (whole wheat)	7.4
White bread	1.9
Cereals	
Bran cereal	35.3
Bran flakes	18.8
Cornflakes	2.0
Oatmeal	10.6
Wheat flakes	9.0
Grains	
Barley, pearled (minus its outer covering), raw	15.6
Cornmeal, whole grain	11.0

Food	Grams of Fiber in a 100-Gram (3.5-Ounce) Serving
De-germed	5.2
Oat bran, raw	6.6
Rice, raw (brown)	3.5
Rice, raw (white)	1.0 – 2.8
Rice, raw (wild)	5.2
Wheat bran	15.0
Fruits	
Apple, with skin	2.8
Apricots, dried	7.8
Figs, dried	9.3
Kiwifruit	3.4
Pear, raw	2.6
Prunes, dried	7.2
Prunes, stewed	6.6
Raisins	5.3
Vegetables	
Beans	
Baked (vegetarian)	7.7
Chickpeas (canned)	5.4
Lima, cooked	7.2
Broccoli, raw	2.8
Brussels sprouts, cooked	2.6
Cabbage, white, raw	2.4
Cauliflower, raw	2.4
Corn, sweet, cooked	3.7
Peas with edible pods, raw	2.6
Potatoes, white, baked, w/skin	5.5
Sweet potato, cooked	3.0
Tomatoes, raw	1.3
Other	
Corn chips, toasted	4.4
Nuts	

(continued)

Table 8-3 *(continued)*

Food	Grams of Fiber in a 100-Gram (3.5-Ounce) Serving
Almonds, oil-roasted	11.2
Coconut, raw	9.0
Hazelnuts, oil-roasted	6.4
Peanuts, dry-roasted	8.0
Pistachios	10.8
Tahini	9.3
Tofu	1.2

Source: Provisional Table on the Dietary Fiber Content of Selected Foods (Washington, D.C.: U.S. Department of Agriculture, 1988).

Fiber and your heart: The continuing saga of oat bran

Oat bran is the second chapter in the fiber fad that started with wheat bran around 1980. Wheat bran, the fiber in wheat, is rich in the insoluble fibers cellulose and lignin.

Oat bran's gee-whiz factor is the soluble fiber beta-glucans. For more than 30 years, scientists have known that eating foods high in soluble fiber can lower your cholesterol, although nobody knows exactly why. Fruits and vegetables (especially dried beans) are high in soluble fiber, but ounce for ounce, oats have more. In addition, beta-glucans are a more effective cholesterol-buster than pectin and gum, the soluble fibers in most fruits and vegetables.

By 1990, researchers at the University of Kentucky reported that people who add ½ cup dry oat bran (*not* oatmeal) to their regular daily diet can lower their levels of low density lipoproteins (LDLs), the particles that carry cholesterol into your arteries, by as much as 25 percent.

Doctors measure your cholesterol level in terms of the number of milligrams (mg) of cholesterol in one deciliter (dl) of blood. (A deciliter is ⅒th of a liter.)

When scientists at the Medical School of Northwestern University funded by Quaker Oats enlisted 208 healthy volunteers whose normal cholesterol readings averaged about 200 mg/dl and fed them oat bran, they were able to reduce the volunteers' total cholesterol levels an average of 9.3 percent with a lowfat, low cholesterol diet supplemented by two ounces of oats or oat bran every day.

About one-third of the cholesterol reduction was credited to the oats.

Oat cereal makers rounded the total loss to 10 percent and the National Research Council said that a 10 percent drop in cholesterol could produce a 20 percent drop in the risk of a heart attack.

Do I have to tell you what happened next? Books on oat bran hit the bestseller list. Cheerios elbowed Frosted Flakes aside to become the number one cereal in America. And people added oat bran to everything from bagels to orange juice.

Today scientists know that while oat bran couldn't hurt, the link between oats and cholesterol levels is no cure-all.

As a general rule, an adult whose cholesterol level is higher than 250 mg/dl is considered to be at "high risk." A cholesterol reading between 200 and 250 mg/dl is considered "moderately risky."

If your cholesterol level is above 250 mg/dl, lowering it 10 percent through a diet that contains oat bran may reduce your risk of heart attack without the use of medication. If your cholesterol level is lower than that to begin with, the effects of oat bran are less dramatic. For example:

✔ If your cholesterol level is below 250 mg/dl, a lowfat, low cholesterol diet alone may push it down 15 points into the "moderately risky" range. Adding oats reduces it another 8 points, but doesn't take you into "safe" territory, under 200 mg/dl.

✔ If your cholesterol is already a "safe" 199 mg/dl or lower, a lowfat, low cholesterol diet plus oats may drop it to 180 mg/dl, but the oats account for only 6 points of your loss.

Recognizing oat bran's benefits, the Food and Drug Administration now permits health claims on oat product labels. For example, the product label might say "Soluble fiber from foods such as oat bran, as part of a diet low in saturated fat and cholesterol, may reduce the risk of heart disease."

By the way, the soluble pectin in apples and the soluble beta-glucans (gums) in beans and peas also lower cholesterol levels. The insoluble fiber in wheat bran does not.

Chapter 9

Alcohol: Another Form of Grape and Grain

*A*lcohol beverages are among mankind's oldest home remedies and simple pleasures, so highly regarded that the ancient Greeks and Romans called wine a "gift from the gods," and when the Gaels — early inhabitants of Scotland and Ireland — first produced whiskey, they named it *uisgebeatha* (whis-key-ba), a combination of the words for water (uisge) and life (beatha). Today, although you may share their appreciation for the product, you know that alcohol beverages may have risks as well as benefits.

By the way, throughout this chapter I refer to beverages made from alcohol as "alcohol beverages." Yes, I know the grammatically correct term is probably "alcoholic beverages," but whenever I write or say those words, I get an immediate image of tipsy beer bottles. So indulge me.

The Many Faces of Alcohol

When micro-organisms (yeasts) digest (ferment) the sugars in carbohydrate foods, they make two by-products: a liquid and a gas. The gas is carbon dioxide. The liquid is ethyl alcohol, also known as ethanol, the intoxicating ingredient in alcohol beverages.

This biochemical process is not an esoteric one. In fact, it happens in your own kitchen every time you make a yeast bread. Remember the faint, beer-like odor in the air while the dough is rising? That odor is from the alcohol the yeasts make as they chomp their way through the sugars in the flour. (Don't worry, the alcohol evaporates when you bake the bread.) As the yeasts digest the sugars, they also produce carbon dioxide, which makes the bread rise.

From now on, whenever you see the word *alcohol* alone in this book, it means ethanol, the only alcohol used in alcohol beverages.

How Alcohol Beverages Are Made

Alcohol beverages are produced either through fermentation or through a combination of fermentation plus distillation.

Fermented alcohol products

Fermentation is a simple process in which yeasts or bacteria are added to carbohydrate starting material. The yeasts used to ferment sugars for alcohol beverages digest the sugars in the food, leaving liquid (alcohol), which is filtered to remove the solids. Adding water dilutes the alcohol producing — voilà — an alcohol beverage.

What other alcohols do you have in your home?

Ethanol is the only alcohol used in food and alcohol beverages, but it isn't the only alcohol used in consumer products. Here are the other alcohols that may be sitting on the shelf in your bathroom or workshop:

Methyl alcohol (methanol): *Methanol* is a poisonous alcohol made from wood. It's used as a *chemical solvent* (a liquid that dissolves other chemicals). During Prohibition, when the sale of beverage alcohol was illegal in the United States, some unscrupulous producers would substitute methanol for ethanol, thus leading to many truly unpleasant results such as blindness and death among people who drank it.

Isopropyl alcohol (rubbing alcohol): *Isopropyl alcohol* is a poisonous alcohol made from *propylene,* a petroleum derivative. This type of alcohol is *denatured* — which means it includes a substance that makes it taste and smell bad so that you won't drink it by mistake.

Denatured alcohol: When ethanol is used in cosmetics such as hair tonic, it, too, is treated to make it smell and taste bad. Treated ethanol is called *denatured alcohol.* Some denaturants (the chemicals used to denature the alcohol) are poisonous, so some denatured alcohol is poisonous. In other words, substituting hair tonic for beverage alcohol is definitely not a good idea.

Beer is made this way. So is wine. *Kumiss,* a fermented milk product, is slightly different because it's made by adding yeasts and friendly bacteria called *lactobacilli* (lacto = milk) to mare's milk. The micro-organisms make alcohol, but it isn't separated from the milk, which turns into a fizzy fermented beverage. *Kefir* is another fermented milk product.

Distilled alcohol products

The second way to make an alcohol beverage is *distillation.*

The process begins with yeasts, which make alcohol from sugars. But yeasts can't thrive in a place where the concentration of alcohol is higher than 20 percent. To concentrate the alcohol and separate it from the rest of the ingredients in the fermented liquid, distillers pour the fermented liquid into a *still,* a large vat with a wide column-like tube on top. The still is heated so that the alcohol, which boils at a lower temperature than everything else in the vat, turns to vapor, which rises through the column on top of the still, to be collected in containers where it condenses back into a liquid.

This alcohol, called *neutral spirits,* is the base for the alcohol beverages called spirits or distilled spirits: gin, rum, tequila, whiskey, and vodka. (Brandy is a special product — fermented wine — which is then distilled. Cognac is distilled grape wine; pear brandy is distilled wine made from pears.)

The foods used to make beverage alcohol

Beverage alcohol can be made from virtually any carbohydrate food. The foods most commonly used are cereal grains, fruit, honey, molasses, or potatoes. All produce alcohol, but the alcohols have slightly different flavors and colors. Table 9-1 shows you which foods are used to produce the different kinds of alcohol beverages.

Check the spelling

Here's an interesting consumer note: Whiskey is spelled with an "e" if it's made in North America or Ireland; without an "e" — whisky — if it comes from another country (Scotland is the best example).

Why? Nobody knows for sure. But a reasonable assumption is that the Scots may simply have dropped the "e" to differentiate their distilled spirits from the spirits distilled in Ireland. Journeying to the United States, Irish immigrants brought their distillation methods and their "e" with them, so that theirs became the name for whiskey made in America.

Table 9-1	Which Food Makes What Beverage?
Start with This Food	*To Get This Alcohol Beverage*
Fruit and fruit juice	
Agave plant	Tequila
Apples	Hard cider
Grapes & other fruits	Wine
Grain	
Barley	Beer, various distilled spirits, kvass
Corn	Bourbon, corn whiskey, beer
Rice	Sake (a distilled product), rice wine
Rye	Whiskey
Wheat	Distilled spirits, beer
Others	
Honey	Mead
Milk	Kumiss (koumiss), kefir
Potatoes	Vodka
Sugar cane	Rum

How Much Alcohol Is in That Bottle?

No alcohol beverage is 100 percent alcohol. It's alcohol plus water, and — if it's a wine or beer — some residue of the foods from which it was made.

The label on every bottle of wine and spirits shows the alcohol content as *alcohol by volume* (ABV). (For reasons too complicated to discuss in fewer than, say, 50 pages, beer containers may carry this information, but United States law does not require it.)

ABV measures the amount of alcohol as a percentage of all the liquid in the container. For example, if your container holds 10 ounces of liquid and one ounce of that is alcohol, the product is 10 percent ABV (the alcohol content — one ounce — divided by the total amount of liquid — 10 ounces).

You may also have seen an older term describing alcohol content: *proof.* Proof is two times the ABV. For example, an alcohol beverage that is 10 percent ABV is 20 proof. (ABV replaced proof in the early 1990s.)

How Alcohol Moves through Your Body

On its own, alcohol provides energy (7 calories per gram) but no nutrients — zero, zilch, zip. Distilled spirits, such as whiskey or plain, unflavored vodka, have no nutrients other than calories. Beer, wine, cider, and other fermented beverages such as kumiss (fermented milk) contain some of the food from which they were made, so they also contain small amounts of proteins and carbohydrates, vitamins, and minerals.

Unlike other foods, which must be digested before they can be absorbed by your cells, alcohol flows directly through your body's membranes into your bloodstream. In fact, alcohol is absorbed so fast and so efficiently that about 20 percent of the alcohol in your drink reaches your brain within seconds after you drink it.

Your blood carries alcohol to nearly every organ in your body. Here's a road map to show you the route traveled by the alcohol in every drink you take.

Down the hatch from mouth to stomach

Alcohol is an *astringent;* it coagulates the proteins on the surface of the lining of your cheeks and makes them "pucker." Some alcohol is absorbed here, some through the lining of your throat; but most spills into your stomach where an enzyme called *gastric alcohol dehydrogenase* (ADH) begins to metabolize it.

Your body makes only a limited amount of gastric ADH. As a result, some unmetabolized alcohol flows through your stomach walls into your bloodstream. The average woman makes less ADH than the average man, so more alcohol flows from her stomach into her blood. As a result, she is likely to become tipsy on smaller amounts of alcohol.

Meanwhile, the alcohol that isn't broken down by gastric ADH moves on to your small intestine.

A short visit to the energy factory

Most alcohol is absorbed through the duodenum (small intestine), and then flows through a large blood vessel (the portal vein) into your liver. In the liver, an enzyme similar to gastric ADH metabolizes the alcohol, which is converted to energy by a coenzyme called *nicotinamide adenine dinucleotide* (NAD). NAD also converts the glucose you get from other carbohydrates to energy; while NAD is being used for alcohol, glucose conversion grinds to a halt.

The normal, healthy liver can process about ½ ounce of pure alcohol (that's 6 to 12 ounces of beer, 5 ounces of wine, or 1 ounce of spirits) in an hour. The rest flows on to your heart.

Time out for air

Entering your heart, alcohol reduces the force with which your heart muscle contracts. You pump out slightly less blood for a few minutes, blood vessels all over your body relax, and your blood pressure goes down temporarily. The contractions soon return to normal, but the blood vessels may remain relaxed and your blood pressure lower for as long as half an hour.

At the same time, alcohol flows in blood from your heart through your pulmonary vein to your lungs. Now you breathe out a tiny bit of alcohol every time you exhale, and your breath "smells of liquor." Then the newly oxygenated, still alcohol-laden blood flows back through the pulmonary artery to your heart, and up and out through the aorta (the major artery that carries blood out to your body).

Rising to the surface

Traveling in your blood, alcohol raises your level of high density lipoproteins, although not necessarily the specific "good" ones that carry cholesterol out of your body. (For more about lipoproteins, see Chapter 7.) Alcohol also makes blood platelets (tiny particles that enable blood to clot) less sticky and reduces the effectiveness of fibrinogen, another blood-clotting agent. This temporarily lowers your risk of blood-clot-related heart attack and stroke.

Alcohol makes blood vessels expand, so more warm blood flows up from the center of your body to the surface of the skin. You feel (temporarily) warmer and, if your skin is fair, you may flush and turn pink. At the same time, tiny amounts of alcohol ooze out through your pores, and your perspiration smells of alcohol.

Curves in the road

Alcohol is a sedative. When it reaches your brain, it slows the transmission of impulses between nerve cells that control thinking as well as movement. That's why your thoughts may be fuzzy, your judgment impaired, your tongue twisted, your vision blurred, and your muscles rubbery.

Do you feel a sudden urge to pee? Alcohol reduces your brain's production of *antidiuretic hormones,* chemicals that keep you from making too much urine. You may lose lots of liquid, plus vitamins and minerals. You're also very thirsty and your urine smells faintly of alcohol. This cycle continues as long as you have alcohol circulating in your blood, or in other words, until your liver can manage to produce enough ADH to metabolize all the alcohol you've consumed. How long is that? Most people need a full hour to metabolize the amount of alcohol (½ ounce) in one drink. But that's only an average: Some people still have alcohol circulating in their blood for as long as two to three hours after they take a drink.

Alcohol and Health

Beverage alcohol has benefits as well as side effects. The benefits seem to be linked to what is commonly called *moderate drinking* — no more than one drink a day for a woman, two drinks a day for a man — consumed with food. The risks generally appear to flow from alcohol abuse.

Moderate drinking: Some benefits, some risks

Moderate amounts of alcohol reduce stress, so it's not surprising that recent well-designed scientific studies on large groups of men and women suggest that moderate drinking is heart-healthy, protecting the cardiovascular system (that's science talk for heart and blood vessels).

✔ The American Cancer Society's Cancer Prevention Study 1 followed more than one million Americans in 25 states for 12 years. Analyzing the lifestyles of 276,802 middle-aged men and the circumstances of those who died during the study period, the researchers concluded that moderate alcohol intake had an "apparent protective effect on coronary heart disease." Translation: Men who drink moderately lower their risk of heart attack — the risk is 21 percent lower for men who have one drink a day than for men who never drink. In addition, men who have one or two drinks a day are 22 percent less likely to die of a stroke.

✔ In January 1999, researchers at New York Presbyterian Hospital-Columbia University published results of a 677-person study suggesting that moderate alcohol consumption by older people also reduces the risk of ischemic stroke (stroke caused by a blood clot blocking a blood vessel in the brain). As always, moderation is the key: Heavy alcohol consumption — more than seven drinks a day — is linked to a higher risk of stroke. People who once drank heavily but cut their consumption to moderate levels cut their risk of stroke as well.

✔ An earlier analysis of data on nearly 600,000 women in the study showed that — like men — women who drink occasionally or have one drink a day are less likely to die of heart attack than women who don't drink at all. Among the more than 80,000 women enrolled in the long-running Nurse Health Study, those who took 400 mg of the B vitamin folate plus 3 mg of vitamin B6 every day had a 50 percent lower risk of heart attack. Adding one drink a day to vitamins reduced the risk by almost 80 percent.

✔ Moderate drinking also seems to raise the level of high density lipoproteins, the "good" cholesterol that lowers your risk of heart disease.

That's the good news. Here's the bad news: The same studies that applaud the effects of moderate drinking on heart-health are less reassuring about the relationship between alcohol and cancer: The American Cancer Society's Cancer Prevention Study 1 study shows that people who take more than two drinks a day have a higher incidence of cancer of the mouth and throat (esophagus). In addition:

✔ Researchers at the University of Oklahoma say that men who drink five or more beers a day double their risk of rectal cancer.

✔ American Cancer Society statistics show a higher risk of breast cancer among women who have more than three drinks a week, but newer studies suggest this effect may apply only to older women using hormone replacement therapy.

For several years, bottles of beer, wine, and spirits have carried label warnings about the risks of alcohol consumption. Recently, winemakers asked the Bureau of Alcohol, Tobacco, and Firearms (BATF), which regulates beverage alcohol products, to grant equal space for a general label statement regarding the potential health benefits of moderate drinking. In the spring of 1999, BATF agreed, and wine bottles may now carry one (or both) of the following statements: "To learn the health effects of wine consumption, send for the federal government's Dietary Guidelines for Americans" or "The proud people who made this wine encourage you to consult your family doctor about the health effects of wine consumption." If spirits and beer companies request the right to use the same label copy, BATF is expected to say yes.

The risks of alcohol abuse

Alcohol abuse is a term generally taken to mean drinking so much that it interferes with your ability to run a normal, productive life.

The short-term effects of excessive drinking are well-known to one and all, especially men who may find that drinking too much decreases sexual desire and makes it impossible to . . . well . . . perform. (No evidence suggests that excessive drinking interferes with female orgasm.)

Excessive drinking can also make you feel terrible the next day. The "morning after" is not fiction. A "hangover" is a miserable physical fact:

✔ You're thirsty because you lost excess water through copious urination.

✔ Your stomach hurts and you're queasy because even small amounts of alcohol irritate your stomach lining, causing it to secrete extra acid and lots of *histamine,* the same immune system chemical that makes the skin around a mosquito bite red and itchy.

✔ Your muscles ache and your head pounds because processing alcohol through your liver requires an enzyme — nicotinamide adenine dinucleotide (NAD) — normally used to convert *lactic acid,* a by-product of muscle activity, to other chemicals that can be used for energy. The extra unprocessed lactic acid piles up painfully in your muscles.

Alcoholism: An addiction disease

Alcoholics are people who can't control their drinking. Untreated alcoholism is a life-threatening disease that can lead to death either from an accident or suicide (both are more common among heavy drinkers) or from a toxic reaction (acute alcohol poisoning that paralyzes body organs, including heart and lungs) or malnutrition.

Alcoholism makes it extremely difficult for the body to get essential nutrients. Here's why:

✔ Alcohol depresses appetite.

✔ An alcoholic may substitute alcohol for food, getting calories but no nutrients.

✔ Even if the alcoholic does eat, the alcohol in his tissues can prevent him from absorbing vitamins (notably the B vitamins), minerals, and other nutrients. It may also reduce his ability to synthesize proteins.

No one knows exactly why some people are able to have a drink once a day or once a month or once a year, enjoy it, and move on, while others become addicted to alcohol. In the past, alcoholism has been blamed on heredity ("bad genes") or "lack of will power" or a bad upbringing. But as science unravels the mysteries of body chemistry, other possible explanations have surfaced.

In 1998, researchers at the University of Washington in Seattle reported that genetically-engineered mice with a lack of a natural chemical called neuropeptide Y (NPY, for short) recover more quickly from the sedative effects of alcohol. They may be up and frisking about when mice with normal amounts of NPY are still "sleeping it off," so they're likely to drink more than normal mice do. Human beings also produce NPY, so the researchers want to find out whether people who make less NPY are also less sensitive to alcohol's sedative effects and therefore more likely to drink to excess.

The NPY story is only one line of investigation into the link between body chemistry and addictive behavior. You can expect to hear more about this line of research in the near future.

Who should not drink

No one should drink to excess. But some people should not drink at all, not even in moderation. For example:

- ✔ **People who plan to drive or to do work that takes both attention and skill.** As noted earlier, alcohol slows reaction time and makes your motor skills — turning the wheel of the car, operating a sewing machine — less precise.

- ✔ **Women who are pregnant or who plan to become pregnant in the near future.** *Fetal alcohol syndrome* (FAS) is a collection of birth defects including low birth weight, heart defects, retardation, and facial deformities documented only in babies born to female alcoholics. No evidence links FAS to casual drinking — that is, one or two drinks during a pregnancy or even one or two drinks a week. But the fact is that about 7 percent of the babies born in the United States each year are born with birth defects independent of any parental behavior. The parents of these children may feel guilty, even though their behavior had absolutely nothing to do with the birth defect. Your decision about alcohol should take into consideration the possibility of (misplaced) lifelong guilt due to having had a drink.

- ✔ **People who take prescription drugs or over-the-counter medication.** Alcohol makes some drugs stronger, increasing the side effects, and renders others less effective. At the same time, some drugs make alcohol a more powerful sedative or slow down alcohol's elimination from your body.

Table 9-2 shows some of the interactions known to occur between alcohol and some common prescription and over-the-counter drugs. This short list gives you an idea of some of the general interactions likely to occur between alcohol and drugs. But the list is far from complete, so if you're taking any medication — over-the-counter or prescription — check with your doctor or pharmacist regarding the possibility of an interaction with alcohol.

Table 9-2	Drugs and Alcohol Don't Mix!
Drug	*Possible Reaction*
Analgesics (Acetaminophen)	Increased liver toxicity
Analgesics (aspirin and other non-steroidal inflammatory drugs — NSAIDs)	Increased stomach bleeding; irritation
Anti-arthritis drugs	Increased stomach bleeding; irritation
Antidepressants	Increased drowsiness/intoxication; high blood pressure (depends on type of drug; check with your doctor)
Antidiabetes drugs	Excessive low blood sugar
Antihypertension drugs	Very low blood pressure
Antituberculosis medication (isoniazid)	Decreased drug effectiveness; higher risk of hepatitis
Diet pills	Excessive nervousness
Diuretics	Low blood pressure
Iron supplements	Excessive absorption of iron
Sleeping pills	Increased sedation
Tranquilizers	Increased sedation

Source: James W. Long and James J. Rybacki, The Essential Guide to Prescription Drugs 1995 (New York: Harper Collins, 1995).

A Word from the Sages: Moderation

Good advice is always current. The folks who wrote Ecclesiastes (a book in the *Bible*) centuries ago might have been speaking to you when they said that "wine is as good as life to man if it be drunk moderately." And it's impossible to improve on this slogan from the Romans (actually, one Roman writer named Terence): "Moderation in all things." Hey, you can't get a message more direct — or more sensible — than that.

The power of purple (and peanuts)

Grape skin, pulp, and seeds contain *resveratrol,* a naturally-occurring plant chemical that seems to reduce the risk of heart disease and some kinds of cancer. The darker the grapes, the higher the concentration of resveratrol.

Dark purple grape juice, for example, has more resveratrol than red grape juice, which has more resveratrol than white grape juice.

Because wine is made from grapes, it, too, contains resveratrol (red wine has more resveratrol than white wine).

But you don't need to drink grape juice or wine to get resveratrol. You can simply snack on peanuts. Yes, peanuts. A 1998 analysis from the USDA Agricultural Research Service in Raleigh, North Carolina, showed that peanuts have 1.7 to 3.7 mcg of resveratrol per gram. Compare that to the 0.6 to 8.0 mcg of resveratrol per gram of red wine.

This fact may explain data from the long-running Harvard University/Brigham and Women's Hospital Nurses Health Study, which shows that women who eat an ounce of nuts a day have a lower risk of heart disease. So let's see — wine, grape juice, peanuts . . . decisions, decisions.

Chapter 10

Vigorous Vitamins

• •

In This Chapter

▶ The value of vitamins

▶ The best food sources for the vitamins you need

▶ What happens if you take too many (or too few) vitamins

▶ When you may need extra vitamins

• •

*V*itamins are *organic chemicals,* substances that contain carbon, hydrogen, and oxygen. They occur naturally in all living things, plants as well as animals: flowers, trees, fruits, vegetables, chicken, fish, cows — and you.

Vitamins regulate a variety of bodily functions. They are essential for building body tissues such as bones, skin, glands, nerves, and blood. They assist in the metabolism of proteins, fats, and carbohydrates, so that you can get energy from food. They prevent nutritional deficiency diseases, promote healing, and encourage good health.

How Your Body Uses Vitamins

Your body needs at least 11 specific vitamins: vitamin A, vitamin D, vitamin E, vitamin K, vitamin C, and the members of the B vitamin family: thiamin (vitamin B1), riboflavin (B2), niacin, vitamin B6, folate, and vitamin B12. Two more B vitamins — biotin and pantothenic acid — are now believed valuable to your well-being as well. You need only miniscule quantities of vitamins for good health. In some cases, the recommended dietary allowances (RDAs), determined by the National Research Council, may be as small as several micrograms ($\frac{1}{1,000,000}$ of a gram).

The father of all vitamins: Casimir Funk

Vitamins are so much a part of modern life you may have a hard time believing they were first discovered less than 90 years ago.

People have long known that certain foods contain something "special."

For example, the ancient Greek physician Hippocrates prescribed liver for *night-blindness* (the inability to see well in dim light). By the end of the 18th century (1795), British Navy ships carried a mandatory supply of limes or lime juice to prevent scurvy among the men, thus earning the Brits once and forever the nickname "Limies." Later on, the Japanese Navy gave their sailors whole grain barley to ward off beriberi.

Everyone knew these "prescriptions" worked, but nobody knew why — until 1912, when

Casimir Funk (1884-1967), a Polish biochemist working first in England and then in the United States, came up with the theory that the "somethings" in food were substances called *vitamines* (*vita* = life; *amines* = nitrogen compounds).

The following year, Funk and a fellow biochemist, Briton Frederick Hopkins, proposed a second theory: Conditions such as scurvy and beriberi were simply deficiency diseases caused by the absence of a specific nutrient in the body. Adding a food with the "missing" nutrient to one's diet would prevent or cure the deficiency disease.

Eureka!

How Vitamins Are Stored in Your Body

Nutritionists classify vitamins as either "fat soluble" or "water soluble," meaning that they dissolve either in fat or in water. If you consume larger amounts of fat-soluble vitamins than your body needs, the excess will be stored in body fat. Excess water-soluble vitamins are eliminated in urine.

Large amounts of fat-soluble vitamins stored in your body may cause problems (see the section "Fat-Soluble Vitamins" in this chapter). With water-soluble vitamins, your body simply shrugs its shoulders, so to speak, and urinates away most of the excess.

Medical students often use mnemonic (pronounced *ne-mon-ik*) devices — "memory joggers" — to remember complicated lists of body parts and symptoms of diseases. Here's one I use to remember which vitamins are fat-soluble and which dissolve in water: "**A**ll **D**ogs **E**at **K**idneys." This saying helps me remember that vitamins A, D, E, and K are fat-soluble. All the rest dissolve in water.

Fat-Soluble Vitamins

Vitamin A, vitamin D, vitamin E, and vitamin K are relatives that have two characteristics in common: all dissolve in fat, and all are stored in your fatty tissues. But like members of any family, they also have distinct "personalities." One keeps your skin moist. Another protects your bones. A third keeps reproductive organs purring happily. And the fourth enables you to make special proteins.

Which does what? Read on.

Vitamin A

Vitamin A is the moisturizing nutrient. This vitamin keeps your skin and *mucous membranes* (the slick tissue that lines the eyes, nose, mouth, throat, vagina, and rectum) smooth and supple. Vitamin A is also the vision vitamin, a constituent of *11-cis retinol,* a protein in the rods (cells in the back of your eye that make it possible for you to see even when the lights are low). Vitamin A promotes the growth of healthy bones and teeth, keeps your reproductive system humming, and encourages your immune system to churn out the cells you need to fight off infection.

Two chemicals provide vitamin A — retinoids and carotenoids. *Retinoids* are compounds whose names all start with *ret-:* retinol, retinaldehyde, retinoic acid, and so on. These fat-soluble substances are found in several foods of animal origin: liver (again!) as well as whole milk, eggs, and butter. Retinoids give you *preformed* vitamin A, the kind of nutrient your body can use right away.

The second form of vitamin A is some of the carotenoids — yellow, red, and dark green coloring agents (pigments) — in fruits and vegetables. *Carotenoids* are vitamin A *precursors,* chemicals your body transforms into retinol-like substances.

So far, scientists have identified at least 500 different carotenoids. Only one in 10 — about 50 altogether — are considered to be a source of vitamin A. The star of the lot is beta-carotene, a pigment found in most bright yellow and deep green fruits and vegetables.

New research suggests that these carotenoids play an important role in vision, preventing or slowing the development of age-related *macular degeneration,* progressive damage to the retina of the eye which can cause the loss of central vision (the ability to see clearly enough to read or do fine work).

Because retinol is the most efficient source of vitamin A, the recommended dietary allowance (RDA) for vitamin A is usually written as retinol equivalents, abbreviated as RE.

TECHNICAL STUFF

Hand in hand: How vitamins help each other

All vitamins have specific jobs in your body. Some have partners. Here are some examples of nutrient cooperation.

Vitamin E keeps vitamin A from being destroyed in your intestines.

Vitamin D enables your body to absorb calcium and phosphorus.

Vitamin C helps folate build proteins.

Vitamin B1 works in digestive enzyme systems with niacin, pantothenic acid, and magnesium.

In addition, taking vitamins with other vitamins may improve body levels of nutrients. In 1993, scientists at the National Cancer Institute and the U. S. Department of Agriculture (USDA) Agricultural Research Service gave one group of volunteers a vitamin E capsule plus a multivitamin pill; a second group, vitamin E alone; and a third group, no vitamins at all. The people getting vitamin E plus the multivitamin had the highest amount of vitamin E in their blood — more than twice as high as those who took plain vitamin E capsules.

Sometimes, one vitamin may even alleviate a deficiency due to the lack of another vitamin. People who do not get enough folate are at risk of a form of anemia in which their red blood cells fail to mature. As soon as they get folate, either by injection or by mouth, they begin to make new healthy cells. That's to be expected. What's surprising is the fact that anemia due to pellagra, the niacin deficiency disease, may also respond to folate treatment.

Isn't nature neat?

Vitamin D

If I say "bones" or "teeth," what nutrient springs most quickly to mind? If you answer calcium, you're only partly right. True, calcium is essential for hardening both teeth and bones. But no matter how much calcium you consume, without vitamin D, your body cannot absorb and use the mineral.

Vitamin D comes in three forms: calciferol, cholecalciferol, and ergocalciferol. *Calciferol* occurs naturally in fish oils and egg yolk; in the United States, it is added to margarines and milk. *Cholecalciferol* is created when sunlight hits your skin and ultraviolet rays react with steroid chemicals in body fat just underneath. *Ergocalciferol* is synthesized in plants exposed to sunlight. Cholecalciferol and ergocalciferol justify vitamin D's nickname: "The sunshine vitamin."

The RDA for vitamin D is measured either in International Units (IUs) or micrograms (mcg) of cholecalciferol: 10 mcg cholecalciferol = 400 IU vitamin D.

Vitamin E

Every animal, including you, needs vitamin E to maintain a healthy reproductive system, nerves, and muscles. In addition, science is beginning to find evidence to show that the long-lived rumors about vitamin E and heart health — once pooh-poohed by the nutrition establishment — are true. For example, a 1996 clinical trial at Cambridge University in England shows that taking 800 IU (International Units) vitamin E, two times the RDA, may reduce the risk of nonfatal heart attacks for people who already have heart disease. And researchers at the University of Minnesota say that post-menopausal women who get at least 10 IU of vitamin E a day from food cut their risk of heart disease by nearly 66 percent.

You get vitamin E from *tocopherols* and *tocotrieonols,* two families of naturally-occurring chemicals in vegetable oils, nuts, whole grains, and green leafy vegetables — your best natural sources of vitamin E. Tocopherols, the more important source, have two sterling characteristics: They are anticoagulants and antioxidants.

Anticoagulants reduce blood's ability to clot and may reduce the risk of clot-related stroke and heart attack. *Antioxidants* prevent free radicals (incomplete pieces of molecules) from hooking up with other molecules or fragments of molecules to form toxic substances that can attack tissues in your body. In the spring of 1996, nutrition scientists at Purdue University released a study showing that vitamin E promotes bone growth by stopping free radicals from reacting with polyunsaturated fatty acids (see Chapter 7 for information on fats) to create molecules that interfere with the formation of new bone cells.

Can tocopherols lower cholesterol? Could be. Tocopherols ride around your body on the back of *lipoproteins,* the fat and protein particles that carry cholesterol either into arteries or out of the body. Some research suggests that the tocopherol passengers may prevent low density lipoproteins (LDLs, the *bad* cholesterol) from glomming onto artery walls and blocking blood vessels — another explanation for vitamin E's link to a healthy heart. For more on cholesterol, see Chapter 7.

Your best sources of vitamin E are vegetables, oils, nuts, and seeds. The RDA is expressed as a-tocopherol equivalents (abbreviated as *a-TE*).

Vitamin K

Vitamin K is a group of chemicals that your body uses to make specialized proteins found in blood *plasma* (the clear fluid in blood), such as prothrombin, the protein chiefly responsible for blood clotting. You also need vitamin K to make bone and kidney tissues.

Like vitamin D, vitamin K is essential for healthy bones. Vitamin D increases calcium absorption; vitamin K activates at least three different proteins that take part in forming new bone cells.

Vitamin K is in dark green leafy vegetables (broccoli, cabbage, kale, lettuce, spinach, and turnip greens), cheese, liver, cereals, and fruits; but most of what you need comes from resident colonies of friendly bacteria in your intestines, an assembly-line of busy bugs churning out the vitamin day and night.

Water-Soluble Vitamins

Vitamin C and the entire roster of B vitamins (thiamin, riboflavin, niacin, vitamin B6, folate, biotin, pantothenic acid) are usually grouped together simply because they all dissolve in water.

The ability to dissolve in water is a very important point. It means large amounts of these nutrients can't be storied in your body. If you take in more than you need to perform specific body tasks, you will simply pee away virtually all the excess. The good news is that these vitamins rarely cause side effects. The bad news is that you have to take enough of these vitamins every day in order to protect yourself against deficiency.

Vitamin C

Vitamin C, a.k.a. ascorbic acid, is essential for the development and maintenance of connective tissue (the fat, muscle, and bone framework of the human body). Vitamin C speeds the production of new cells in wound healing, and — like vitamin E — it is an antioxidant that keeps free radicals from hooking up with other molecules to form damaging compounds that might attack your tissues, which may explain the results of several studies showing that taking vitamin C supplements (400-700 mg/day) for longer than 10 years slows the development of cataracts. Vitamin C protects your immune system, helps you fight off infection, reduces the severity of allergic reactions, and plays a role in the synthesis of hormones and other body chemicals.

After years of wrangling, the National Institute of Health has proposed increasing the RDA for vitamin C (currently 60 mg) to 200 mg for healthy adults. You can easily obtain this amount, which may make it into the next version of the RDAs, by consuming five daily servings of fruits and vegetables such as broccoli, citrus fruits (oranges, lemons, limes, and grapefruit), green peppers, strawberries, and tomatoes.

Lemons, limes, oranges — and bacon?

Check the label. There it is. Vitamin C in the form of *sodium ascorbate* or *isoascorbate*.

The Food and Drug Administration says it has to be there because vitamin C does for meat exactly what it does for your body: prevents free radicals from hooking up with each other to form damaging compounds, in this case *carcinogens* (substances that cause cancer).

Processed meats such as bacon and sausages are preserved with sodium nitrite, which protects the meat from *Clostridium botulinum,* micro-organisms that cause the potentially fatal food poisoning known as botulism. On its own, sodium nitrite reacts at high temperatures with compounds in meat to form carcinogens called nitrosamines.

But, like the Lone Ranger, antioxidant vitamin C rides to the rescue, preventing the chemical reaction and keeping the sausage and bacon safe to eat. How's that for healthy eating, *kemosabe?*

Thiamin (vitamin B1)

Call it thiamin. Call it B1. Just don't call it late for lunch (or any other meal). This sulfur *(thia)* and nitrogen *(amin)* compound, the first of the B vitamins to be isolated and identified, helps ensure a healthy appetite. It acts as a *coenzyme* (a substance that works along with other enzymes) essential to at least four different processes by which your body extracts energy from carbohydrates. And thiamin is also a mild diuretic (something that makes you urinate more).

Although thiamin is found in every body tissue, the highest concentrations are in your organs — heart, liver, and kidneys.

The richest dietary sources of thiamin are unrefined cereals and grains, lean pork, beans, nuts, and seeds. In the United States, refined flours, stripped of their thiamin, are a nutritional reality so most Americans get most of their thiamin from breads and cereals enriched with additional B1.

Riboflavin (vitamin B2)

Riboflavin (vitamin B2), the second B vitamin to be identified, was once called "vitamin G." Its present name derives from its chemical structure, a carbon-hydrogen-oxygen skeleton that includes *ribitol* (a sugar) attached to a *flavonoid* (a substance from plants containing a pigment called flavone).

Like thiamin, riboflavin is a co-enzyme. Without it, your body cannot digest and use proteins and carbohydrates. Like vitamin A, it protects the health of mucous membranes — the moist tissues that line the eyes, mouth, nose, throat, vagina, and rectum.

You get riboflavin from foods of animal origin (meat, fish, poultry, eggs, and milk), whole or enriched grain products, brewers yeast, and dark green vegetables (broccoli and spinach are good examples).

Niacin

Niacin is one name for a pair of naturally occurring nutrients, nicotinic acid and nicotinamide. Niacin is essential for proper growth, and like other B vitamins, it is intimately involved in enzyme reactions. In fact, it is an integral part of an enzyme that allows oxygen to flow into body tissues. Like thiamin, it gives you a healthy appetite and participates in the metabolism of sugars and fat.

Niacin is available either as a preformed nutrient or via the conversion of the amino acid tryptophane. Preformed niacin comes from meat; tryptophane, from milk and dairy foods. Some niacin is in grains, but your body cannot absorb it efficiently unless the grain has been treated with lime — the mineral, not the fruit. This is a common practice in Central American and South American countries where lime is added to corn meal in making tortillas. In the United States, breads and cereals are routinely fortified with niacin. The added niacin is easily absorbed by your body.

The term used to describe the niacin RDA is NE (niacin equivalent); 60 mg tryptophane = 1 mg niacin = 1 niacin equivalent (NE).

Vitamin B6 (Pyridoxine)

Vitamin B6 is another multiple compound, this one comprising three related chemicals: pyridoxine, pyridoxal, and pyridoxamine. Vitamin B6, a component of enzymes that metabolize proteins and fats, is essential for getting energy and nutrients from food. It plays an important role in removing excess amounts of homocysteine (see Chapter 6) from your blood. According to the American Heart Association, a high level of *homocysteine,* an amino acid produced when you digest proteins, is an independent risk factor for heart disease, perhaps as important as your cholesterol levels.

The best food sources of vitamin B6 are liver, chicken, fish, pork, lamb, milk, eggs, unmilled rice, whole grains, soy beans, potatoes, beans, nuts, seeds, and dark green vegetables such as turnip greens. In the United States, bread and other products made with refined grains have added vitamin B6.

Folate

Folate is an essential nutrient for human beings and other *vertebrates* (animals with a backbone). Folate takes part in the synthesis of DNA, the metabolism of proteins, and the subsequent synthesis of amino acids used to produce new body cells and tissues. Folate is vital for normal growth and wound healing. An adequate supply of the vitamin is essential for pregnant women to enable them to create new maternal tissue as well as fetal tissue. In addition, an adequate supply of folate dramatically reduces the risk of spinal cord birth defects. Beans, dark green leafy vegetables, liver, yeast, and various fruits are excellent food sources of folate, and all multivitamin supplements must now provide 400 mcg of folate.

Vitamin B12

Vitamin B12 (cyanocobalamin) makes healthy red blood cells. Vitamin B12 protects *myelin,* the fatty material that covers your nerves and enables you to transmit electrical impulses ("messages") between nerve cells. These messages make it possible for you to see, hear, think, move, and do all the things a healthy body does each day.

Vitamin B12 is unique. First, it is the only vitamin that contains a mineral, cobalt. (Cyanocobalamin, a cobalt compound, is commonly used as "vitamin B12" in vitamin pills and nutritional supplements.) Second, it is a vitamin that cannot be made by higher plants (the ones that give us fruits and vegetables). Like vitamin K, vitamin B12 is made by beneficial bacteria living in your small intestine. Meat, fish, poultry, milk products, and eggs are good sources of vitamin B12. Grains do not contain vitamin B12 naturally, but like other B vitamins, it is added to grain products in the United States.

Biotin

Biotin is a B-vitamin, a component of enzymes that ferry carbon and oxygen atoms between cells. Biotin helps to metabolize fats and carbohydrates and is essential for synthesizing fatty acids and amino acids needed for healthy growth. And it seems to prevent a buildup of fat deposits that might interfere with the proper functioning of liver and kidneys. (No, biotin won't keep fat from settling in more visible places, such as your hips.)

Your best food sources of biotin are liver, egg yolk, yeast, nuts, and beans. If your diet doesn't give you all the biotin you need, bacteria in your gut will synthesize enough to make up the difference. No RDA exists for biotin, but the Food and Nutrition Board has established an estimated safe and effective daily dietary intake.

Pantothenic acid

Pantothenic acid, another B-vitamin, is vital to enzyme reactions that make it possible for you to use carbohydrates and create steroid biochemicals such as hormones. Pantothenic acid also helps stabilize blood sugar levels, defends against infection, and protects *hemoglobin* (the protein in red blood cells that carries oxygen through the body), as well as nerve, brain, and muscle tissue. You get pantothenic acid from meat, fish and poultry, beans, whole grain cereals, and fortified grain products. As with biotin, the Food and Nutrition Board has an estimated safe and effective daily dietary intake for pantothenic acid.

Get Your Vitamins Here!

One reasonable set of guidelines for good nutrition is the list of Recommended Dietary Allowances (RDAs) established by the National Research Council's Food and Nutrition Board. The RDAs present safe and effective doses for healthy people.

You can find the entire chart in Chapter 4. It is very, very long, with RDAs for 18 different groups of people (men, women, old, young) for 18 specific vitamins and minerals, plus protein. I couldn't possibly ask you to read through it again here. Personally, just the thought of retyping the whole thing gives me hives.

Table 10-1 is the easy alternative: It gives you the RDAs for adult men and women (age 19 to 50) plus a quick, no-brainer guide to food portions that give you at least 25 percent of the recommended dietary allowance (RDA) of vitamins for healthy adult men and women, age 25 to 50.

Photocopy this chart. Pin it on your fridge. Tape it to your organizer or appointment book. Stick it in your wallet. Think of it as the truly simple way to see how easy it is to eat healthy.

Table 10-1	Reasonable Servings that Provide 25 Percent — or More — of the RDA
Food	*Serving = 25% RDA*
VITAMIN A	**RDA: Women 800 mcg RE, Men 1,000 mcg RE**
Breads, cereals, grains	
Oatmeal, instant, fortified	2⅓ cup
Cold cereals	1 ounce

Food	Serving = 25% RDA
Fruits	
Apricots (dried, cooked)	½ cup
Cantaloupe, raw	½ cup
Mango, raw	½ medium
Vegetables	
Carrots, kale, peas & carrots, pepper (sweet, red) — all cooked	1/2 cup
Meat, poultry, fish	
Liver (beef, calf, pork)	3 ounces (diced)
Liver (chicken, turkey)	½ cup (diced)
Dairy products	
Milk, lowfat or skim	2 cups
VITAMIN D	**RDA: Women 5 mcg/200 IU, Men 5 mcg/200 IU**
Meat, poultry, fish	
Salmon, canned	1½ ounces
Tuna, canned	2 ounces
Dairy products	
Eggs	3 medium
Milk, enriched	1 cup
VITAMIN E	**RDA: Women 8 mg a-TE, Men 10 mg a-TE**
Breads, cereals, grains	
Cold cereal	1 ounce
Wheat germ, plain	2 tbsp.
Fruits	
Apricots, peaches (canned)	1 cup
Vegetables	
Greens (dandelion, mustard, turnip), cooked	1 cup
Meat, poultry, fish	
Shrimp	3 ounces
Other	
Almonds, hazelnuts (filberts)	2 tbsp.

(continued)

Table 10-1 *(continued)*

Food	*Serving = 25% RDA*
Peanut butter	2 tbsp.
Sunflower seeds	2 tbsp.
VITAMIN C	**RDA: Women 60 mg, Men 60 mg**
Breads, cereals, grains	
Cold cereals	1 ounce
Fruits	
Cantaloupe	½ cup, diced
Grapefruit	½
Mango, raw	½ medium
Orange	1 medium
Strawberries	½ cup
Grape, orange, tomato juice	¼ cup
Vegetables	
Asparagus, broccoli, brussels sprouts, kale, kohlrabi, sweet peppers, snow peas (cooked)	½ cup
Sweet potato	1 medium
Meat, poultry, fish	
Liver (beef, pork)	3 ounces
THIAMIN (VITAMIN B1)	**RDA: Women 1.1 mg, Men 1.5 mg**
Breads, cereals, grains	
Bagel, English muffin, roll	2 whole
Bread	4 slices
Farina, grits	⅓ cup
Oatmeal, instant, fortified	⅓ cup
Fruits	
Cantaloupe, honeydew	1 cup
Vegetables	
Corn, peas, peas & carrots, cooked	1 cup

Food	Serving = 25% RDA
Meat, poultry, fish	
Ham, roast, smoked, cured, lean	3 ounces
Liver (beef, pork)	3 ounces
Pork (all varieties except sausage)	3 ounces
Other	
Sunflower seeds, hulled, unroasted	2 tbsp.
RIBOFLAVIN (VITAMIN B2)	**RDA: Women 1.3 mg, Men 1.7 mg**
Breads, cereals, grains	
Bagel, English muffin, pita	2 whole
Cold cereal	1 ounce
Meat, poultry, fish	
Liver (beef, calf, pork)	3 ounces
Liver (chicken, turkey)	½ cup, diced
Liverwurst	1 ounce
Dairy products	
Milk (all varieties)	2 cups
Yogurt (lowfat, nonfat)	1 cup
NIACIN	**RDA: Women 15 mg NE, Men 19 mg NE**
Breads, cereals, grains	
Bagel, bran muffin, English muffin, pita, roll	2 whole
Cold cereal (fortified)	1 ounce
Meat, poultry, fish	
Lamb, pork, veal (lean)	3 ounces
Liver (beef, calf, pork)	3 ounces
Chicken (no skin)	3 ounces (½ breast)
Mackerel, mullet, salmon, swordfish	3 ounces
Other	
Peanuts, peanut butter	4 tbsp.

(continued)

Table 10-1 *(continued)*

Food	Serving = 25% RDA
VITAMIN B6	**RDA: Women 1.6 mg, Men 2.0 mg**
Breads, cereals, grains	
Oatmeal, instant, fortified	⅓ cup
Cold cereal	1 ounce
Fruits	
Banana, raw	1 medium
Prunes, dried, cooked	1 cup
Vegetables	
Plantain, boiled	1 medium
Meat, poultry, fish	
Chicken, roasted, no skin	½ breast
Lamb (lean only)	1 chop
Liver (beef)	3 ounces
FOLATE	**RDA: Women 180 mcg, Men 200 mcg**
Breads, cereals, grains	
Whole wheat English muffin, pita	2 whole
Cold cereal	1 ounce
Vegetables	
Asparagus, beets, broccoli, brussels sprouts, cauliflower, Chinese cabbage, corn (creamed), spinach (cooked)	1 cup
Beans, dry (black-eyed peas, lentils, red kidney) cooked	½ cup
Greens (mustard, turnip), cooked	1 cup
Meat, poultry, fish	
Liver (beef, calf, pork)	3 ounces

Food	Serving = 25% RDA
VITAMIN B12	**RDA: Women 2.0 mcg, Men 2.0 mcg**
Meat, poultry, fish	
Beef, pork, lamb, veal	3 ounces
Liver (beef, calf, pork)	3 ounces
Liver (chicken, turkey)	½ cup, diced
Catfish, crabmeat, croaker, lobster, mackerel, mussels, oysters, scallops, swordfish, trout, tuna	3 ounces
Dairy products	
Eggs	2 large
Milk (whole, lowfat, skim)	2 cups
Yogurt	2 cups

Source: "Good Sources of Nutrients" (Washington D.C.: U.S. Department of Agriculture/Human Nutrition Service, 1990); "Nutritive Value of Food" (Washington D.C.: U.S. Department of Agriculture, 1991).

Too Much or Too Little: Two Ways to Go Wrong with Vitamins

RDAs are broad enough to prevent vitamin deficiencies and avoid the side effects associated with very large doses of some vitamins. If your diet doesn't meet these guidelines, or if you take very large amounts of vitamins as supplements, you could be in for trouble.

Vitamin deficiencies

The good news is that vitamin deficiencies are rare among people who have access to a wide variety of foods and know how to put together a balanced diet. For example, the only people likely to experience a vitamin E deficiency are premature and/or low-birth-weight infants and people with a metabolic disorder that keeps them from absorbing fat. A healthy adult may go as long as 10 years on a vitamin-E–deficient diet without developing any signs of a problem.

Aha, you say, but what's this subclinical deficiency I hear so much about?

Nutritionists use the term *subclinical deficiency* to describe a nutritional deficit not yet far enough advanced to produce obvious symptoms. In lay terms, however, the phrase has become a handy explanation for such common but hard-to-pin-down symptoms such as fatigue, irritability, nervousness, emotional depression, allergies, and insomnia. And it's a dandy way to increase the sale of nutritional supplements.

Simply put, the RDAs protect you against deficiency. If your odd symptoms linger even after you take reasonable amounts of vitamin supplements, probably something other than a lack of any one vitamin is to blame. Don't wait until your patience or your bank account has been exhausted to find out. Get a second opinion as soon as you can. Table 10-2 lists the symptoms of various vitamin deficiencies.

Table 10-2	Vitamin Alert: What Happens When You Don't Get the Vitamins You Need
A Diet Low in This Vitamin	*May Produce These Signs of Deficiency*
Vitamin A	Poor night vision; dry, rough or cracked skin; dry mucous membranes including the inside of the eye; slow wound healing; nerve damage; reduced ability to taste, hear and smell; inability to perspire; reduced resistance to respiratory infections
Vitamin D	*In children:* rickets (weak muscles, delayed tooth development, and soft bones, all due to the inability to absorb minerals without vitamin D). *In adults:* osteomalacia (soft, porous bones that fracture easily)
Vitamin E	Inability to absorb fat
Vitamin K	Blood fails to clot
Vitamin C	Scurvy (bleeding gums; tooth loss; nosebleeds; bruising; painful or swollen joints; shortness of breath; increased susceptibility to infection; slow wound healing; muscle pains; skin rashes)
Thiamin (vitamin B1)	Poor appetite; unintended weight loss; upset stomach; gastric upset (nausea, vomiting); mental depression; an inability to concentrate
Riboflavin (vitamin B2)	Inflamed mucous membranes, including cracked lips, sore tongue and mouth, "burning" eyes; skin rashes; anemia

A Diet Low in This Vitamin	May Produce These Signs of Deficiency
Niacin	Pellagra (diarrhea; inflamed skin and mucous membranes; mental confusion and/or dementia)
Vitamin B6	Anemia; convulsions similar to epileptic seizures; skin rashes; upset stomach; nerve damage (infants)
Folate	Anemia (immature red blood cells)
Vitamin B12	Pernicious anemia (destruction of red blood cells, nerve damage, increased risk of stomach cancer due to damaged stomach tissue, neurological/psychiatric symptoms due to nerve cell damage)
Biotin	Loss of appetite; upset stomach; pale, dry, scaly skin; hair loss; emotional depression; skin rashes (infants younger than 6 months)

Big trouble: Vitamin megadoses

Can you get too much of a good thing? Darned right, you can. Some vitamins are toxic if taken in the very large amounts popularly known as *megadoses*. How much is a megadose? Nobody knows for sure. The general consensus is that a megadose is several times the RDA, but the term is so vague it's not in either my medical dictionary or the dictionary on my computer.

- Megadoses of vitamin A (as retinol) may cause symptoms that make you think you have a brain tumor.

- Taken by a pregnant woman, megadoses of vitamin A may damage the fetus.

- Megadoses of vitamin D may cause kidney stones and hard lumps of calcium in soft tissue (muscles and organs).

- Megadoses of niacin (sometimes used to lower cholesterol levels) can damage liver tissue.

- Megadoses of vitamin B6 can cause (temporary) damage to nerves in arms and legs, fingers and toes.

But here's an interesting fact: With one exception, the likeliest way to get a megadose of vitamins is to take supplements. It's pretty much impossible for you to cram down enough food to overdose on vitamin D, E, K, C, and all the Bs. Did you notice the exception? Right: vitamin A.

Liver and fish liver oils are concentrated sources of preformed vitamin A (retinol), the potentially toxic form of vitamin A. Liver contains so much retinol that early 20th explorers to the South Pole made themselves sick on seal and whale liver. There have also been cases of vitamin A toxicity reported among children given daily servings of chicken liver.

On the other hand, even very large doses of vitamin E, vitamin K, thiamin (vitamin B1), riboflavin (vitamin B2), folate, vitamin B12, biotin, and pantothenic acid appear safe for human beings. Table 10-3 lists the effects of vitamin overdoses.

Table 10-3	Vitamin Overdoses: How Much Is Too Much For Healthy People?
Vitamin	*Overdose*
Vitamin A	15,000 to 25,000 IU retinoids a day for adults (2,000 IU or more for children) may lead to liver damage, headache, vomiting, abnormal vision, constipation, loss of hair, loss of appetite, low-grade fever, bone pain, sleep disorder, dry skin and mucous membranes. A pregnant woman who takes more than 10,000 IU a day doubles her risk of giving birth to a child with birth defects.
Vitamin D	2,000 IU a day can cause irreversible damage to kidneys and heart. Smaller doses may cause muscle weakness, headache, nausea, vomiting, high blood pressure, retarded physical growth and mental retardation in children, and fetal abnormalities.
Vitamin E	Large amounts (more than 400 – 800 IU a day) may cause upset stomach or dizziness.
Vitamin C	1,000 mg or higher may cause upset stomach, diarrhea, or constipation.
Niacin	Doses higher than the RDA raise the production of liver enzymes and blood levels of sugar and uric acid, leading to liver damage and an increased risk of diabetes and gout.
Vitamin B6	50 mg a day may (temporarily) damage nerves in arms and legs, hands and feet.

Who Needs Extra Vitamins?

Maybe you. The RDAs are designed to protect healthy people from deficiencies, but sometimes the circumstances of your life (or your lifestyle) mean that you need something extra. Are you taking medication? Do you smoke? Are you on a restrictive diet? Are you pregnant? Are you a nursing mother? Are you approaching menopause? Answer "yes" to any of these questions, and you may be a person who needs larger amounts of vitamins than the RDAs provide.

I'm taking medication

Many valuable medicines interact with vitamins. Some drugs increase or decrease the effectiveness of vitamins; some vitamins increase or decrease the effectiveness of drugs. For example, a woman who is using birth control pills may absorb less than the customary amount of the B vitamins. For more about vitamin and drug interactions, see Chapter 25.

I'm a smoker

It's a fact. You probably have abnormally low blood levels of vitamin C. More trouble: chemicals from tobacco smoke create more free radicals in your body. Even the National Research Council, which is tough on vitamin overdosing, says that regular smokers should take about 66 percent more vitamin C — up to 100 mg a day — than non-smokers.

Help! I'm turning orange

Because you store retinol in your liver, megadoses of preformed vitamin A can build up to toxic levels. Not so with carotenoids. They aren't stored in the liver, so these red, green, and yellow pigments in fruits and vegetables are safe even in very large amounts.

But that doesn't mean that they have no side effects. Carotenoids, like retinoids, are stored in body fat. If you wolf down large quantities of carotenoid-rich foods like carrots and tomatoes every day, day after day, for several weeks, your skin — particularly the palms of your hands and the soles of your feet — will turn a nifty shade of dusty orange, brighter if your skin is naturally light, darker if it is naturally dark. It sounds fantastic, but it has actually happened to people eating two cups of carrots and two whole tomatoes a day for several months. When they cut down on the carrots and tomatoes, the color faded.

Now, let's see, it's September 1, and you've been invited to a Halloween party. Maybe this year you'll go as a pumpkin. If you start packing in the carrots and tomatoes right now. . . .

TECHNICAL STUFF

A special case: The continuing saga of Vitamin C

In 1970, chemist Linus Pauling published *Vitamin C and the Common Cold,* a small book (just about 100 pages) made weightier by the fact that Pauling had not one, but two Nobel prizes on his shelf — one for chemistry and one for peace.

Ever since, people have been fighting over Pauling's message that very large doses of vitamin C — called *gram doses* because they provide more than 1,000 mg/1 gram — prevent or cure the common cold. (Later on, Pauling said that large doses may also cure advanced cancer. Based on current research, though, Pauling's theory was unfounded.)

In experiment after experiment, volunteers have taken varying amounts of vitamin C, all the way up to 10,000 mg (10 grams). This is what researchers found: Taking vitamin C doesn't prevent a cold, but people who take the vitamin once they get sick may recover only a few hours to a few days sooner than people who don't take the vitamin. Those are the facts, and I am honor-bound to report them to you. But I also have to tell you that when I have a cold, I take extra vitamin C. For two or three days I step up from my regular 500 mg a day to 1,000 mg. My brain tells me it won't do very much good, but my heart says, "Give me a break! You can't just sit there and feel rotten without trying to do something about it."

Actually, if my organs are going to give me nutritional advice, they may be on stronger ground

arguing that vitamin C protects heart health. Recent studies strongly suggest (but do not prove) that for some people, large amounts of vitamin C may raise blood levels of high density lipoproteins (HDLs), the *good* fat and protein particles that carry cholesterol and fat out of the body. (Check out the chapter on fats, Chapter 7.)

However, large amounts of vitamin C cause kidney stones in some people or can upset your stomach. And if you take megadoses for a while and then quit, you can end up with *rebound scurvy,* a temporary deficiency.

Here's what happens: Your body normally produces an enzyme that breaks down vitamin C so that you can eliminate any excess through urinating. When you take larger and larger doses of vitamin C, your body makes more and more of this enzyme. If you suddenly cut back on your vitamin C, your body will continue to produce extra enzymes for a while so that you continue to urinate away lots of vitamin C, maybe more than you take in. This reaction, which ends as soon as enzyme production drops back to normal, can cause deficiency in newborns whose mothers took very large doses of vitamin C while pregnant. The kids are born requiring higher-than-normal doses for a while. Eventually, they, too, slip back to normal.

I never eat animals

On the other hand, if you are nuts for veggies but follow a vegan diet — one that shuns all foods from animals (including milk, cheese, eggs, and fish oils) — you simply cannot get enough vitamin D without taking supplements.

Vegans also benefit from extra vitamin C because it increases their ability to absorb iron from plant food. And vitamin-B12-enriched grains or supplements are a must to supply the nutrient found only in fish, poultry, milk, cheese and eggs.

I'm a couch potato who plans to start working out

When you do head for the gym, take it slow, and take an extra dose of vitamin E. A study at the USDA Center for Human Nutrition at Tufts University (Boston) suggests that an 800 mg vitamin E supplement every day for the first month after you begin exercising minimizes muscle damage by preventing reactions with free radicals that cause inflammation. After that, you're on your own: The vitamin doesn't help conditioned athletes, however, whose muscles have adapted to workout stress.

I'm pregnant

Keep in mind that "eating for two" means that you are the sole source of nutrients for the growing fetus, not that you should double the amount of food you eat. If you don't get the vitamins you need, neither will your baby.

The RDAs for vitamin A, vitamin D, and the B vitamins thiamin (B1) and B12 are exactly the same as those for women who are not pregnant. But when you're pregnant, you need extra

- ✔ **Vitamin E:** To create all that new tissue (the woman's as well as the baby's), a pregnant woman needs an extra 2 mg a-TE, the approximate amount in one egg.

- ✔ **Vitamin C:** The level of vitamin C in your blood falls as your vitamin C flows across the placenta to your baby, who may — at some point in the pregnancy — have vitamin C levels as much as 50 percent higher than yours. So you need an extra 10 mg vitamin C (½ cup cooked zucchini or 2 stalks of asparagus).

- ✔ **Riboflavin:** To protect the baby against structural defects such as cleft palate or a deformed heart, a pregnant woman needs an extra 0.3 mg riboflavin (slightly less than 1 ounce of ready-to-eat cereal).

- ✔ **Folate:** To protect the child against cleft palate and neural tube (spinal cord) defects. As many as two of every 1,000 babies born each year in the United States have a neural tube (spinal cord) defect such as spina bifida because their mothers did not get enough folate to meet the RDA standard. The accepted increase in folate for pregnant women has been

200 mcg (slightly more than the amount in 8 ounces of orange juice). But new studies show that taking 400 mg folate before becoming pregnant and through the first two months of pregnancy significantly lowers the risk of giving birth to a child with cleft palate. Taking 400 mg folate through an entire pregnancy reduces the risk of neural tube defect.

✔ **Vitamin B12:** To meet the demands of the growing fetus, a pregnant woman needs an extra 0.2 mcg vitamin B12 (3 ounces of roast chicken).

I'm breast-feeding

You need extra vitamin A, vitamin E, thiamin, riboflavin, and folate to produce sufficient quantities of nutritious breast milk, about 750 ml (¾ liter) each day. You need extra vitamin D, vitamin C, and niacin as insurance to replace the vitamins you "lose" — that is, transfer to your child in your milk.

I'm approaching menopause

Information about the specific vitamin requirements of older women is as hard to find as, well, information about the specific vitamin requirements about older men. It's enough to make you wonder what's going on with the people who set the RDAs. Don't they know that everyone gets older? Right now, just about all anybody can say for sure about the nutritional needs of older women is that they require extra calcium to stem the natural loss of bone that occurs when women reach menopause and their production of the female hormone estrogen declines. They may also need extra vitamin D to enable their bodies to absorb and use the calcium.

Adding vitamin D supplements to calcium supplements increases bone density in older people. The current RDA for vitamin D is set at 5 mcg/200 IU for all adults, but the new AI (adequate intake) for vitamin D is 10 mcg/400 IU for people age 51 to 70, and 15 mcg/600 IU for people 71 and older. Some researchers suggest that even these amounts may be too low to guarantee maximum calcium absorption.

Check with your doctor before adding vitamin D supplements. In very large amounts, this vitamin can be toxic.

Chapter 11

Mighty Minerals

• •

In This Chapter

▶ How your body uses minerals

▶ Foods that give you the minerals you need

▶ What happens when you don't get enough minerals (or get too much of them)

▶ How to tell if you need extra minerals

• •

*M*inerals are substances that occur naturally in non-living things such as rocks and metal ores. Minerals are also present in plants and animals, but they are imported: Plants get minerals from soil; animals get minerals by eating the plants.

Most minerals have names reflecting the place they are found or characteristics such as their color. For example, the word calcium comes from *calx,* the Greek word for lime (chalk); chlorine comes from *chloros,* the Greek word for greenish-yellow.

Minerals are *elements,* substances composed of only one kind of atom. Minerals are inorganic; unlike vitamins, they usually do not contain the carbon, hydrogen, and oxygen atoms found in all organic compounds.

How Your Body Uses Minerals

Think of your body as a house. Vitamins are like tiny little maids and butlers, scurrying about to turn on the lights and make sure that the windows are closed to keep the heat from escaping. Minerals are more sturdy stuff, the mortar and bricks that strengthen the frame and the current that keeps the lights running.

Nutritionists classify the minerals essential for human life as either major minerals (including the principal electrolytes; see Chapter 13) or trace elements. Major minerals and trace elements are both minerals. The difference between them, nutritionally speaking, is how much you have in your body and how much you need to take in to maintain a steady supply.

An elementary guide to minerals

The early Greeks thought that all material on earth was constructed of a combination of four basic elements: earth, water, air, and fire. Wrong. Centuries later, alchemists looking for the formula for precious metals, such as gold, decided that the essential elements were sulfur, salt, and mercury. Wrong again.

In 1669, a group of German chemists isolated phosphorus, the first mineral element to be accurately identified. After that, things moved a bit more swiftly. By the end of the 19th century, scientists knew the names and chemical properties of 82 elements. Today, 109 elements have been identified. Nutrition scientists consider 16 minerals to be essential nutrients for human beings.

Many recently discovered elements have names that reflect where they were found or honor an important scientist: Americium, Curium, Berkelium, Californium, Fermium, and Nobelium.

The classic guide to chemical elements is the periodic table, a chart devised in 1869 by Russian chemist Dmitri Mendeleev (1834–1907), for whom Mendelevium was named. The table was revised by British physicist Henry Moseley (1887–1915), who came up with the concept of atomic numbers, numbers based on the number of protons (positively charged particles) in an elemental atom.

The periodic table is a clean, crisp way of characterizing the elements, and if you are now or ever were a chemistry, physics, or pre-med student, you can testify firsthand to the joy (maybe that's not the best word?) of memorizing the information it provides. Personally, I'd rather be forced to watch reruns of The Dating Game.

Your body stores various amounts of minerals but more than 5 grams (about one-sixth of an ounce) of each of the major minerals and principal electrolytes; it needs more than 100 milligrams a day of each to maintain a steady supply and to make up for losses. You store less than 5 grams of each of the trace elements and need to take less than 100 milligrams a day.

The following shows how nutritionists classify the minerals essential for human beings. The major minerals include

- Calcium
- Phosphorus
- Magnesium
- Sulfur
- Sodium
- Potassium
- Chloride

Note: Sodium, potassium, and chloride are also known as the principal electrolytes. I discuss them in Chapter 13.

Although sulfur, a major mineral, is an essential nutrient for human beings, it is almost never included in nutritional books and/or charts. Why? Because it is an integral part of all proteins; any diet that provides adequate protein also provides adequate sulfur.

Trace elements include

- Iron
- Zinc
- Iodine
- Selenium
- Copper
- Manganese
- Fluoride
- Chromium
- Molybdenum

Calcium

When you step on the scale in the morning, you can assume that about three pounds of your body weight is calcium, most of it packed into your bones and teeth.

Calcium is also present in extracellular fluid (the liquid around body cells), where it performs the following duties:

- Regulates fluid balance by controlling the flow of water in and out of cells
- Makes it possible for cells to send messages back and forth from one to another
- Keeps muscles moving smoothly and prevents cramping

An adequate amount of calcium is important to controlling high blood pressure — and not just for the person who takes the calcium directly. At least one study shows that when a pregnant woman gets a sufficient amount of calcium, her baby's blood pressure stays lower than average for at least the first seven years of life, meaning a lower risk of developing high blood pressure later on.

Getting enough calcium also seems to lower your risk of cancer of the colon and rectum. The evidence is still inconclusive, but calcium decreases the growth of cells in the colon and reduces the chance that developing cells may become cancerous.

Your best food sources of calcium are milk and dairy products, plus fish such as canned sardines and salmon. Calcium is also found in dark green, leafy vegetables, but the calcium in plant foods is bound into compounds less easily absorbed by your body.

Phosphorus

Like calcium, phosphorus is essential for strong bones and teeth. You also need phosphorus to transmit the genetic code (genes and chromosomes that carry information about your special characteristics) from one cell to another when cells divide and reproduce. In addition, phosphorus

- ✔ Helps maintain the pH balance of blood (that is, keeps it from being too acidic or too alkaline)
- ✔ Is vital for metabolizing carbohydrates, synthesizing proteins, and ferrying fats and fatty acids among tissues and organs
- ✔ Is part of *myelin,* the fatty sheath that surrounds and protects each nerve cell

Phosphorus is in almost everything you eat, but the best sources are high-protein foods such as meat, fish, poultry, eggs, and milk. These foods provide more than half the phosphorus in a nonvegetarian diet; grains, nuts, seeds, and dry beans also provide respectable amounts.

Magnesium

Your body uses magnesium to make body tissues, especially bone; the adult human body has about an ounce of magnesium, three-quarters of it in the bones. Magnesium is also part of more than 300 different enzymes that trigger chemical reactions throughout your body.

You use magnesium to

- ✔ Move nutrients in and out of cells
- ✔ Send messages between cells
- ✔ Transmit the genetic code (genes and chromosomes) when cells divide and reproduce

A nutritional balancing act: Calcium and phosphorus

Imagine a pair of contentious business partners. That's calcium and phosphorus. Each needs the other and resents this fact mightily.

For tip-top nutritional performance, you need about twice as much calcium as phosphorus. Nature recognizes this by producing human breast milk with a nearly perfect calcium-to-phosphorus ratio, 2.3 parts calcium to 1 part phosphorus. (Cows' milk is 1.3 parts calcium to 1 part phosphorus.)

Change the ratio by taking in more phosphorus than calcium, and confusion reigns. You excrete extra calcium in your urine. You have less calcium circulating in your blood. And in self-defense, your body begins to pull the calcium it needs from what's stored in your bones.

Luckily, the normal American diet isn't abnormally high in phosphorus. The exception is a high-protein diet, sometimes used for weight loss. High-protein foods such as meat, fish, and poultry are high in phosphorus, but very low in calcium. Without high-calcium foods to set a balance, a high-protein diet can trip you into the reversed phosphorus-to-calcium ratio that spells d-a-n-g-e-r to your bones. To avoid the problem, lower the meat, fish, and poultry; raise the milk, cheese, and leafy greens.

An adequate supply of magnesium is also heart-healthy because it enables you to convert food to energy using less oxygen.

Bananas are a good source of magnesium and so are many other plant foods, including dark green fruits and vegetables (magnesium is part of chlorophyll, the green pigment in plants), whole seeds, nuts, beans, and grains.

Iron

Iron is an essential constituent of hemoglobin and myoglobin, two proteins that store and transport oxygen. You find hemoglobin in red blood cells (it's what makes them red). Myoglobin (myo = muscle) is in muscle tissue. Iron is also part of various enzymes.

Your best food sources of iron are organ meats (liver, heart, kidneys), red meat, egg yolks, wheat germ, and oysters. These foods contain heme (heme = blood) iron, a form of iron that your body can easily absorb.

Whole grains, wheat germ, raisins, nuts, seed, prunes (juice), and potato skins contain nonheme iron. Because plants contain substances called *phytates* that bind this iron into compounds, your body has a hard time getting at the iron. Eating plant foods with meat or with foods that are rich in vitamin C (like tomatoes) increases your ability to split away the phytates and get iron out of plant foods.

Zinc

Zinc protects nerve and brain tissue and bolsters the immune system, and is essential for healthy growth. Zinc is part of the enzymes (and hormones such as insulin) that metabolize food, and you can fairly call it the macho male mineral.

The largest quantities of zinc in the human body are in the testes, where it is used in making a continuous supply of testosterone, the hormone a man needs to produce plentiful amounts of healthy, viable sperm. Without enough zinc, male fertility falters. So, yes, the old wives' tale is true: Oysters — a rich source of zinc — are useful for men.

Other good sources of zinc are meat, liver, and eggs. Plenty of zinc is in nuts, beans, miso, pumpkin and sunflower seeds, whole-grain products, and wheat germ. But the zinc in plants, like the iron in plants, occurs in compounds that your body absorbs less efficiently than the zinc in foods from animals.

Iodine

Iodine is a component of the thyroid hormones thyroxin and triiodothyronine, which help regulate cell activities. These hormones are also essential for protein synthesis, tissue growth (including the formation of healthy nerves and bones), and reproduction.

The best natural sources of iodine are seafood and plants grown near the ocean, but modern Americans are most likely to get the iodine they need from iodized salt (plain table salt with added iodine). And here's an odd nutritional note: You may get substantial amounts of iodine from milk. Are the cows consuming iodized salt? No. The milk is processed and stored in machines and vessels kept clean and sanitary with iodates and *iodophors,* iodine-based disinfectants. Tiny trace amounts get into the products sent to the stores. Iodates are also used as dough conditioners (additives that make dough more pliable), so you will also find some iodine in most bread sold in supermarkets.

Selenium

Selenium was identified as an essential human nutrient in 1979 when Chinese nutrition researchers discovered, almost by accident, that people with low body stores of selenium were at increased risk of *Keshan disease,* a disorder of the heart muscle whose symptoms include rapid heartbeat, enlarged heart, and (in severe cases) heart failure, a consequence most common among young children and women of child-bearing age.

How does selenium protect your heart? One possibility is that it works as an antioxidant in tandem with vitamin E. A second possibility, raised by U.S. Department of Agriculture studies with laboratory rats, is that it prevents viruses from attacking heart muscle.

Here is some exciting news. The results of a four-year study involving 1,312 patients previously treated for skin cancer strongly suggests that daily doses of selenium three times the current RDA for men (70 mcg) may reduce the incidence of cancers of the lung, prostate, colon, and rectum. The study, led by University of Arizona epidemiologist Larry C. Clark, was designed to see if taking selenium lowered the risk of skin cancer. It didn't. But among the patients who got selenium rather than a placebo, there were 45 percent fewer lung cancers, 58 percent fewer colon and rectal cancers, 63 percent fewer prostate cancers, and a 50-percent lower death rate from cancer overall. Now a follow-up study will see if these results hold up.

Although fruits and vegetables grown in selenium-rich soils are themselves rich in this mineral, the best sources of selenium are seafood, meat and organ meats (liver, kidney), eggs, and dairy products.

Copper

Copper is an antioxidant found in enzymes that deactivate free radicals and make it possible for your body to use iron. Copper also

✔ Promotes the growth of strong bones

✔ Protects the health of nerve tissue

✔ Prevents your hair from turning gray prematurely

No, no, a thousand times, no: Large amounts of copper absolutely, repeat absolutely, will not turn gray hair back to its original color. Besides, megadoses of copper are potentially toxic.

You can get the copper you need from organ meats (such as liver and heart), seafood, nuts, and dried beans, including cocoa beans (the beans used to make chocolate).

Manganese

Most of the manganese in your body is in glands (pituitary, mammary, pancreas), organs (liver, kidneys, intestines), and bones. Manganese is an essential constituent of the enzymes that metabolize carbohydrates and synthesize fats (including cholesterol). Manganese is important for a healthy reproductive system. During pregnancy, manganese speeds the proper growth of fetal tissue, particularly bones and cartilage.

You get manganese from whole grains, cereal products, fruits, and vegetables. Tea is also a good source of manganese.

Fluoride

Fluoride is the form of fluorine (an element) in drinking water. Your body stores fluoride in bones and teeth. While researchers still have some question as to whether fluoride is an essential nutrient, it's clear that it hardens dental enamel, reducing your risk of cavities. In addition, some nutrition researchers suspect (but cannot prove) that some forms of fluoride strengthen bones.

Small amounts of fluoride are in all soil, water, plants, and animal tissues. You also get a steady supply of fluoride from fluoridated drinking water.

Chromium

Very small amounts of *trivalent chromium,* a digestible form of the very same metallic element that decorates your car and household appliances, are essential for several enzymes you need in order to metabolize fat.

Chromium is also a necessary partner for glucose tolerance factor (GTF), a group of chemicals that enables insulin (an enzyme from the pancreas) to regulate your use of glucose, the end product of metabolism and the basic fuel for every body cell (see Chapter 8). In a recent joint study by USDA and the Beijing Medical University, adults with non-insulin-dependent diabetes who took chromium supplements had lower blood levels of sugar, protein, and cholesterol. In a related study, chromium reduced blood pressure in laboratory rats bred to develop hypertension, a common complication in diabetes.

Right now, very little information exists about the precise amounts of chromium in specific foods. Nonetheless, yeast, calves' liver, American cheese, wheat germ, and broccoli are regarded as valuable sources of this trace element.

Molybdenum

Molybdenum is part of several enzymes that metabolize proteins. You get molybdenum from beans and grains. Cows eat grains, so milk and cheese have some molybdenum. Molybdenum also leeches into drinking water from surrounding soil. The molybdenum content of plants and drinking water depends entirely on how much molybdenum is in the soil.

Table 11-1 is a handy guide to foods that provide the minerals and trace elements your body needs. This chart is the easy way to figure out which foods (and how much) give you 25 percent or more of the recommended dietary allowance (RDA) for adults (age 25–50).

No muss, no fuss, no calculators. Just photocopy these pages and stick them on the fridge. What an easy way to eat right!

Table 11-1	Get Your Minerals Here!
Food	Serving
Calcium and Phosphorus	*DA: Calcium — Men and women 800 mg (Current); 1,000 mg (Recommended) Phosphorus — Men and women 800 mg (Current), 700 mg (Recommended)*
Breads, cereals, grains	
Bran muffin, English muffin	2 whole
Vegetables	
Broccoli, spinach, turnip greens, cooked	1 cup
Dairy products	
Natural Gruyere, Swiss, Parmesan	1 ounce Romano cheeses
Processed Cheddar or Swiss cheeses	1½ ounces
Natural blue, brick, Camembert, Feta, Gouda, Monterey, mozzarella, Muenster, Provolone, Roquefort cheeses	2 ounces
Ricotta	½ cup
Ice cream/ice milk	1 cup
Milk (all varieties, including chocolate)	1 cup
Yogurt (all varieties)	1 cup (8 ounces)
Other	
Tofu	½ cup, cubed

(continued)

Table 11-1 (continued)

Food	Serving
Magnesium	**RDA: Men 350 mg, women 280 mg**
Breads, cereals, grains	
Bread (whole wheat)	4 slices
Bran muffin, English muffin, pita (whole wheat)	2 whole
Cold cereal	2 ounces
Vegetables	
Artichoke	2 medium
Black-eyed peas, chickpeas, soybeans, white beans (dry, cooked)	1 cup
Dairy products	
Milk (chocolate, made with skim milk)	2 cups
Yogurt (plain nonfat)	2 cups
Other	
Nuts and seeds	2 tbsp.
Tofu	½ cup cubed
Iron	**RDA: Men 10 mg, women 15 mg**
Breads, cereals, grains	
Bagel, bran muffin, pita	2 whole
Farina, oatmeal (instant, fortified)	⅓ cup
Cold cereal	1 ounce
Fruits	
Apricots (dried, cooked)	1 cup
Vegetables	
Black-eyed peas, chickpeas, lentils, red & white beans (dried, cooked)	1 cup
Soybeans (cooked)	½ cup
Meat, poultry, fish	
Liver (beef, pork)	3 ounces
Liver (chicken, turkey)	1 cup, diced
Clams (raw, meat only)	3–4 ounces
Oysters (raw, meat only)	1–2 ounces
Other	
Pine nuts, pumpkin or squash seeds	4 tbsp.

Food	Serving
Zinc	**RDA: Men 15 mg, women 12 mg**
Breads, cereals, grains	
Cold cereals (fortified)	2 ounces
Meat, poultry, fish	
Beef (all varieties, lean)	3 ounces
Lamb (all varieties, lean)	3 ounces
Tongue (braised)	3 ounces
Veal (roast, lean only)	3 ounces
Chicken (without skin)	2 legs
Oysters	3 ounces
Dairy products	
Yogurt (all varieties)	2 cups
Other	
Pumpkin or squash seeds	4 tbsp.
Copper	**ESADDI Men and women 1.5 to 3.0 mg**
Breads, cereals, grains	
Barley (cooked)	⅓ cup
Bran muffin, English muffin, pita	2 whole
Fruits	
Prunes (dried, cooked)	1 cup
Vegetables	
Black-eyed peas, lentils, soybeans (cooked)	1 cup
Meat, poultry, fish	
Liver (beef, calf)	3 ounces
Liver (chicken, turkey)	½ cup, diced
Crabmeat, lobster, oysters, shrimp	3 ounces
Other	
Almonds, Brazil nuts, cashews, filberts, peanuts, pistachios, walnuts, mixed nuts	4 tbsp.
Pumpkin, sesame, squash, sunflower seeds	4 tbsp.

Sources: Good Sources of Nutrients (Washington, D.C.: U.S. Department of Agriculture/Human Nutrition Service, 1990); Nutritive Value of Food (Washington, D.C.: USDA, 1991).

Did you notice something missing from this list? Right you are. There are no entries for the essential trace elements chromium, fluoride, iodine, molybdenum, and selenium because a healthful, varied diet provides sufficient quantities of these nutrients. Iodized salt and fluoridated water are extra insurance.

Too Much and Too Little

The RDAs and Estimated Safe and Adequate Daily Dietary Intakes for minerals and trace elements are generous allowances, large enough to prevent deficiency but not so large that they trigger toxic side effects. What happens if you don't get enough minerals and trace elements? Some minerals, such as phosphorus and magnesium, are so widely available in food that deficiencies are rare to nonexistent. No nutrition scientist has yet been able to identify a naturally occurring deficiency of sulfur, manganese, chromium, or molybdenum in human beings who follow a sensible diet. Most drinking water contains adequate fluoride, and Americans get so much copper (can it be from chocolate bars?) that deficiency is practically unheard of in the United States.

But other minerals are more problematic.

Without enough **calcium,** a child's bones and teeth will not grow strong and straight; an adult's bones will not hold onto their minerals. Calcium is a team player. To protect against deficiency, you also need adequate amounts of vitamin D (so that you can absorb the calcium you get from food or supplements) and estrogen (the hormone that helps hold minerals in bone). Milk fortified with vitamin D has done much to eliminate rickets (see Chapter 10 on vitamins), and the use of estrogen replacement therapy — while controversial — does help maintain healthy bones.

"Iron deficiency anemia" is not just an old advertising slogan. Lacking sufficient **iron,** your body cannot make the hemoglobin it requires to carry energy-sustaining oxygen to every tissue; you are often tired and feel weak. Mild iron deficiency may also inhibit intellectual performance. In one Johns Hopkins study, high school girls scored higher verbal, memory, and learning test scores when they took supplements providing RDA amounts of iron.

Check with your doctor before downing iron supplements or cereals fortified with 100% of your daily iron requirement, warns the Environmental Nutrition newsletter. Hemochromatosis, a common but often-undiagnosed genetic defect affecting one of every 250 Americans, can lead to iron overload, an increased absorption of the mineral linked to arthritis, heart disease, diabetes, and an increased risk of infectious diseases and cancer (viruses and cancer cells thrive in iron-rich blood).

An adequate supply of **zinc** is vital for making testosterone and healthy sperm. Men who do not get enough zinc may be temporarily infertile. Zinc deprivation can make you lose your appetite — and your ability to taste food. It may also weaken your immune system, increasing your risk of infections. Wounds heal more slowly when you don't get enough zinc. That includes the tissue damage caused by working out. In plain language: If you don't get the zinc you need, your charley horse may linger longer. And, yes, zinc may fight the common cold. To date, several studies have confirmed that sucking on lozenges containing one form of zinc (zinc gluconate) cuts the length of colds in half. At the start of 1999, scientists were awaiting proof that zinc acetate, a second form of zinc, also goes after a cold.

These results are for adults, not children, and the zinc tablets are meant just for the several days of your cold. To find out more about zinc excess, see the section "How much is too much?" later in this chapter.

A moderate **iodine** deficiency leads to goiter (a swollen thyroid gland) and reduced production of thyroid hormones. A more severe deficiency early in life may cause a form of mental and physical retardation called *cretinism*.

Not enough **selenium** in your diet? Watch out for muscle pain or weakness. To protect against selenium problems, make sure that you get plenty of vitamin E. Some animal studies show that a selenium deficiency responds to vitamin E supplements. And vice versa, too.

Table 11-2 lists some of the known results of mineral deficiencies.

Table 11-2	What Happens if You Do Not Get the Minerals You Need?
People Who Do Not Get Enough of This Mineral	***May Experience These Symptoms***
Calcium	*Children:* stunted growth, higher risk of cavities, rickets; *Adults:* weakened bones, increased risk of osteoporosis, and high blood pressure; *Both:* impaired blood clotting
Phosphorus*	Fragile bones and weak muscles
Magnesium*	Muscle weakness, cramps, tremor, irregular heartbeat; central nervous system problems (memory loss, confusion, hallucinations)
Iron	Iron deficiency anemia, fatigue caused by lower hemoglobin levels, greater sensitivity to cold temperatures

(continued)

Table 11-2 *(continued)*	
People Who Do Not Get Enough of This Mineral	**May Experience These Symptoms**
Zinc	Loss of appetite, reduced ability to taste food, higher susceptibility to infection, reduced tissue growth and slower wound healing; infertility (male)
Iodine	Goiter (swollen thyroid gland), mental and physical retardation, slow learning
Selenium	Muscle pain and weakness (including the heart)
Copper*	Anemia, impaired immune function, greater susceptibility to infection, abnormal heartbeat
Manganese**	No known effects in human beings
Fluoride	Higher risk of cavities
Chromium**	Involuntary weight loss, abnormalities of the central nervous system
Molybdenum**	Breathing difficulties, abnormal (fast) heartbeat, vomiting

 * Rare in the United States.
** No naturally-occurring deficiency observed in human beings.
Source: National Research Council, Recommended Dietary Allowances, 10th ed. (Washington, D.C.: National Academy Press, 1989).

How much is too much?

Like some vitamins, some minerals are potentially toxic in large doses.

Calcium, though clearly beneficial in amounts higher than the current RDAs, is not problem-free:

- ✔ Constipation, bloating, nausea, and intestinal gas are common side effects among healthy people taking supplements equal to 1,500 to 4,000 milligrams of calcium a day.
- ✔ Doses higher than 4,000 milligrams a day may be linked to kidney damage.
- ✔ Megadoses of calcium can bind with iron and zinc, making it harder for your body to absorb these two essential trace elements.

Too much **phosphorus** can lower your body stores of calcium. Megadoses of **magnesium** appear safe for healthy people, but if you have kidney disease, the magnesium overload can cause weak muscles, breathing difficulty, irregular heartbeat and/or cardiac arrest (your heart stops beating).

Overdosing on **iron** supplements can be deadly, especially for young children. The lethal dose for a young child may be as low as 3 grams (3,000 milligrams) elemental iron at one time. This is the amount in 60 tablets with 50 milligrams elemental iron each. For adults, the lethal dose is estimated to be 200 to 250 milligrams elemental iron per kilogram (2.2 pounds) of body weight. That's about 13,600 milligrams for a 150-pound person — the amount you'd get in 292 tablets with 50 milligrams elemental iron each. New FDA rules require individual blister packaging for supplements containing more than 30 mg iron to foil tiny fingers and prevent accidental overdoses.

Moderately high doses of **zinc** (up to 25 milligrams a day) can make it hard for your body to absorb copper. Doses 20 times the RDA (15 milligrams) can interfere with your immune function and make you more susceptible to infection, the very thing that normal doses of zinc protect against. Gram doses (2,000 milligrams or 2 grams) of zinc cause symptoms of zinc poisoning: vomiting, gastric upset, and irritation of the stomach lining.

Iodine overdoses cause exactly the same problems as iodine deficiency: goiter. How can that be? When you consume very large amounts of iodine, the mineral stimulates your thyroid gland, which swells in a furious attempt to step up its production of thyroid hormones. This reaction may occur among people who eat lots of dried seaweed for long periods of time.

In China, nutrition researchers have linked doses as high as 5 milligrams of **selenium** a day (70 to 99 times the RDA) to thickened but fragile nails, hair loss, and perspiration with a garlicky odor. In the United States, a small group of people who had accidentally gotten a supplement that mistakenly contained 27.3 milligrams selenium (400 to 500 times the RDA) fell victim to "selenium intoxication" — fatigue, abdominal pain, nausea and diarrhea, and nerve damage. The longer they used the supplements, the worse their symptoms were.

Despite decades of argument, no scientific proof exists that the **fluorides** in drinking water increase the risk of cancer in human beings. But there's no question that large doses of fluoride — unlikely to consume unless you drink well or ground water in the western United States— causes fluorosis (chalky-white patches on the teeth that eventually turn brown), brittle bones, fatigue, and muscle weakness. Over long periods of time, high doses of fluoride may also cause *out-croppings* (little bumps) of bone on the spine.

Fluoride levels higher than 6 milligrams a day are considered hazardous.

Doses of **molybdenum** two to seven times the Estimated Safe and Adequate Daily Dietary Intake dose can increase the amount of copper you excrete in urine.

Mineral madness

Omigosh. Here's another reason not to gulp down megadoses: Taking too much of one mineral can affect your elimination of, or make it difficult (maybe even impossible) for your body to use, one or more other minerals.

This list shows which mineral megadoses can affect your ability to absorb and use other minerals and trace elements.

If You Get Too Much of This Mineral	Your Body May Not Be Able to Absorb or Use This One
Calcium	Magnesium, iron, zinc
Copper	Zinc
Iron	Phosphorus, zinc
Manganese	Iron
Molybdenum	Zinc, copper
Phosphorus	Calcium
Sulfur (protein)	Molybdenum
Zinc	Copper

Who Needs Extra Minerals?

If your diet provides enough minerals to meet the RDAs, you're in pretty good shape, most of the time.

But a restrictive diet, the circumstances of your reproductive life, and just plain getting older can increase your need for minerals. Here are some scenarios.

I'm a strict vegetarian

Vegetarians who pass up fish as well as meat and poultry must get their iron from fortified whole-grain products, like wheat germ, seeds, nuts, blackstrap molasses, raisins, prune juice, potato skins, green leafy vegetables, tofu, miso, and brewer's yeast. Because the iron in plant foods is bound into compounds difficult for the human body to absorb, iron supplements are pretty much standard fare.

Vegans — vegetarians who avoid all foods from animals, including dairy products — have a similar problem getting the calcium they need. Calcium is in vegetables, but it, like iron, is bound into hard-to-absorb compounds. So vegans need calcium-rich substitutes. Good food choices are soy milk fortified with calcium, orange juice with added calcium, and tofu processed with calcium sulfate.

I live inland, away from the ocean

Now here's a story of 20th century nutritional success. Seafood and plants grown near the ocean are exposed to iodine-rich seawater. Freshwater fish, plants grown far from the sea, and the animals that feed on these fish and plants are not exposed to iodine. So people who live inland and get all their food from local gardens and farms cannot get the iodine they need from food.

American savvy and technology rode to the rescue in 1924 with the introduction of iodized salt. Then came refrigerated railroad cars and trucks to carry food from both coasts to every inland city and state. Together, modern salt and efficient shipment virtually eliminated the iodine deficiency disease goiter in this country. Nonetheless, millions of people worldwide still suffer from chronic iodine deficiency.

I'm a man

Just as women lose iron during menstrual bleeding, men lose zinc at ejaculation. Men who are extremely active sexually may need extra zinc. The trouble is, no one has ever written down standards for what constitutes "extremely active." Check this one out with your doctor.

Men who take a daily supplement of 200 micrograms selenium seem to cut their risk of prostate cancer by two-thirds. The selenium supplement also produces an overall drop in cancer mortality, plus a significantly lower risk of prostate cancer, colon cancer, and lung cancer in both men and women.

I'm a woman

The average woman loses about 2 to 3 teaspoons of blood during each menstrual period, a loss of 1.4 milligrams of iron. Women whose periods are very heavy lose more blood and more iron. Because getting the iron you need from a diet providing fewer than 2,000 calories a day may be virtually impossible, you may develop a mild iron deficiency. To remedy this, some doctors prescribe a daily iron supplement.

NUTRITION SPEAK

I'm looking for an iron supplement. What's this "ferrous" stuff?

The iron in iron supplements comes in several different forms, each one composed of elemental iron (the kind of iron your body actually uses) coupled with an organic acid that makes the iron easy to absorb.

The iron compounds commonly found in iron supplements are

- Ferrous citrate (iron plus citric acid)

- Ferrous fumarate (iron plus fumaric acid)

- Ferrous gluconate (iron plus a sugar derivative)

- Ferrous lactate (iron plus lactic acid, an acid formed in the fermentation of milk)

- Ferrous succinate (iron plus succinic acid)

- Ferrous sulfate (iron plus a sulfuric acid derivative)

In your stomach, these compounds dissolve at different rates, yielding different amounts of elemental iron. So supplement labels list the compound and the amount of elemental iron it provides, like this:

Ferrous gluconate 300 milligrams

Elemental iron 34 milligrams

This tells you that the supplement has 300 milligrams of the iron compound ferrous gluconate, which gives you 34 milligrams of usable elemental iron. If the label just says "iron," that's shorthand for elemental iron. This last number is what you look for in judging the iron content of a vitamin/mineral supplement.

Women who use an IUD may also be given a prescription for iron supplements because IUDs irritate the lining of the uterus and cause a small but significant loss of blood and iron.

I'm pregnant

The news about pregnancy is that women may not need extra calcium. This finding, released late in 1998, is so surprising that it probably pays to stay tuned for more — and definitely check with your own doctor. Meanwhile, pregnant women still need supplements to build fetal tissues, as well as new tissues and blood vessels in their own bodies. Animal studies suggest (but do not prove) that you may also need extra copper to protect nerve cells in the fetal brain. Nutritional supplements for pregnant women are specifically formulated to provide the extra nutrients they need.

I'm breast-feeding my newborn

Nursing mothers need extra calcium, phosphorus, magnesium, iron, zinc, and selenium to protect their own body while producing nutritious milk. The same supplements that provide extra nutrients for pregnant women will meet a nursing mother's needs.

Wow — I think that was a hot flash

Then you need extra calcium. At menopause, your body begins producing less of the bone-protecting hormone estrogen, and you begin to lose bone tissue. Severe loss of bone density can lead to osteoporosis and an increased risk of bone fractures. Women of Caucasian and Asian ancestry are more likely than women of African ancestry to develop osteoporosis. (Men also lose bone tissue as they grow older, but their bones start out heavier and denser, and they lose bone tissue less rapidly than women do.)

Twenty years ago, nutritionists thought that you couldn't do anything about age-related loss of bone density — that your body stopped absorbing calcium when you passed your mid-20s. Today, everybody knows that increasing your calcium consumption can slow the loss of bone tissue no matter what your age is.

Minerals and Medicines

Some minerals interact with other minerals or with medical drugs. For example, calcium binds the antibiotic tetracycline into compounds your body cannot break apart so that the antibiotic moves out of your digestive tract, unabsorbed and unused. That's why your doctor will warn you off milk and dairy products when you are taking this antibiotic.

For more about interactions between minerals and medicines, turn to Chapter 25.

NUTRITION SPEAK

Calcium supplements: What kind of calcium is in that pill?

Calcium-rich foods give you calcium paired with natural organic acids, a combination that your body easily digests and absorbs.

The form of calcium most commonly found in supplements, however, is calcium carbonate, the kind of calcium that occurs naturally in limestone and oyster shells.

Calcium carbonate is a versatile compound. Not only does it build strong bones and teeth, it also neutralizes stomach acid and relieves "heartburn." Calcium carbonate antacids can be used as calcium supplements. They are nutritionally sound and generally cost less than products designed solely as nutritional supplements.

Some calcium supplements contain compounds that mix calcium with an organic acid. Calcium lactate is calcium plus lactic acid, the combination that occurs naturally in milk. Calcium citrate is calcium plus citric acid, an acid found in fruits.

These compounds are easier to digest, but they are sometimes more expensive than calcium carbonate products. Calcium carbonate is nearly half calcium, a very high percentage. But unless your stomach is very acidic, it is hard for your digestive system to break the compound open and get at the elemental calcium (the kind of calcium your body can use). You can increase your absorption of calcium from calcium carbonate by taking the tablets with meals.

Because different calcium compounds yield different amounts of elemental calcium, the label lists both the calcium compound and the amount of elemental calcium provided, like this:

Calcium carbonate, 500 milligrams, providing 200 milligrams elemental calcium.

Any time you see the word calcium alone, it stands for elemental calcium.

The human body absorbs calcium most efficiently in amounts of 500 milligrams or less. You get more calcium from one 500-milligram calcium tablet twice a day than one 1,000-milligram tablet. If the 1,000 tablets are a better buy, break them in half.

Warning: Not all antacids double as dietary supplements. Antacids containing magnesium or aluminum compounds are safe for neutralizing stomach acid, but they will not work as supplements. In fact, just the opposite is true. Taking magnesium antacids reduces your absorption of calcium, and taking aluminum antacids reduces your absorption of phosphorus. Because manufacturers sometimes change the ingredients in their products without notice, you should always read the product label before assuming that an antacid can double as a calcium supplement.

Chapter 12

Phabulous Phytochemicals

• •

In This Chapter

▶ What phytochemicals are

▶ Why phytochemicals are important

▶ The accelerating research on phytochemicals

▶ The phytochemicals you already use

• •

*J*ust when you think you have a handle on a big issue like nutrition, The Guys In Charge of Everything toss something new on the table.

I thought I included something about every aspect of food and health in the first edition of *Nutrition for Dummies.* Then a new word started showing up in nutrition articles and reports. The word is *phytochemicals,* a five-syllable mouthful meaning chemicals from plants.

Phytochemicals (chemicals manufactured only in plants) are the substances that produce the beneficial effects of a diet that includes lots of fruits, vegetables, beans, and grains. This chapter gives you a brief summary of the nature of phytochemicals, tells where to find them, and explains how they work. For details on how to use phytochemical-rich foods to prevent or alleviate specific medical conditions, check out Chapter 26.

Phytochemicals Are Everywhere

Did you take French literature in high school or college? Then you are familiar with Moliere's Bourgeoise Gentleman, a lovable but pompous fellow who's surprised to discover he's been speaking prose all his life without knowing it.

Our relationship with phytochemicals is something like that. We have been eating them all our lives without knowing it. The following are all phytochemicals:

- ✔ Vitamin C
- ✔ Carotenoids (the pigments that make fruits and vegetables orange, red, yellow, and green)
- ✔ Thiocyanates, the smelly sulfur compounds that make you turn up your nose at the aroma of boiling cabbage
- ✔ Daidzein and genistein (hormone-like compounds in many fruits and vegetables)
- ✔ Actein (a hormone-like compound in black cohosh, a native North American herb used by Native Americans and some modern herbalists as a remedy for "female troubles" such as hot flashes and other signs of menopause)
- ✔ Dietary fiber

These and other phytochemicals perform beneficial housekeeping chores in your body. They

- ✔ Keep your cells healthy
- ✔ Slow down tissue degeneration
- ✔ Prevent the formation of carcinogens
- ✔ Stop cancer cells from growing
- ✔ Reduce cholesterol levels
- ✔ Protect your heart
- ✔ Maintain your hormone balance
- ✔ Keep your bones strong

The undeniable value of phytochemicals is one reason the U.S. Department of Agriculture/Health and Human Services Dietary Guidelines for Americans urges you to have least five servings of fruits and vegetables and several servings of grains every day.

Did you notice that no minerals appear in the list of phytochemicals? The omission is deliberate. Plants don't manufacture minerals; they absorb them from the soil. Therefore, minerals aren't phytochemicals.

The Different Kinds of Phytochemicals

The most interesting phytochemicals in plant foods appear to be antioxidants, plant hormones, and enzyme-activating sulfur compounds. Each group plays a specific role in maintaining health and reducing your risk of certain illnesses.

Antioxidants

Antioxidants are named for their ability to prevent a chemical reaction called *oxidation* which enables molecular fragments called *free radicals* to join together, forming potentially carcinogenic compounds in your body.

Antioxidants also slow the normal wear-and-tear on body cells, so a diet rich in plant foods (fruits, vegetables, grains, and beans) is known to reduce the risk of heart disease and may reduce the risk of some kinds of cancer. For example, consuming lots of lycopene (the red carotenoid in tomatoes) has been linked to a lower risk of prostate cancer — as long as the tomatoes are mixed with a dab of oil, which makes the lycopene easy to absorb. Think spaghetti sauce. Or even catsup.

Table 12-1 lists the classes of antioxidant chemicals in plant foods.

Table 12-1	Antioxidants in plants
Chemical group	*Found in*
Vitamins	
Ascorbic acid (vitamin C)	Citrus fruits, other fruits and vegetables
Tocopherols (vitamin E)	Nuts, seeds, vegetable oils
Carotenoids (pigments)	
Alpha carotene and beta carotene	Yellow and deep-green fruits and vegetables
Lycopene	Tomatoes
Flavonoids	
Resveratrol	Grapes, peanuts, tea, wine

Plant hormones

Many plants contain hormone-like chemicals called phytoestrogens ("plant estrogen"). The three kinds of phytoestrogens are

- Isoflavones, in fruits, vegetables, and beans
- Lignans, in grains
- Coumestans, in sprouts, and alfalfa

The most valuable phytoestrogens appear to be the isoflavones daidzein and genistein, two compounds with a chemical structure similar to estradiol (the estrogen produced by mammalian ovaries).

Like natural or synthetic estrogens, daidzein and genistein hook onto sensitive spots in reproductive tissue (breast, ovary, uterus, prostate) called estrogen receptors. But phytoestrogens have weaker estrogenic effects than natural or synthetic estrogens. It takes about 100,000 molecules of daidzein or genistein to produce the same estrogenic effect as one molecule of estradiol. Every phytoestrogen molecule that hooks onto an estrogen receptor displaces a stronger estrogen molecule. As a result, many researchers believe that consuming isoflavone-rich foods may give women the benefits of estrogen (lower cholesterol levels, healthy heart, stronger bones, and relief from hot flashes) without the higher risk of reproductive cancers (of the breast, ovary, or uterus) associated with estrogen therapy.

The best food sources of daidzein and genistein are soybeans and soy products, but these aren't the only foods that contain isoflavones. For example, the active ingredient in red clover, a traditional folk remedy for "female troubles" (in this case, hot flashes) is formononetin, an isoflavone your body converts to daidzein. The active ingredient in black cohosh, another folk remedy, is also an isoflavone.

Research has demonstrated the value of isoflavones and lignans for human beings. Coumestans, on the other hand, haven't proven to be useful and my be hazardous.

These common foods provide isoflavones:

✔ Apples	✔ Carrots	✔ Soybeans
✔ Cherries	✔ Fennel	✔ Parsley
✔ Dates	✔ Garlic	✔ Red clover
✔ Pomegranates	✔ Potatoes	

These foods provide lignans:

- ✔ Rice
- ✔ Wheat

Source: "Environmental estrogens and other hormones," *CBR*, Tulane, and Xavier Universities, New Orleans, 1997

Sulfur compounds

Slide an apple pie in the oven and soon the kitchen fills with a yummy aroma that makes your mouth water and your digestive juices flow. But boil some cabbage and — yuck! What is that awful smell? Sulfur, the same chemical that identifies rotten eggs.

Cruciferous vegetables (which get their name from the Latin word for cross, in reference to their X-shaped blossoms) such as broccoli, Brussels sprouts, cauliflower, kale, kohlrabi, mustard seed, onions, radishes, rutabaga, turnips, and watercress all contain stinky sulfur compounds and non-nutrient substances that seem to tell your body to rev up its production of enzymes that inactivate and help eliminate carcinogens.

The presence of these smelly sulfurs is thought to explain why people who eat lots of cruciferous veggies generally have a lower risk of cancer. This theory is bolstered by a laboratory experiment in which rats given chemicals known to cause breast tumors were less likely to develop tumors when they were given sulforathane, one of the odoriferous sulfur compounds in cruciferous veggies. Other sulfur compounds in cruciferous vegetables are glucobrassicin, gluconapin, gluconasturtin, neoglucobrassicin, and sinigrin.

And don't forget fiber

Dietary fiber is a special bonus found only in plant foods. You can't get it from meat or fish or poultry or eggs or diary foods.

Soluble dietary fiber, such as the pectins in apples and the gums in beans, mops up cholesterol and lowers your risk of heart disease. Insoluble dietary fiber such as the cellulose in fruit skins bulks up stool and prevents constipation, moving food more quickly through your gut so that there is less time for food to create substances thought to trigger the growth of cancerous cells. (Turn to Chapter 8 to find out everything you ever wanted to know about dietary fiber — maybe even more than you ever wanted to know.)

The Phuture of Phytochemicals

Yes, I know that misspelling "future" as "phuture" is gross. I know I already named this chapter Phabulous Phytochemicals and that should have been enough, but I just couldn't resist the tempting play on words.

Please don't let my lack of semantic restraint turn you away from the fact that phytochemical research is serious stuff that should eventually enable us to identify biochemical reactions that trigger — or prevent — specific medical conditions.

While you're waiting for final analyses, the best nutrition advice is to dig into those veggies, fruits, and grains — and turn to Chapter 13 to find out why you should wash them down with lots of cold, clear water.

Chapter 13

Water Works

*Y*our body is mostly (50 to 70 percent) water. Exactly how much water depends on how old you are and how much muscle and fat you have. Muscle tissue has more water than fat tissue. Because the average male body has proportionately more muscle than the average female body, it also has more water. For the same reason — more muscle — a young body has more water than an older one.

You definitely won't enjoy the experience, but if you have to, you can live without food for weeks at a time, getting subsistence levels of nutrients by digesting your own muscle and fat. But water's different. Without it, you'll die in a matter of days — more quickly in a place warm enough to make you perspire and lose water faster.

How Your Body Uses Water

Water is a solvent. It dissolves other substances and carries nutrients and other material (such as blood cells) around the body, making it possible for every organ to do its job. You need water to

✔ Digest food, dissolve nutrients so that they can pass through the intestinal cell walls into your bloodstream, and move food along through your intestinal tract

✔ Carry waste products out of your body

✔ Provide a medium in which biochemical reactions such as metabolism occur

Fluoridated water: The real Tooth Fairy

Except for the common cold, dental cavities are the most common human medical problem.

You get cavities from *mutans streptococci,* bacteria that live in dental plaque. The bacteria digest and ferment carbohydrate residue on your teeth (plain table sugar is the worst offender) leaving acid that eats away at the mineral surface of the tooth. This eating away is called decay. When the decay gets past the enamel to the softer inside of the tooth, your tooth hurts. And you head for the dentist even though you hate it so much you'd almost rather put up with the pain. But "almost" doesn't count, so off you go.

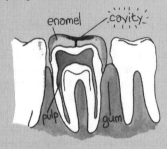

Brushing and flossing help prevent cavities by cleaning your teeth so that bacteria have less to feast on. Another way to reduce your susceptibility to cavities is to drink fluoridated water — water containing the mineral fluorine.

Fluoride — the form of fluorine found in food and water — combines with other minerals in teeth and makes the minerals less soluble (harder to dissolve). You get the most benefit by drinking water containing 1 part fluoride to every million parts water (1ppm) from the day you are born until the day you get your last permanent tooth, usually around age 11 to 13.

Some drinking water, notably in the American southwest, is fluoridated naturally when it flows through rocks containing fluorine. Sometimes so much fluoride is in this water that it causes a brownish spotting ("mottling") that occurs while teeth are developing and accumulating minerals. This effect does not occur with drinking water artificially supplemented with fluoride at the approved standard of one part fluoride to every million parts water.

Because fluorides concentrate in bones, some people believe that drinking fluoridated water raises the risk of bone cancers, but there has never been any evidence in human beings to support this claim. However, in 1990, a U.S. Public Health Service's National Toxicology Program (NTP) study of the long-term effects of high fluoride consumption on laboratory rats and mice added fuel to the fire: Four of the 1,044 laboratory rats and mice fed high doses of fluoride for two years developed *osteosarcoma,* a form of bone cancer.

The study sent an immediate *frisson* (shiver of fear) through the health community, but within a year, federal officials reviewing the study issued an opinion endorsing the safety and effectiveness of fluoridated water.

Here's why. First, the number of cancers among the laboratory animals was low enough to have occurred simply by chance. Second, the cancers occurred only in male rats; no cases were reported in female rats or mice of either sex. Finally, the amount of fluorides the animals got was 50 to 100 times higher than what we get in drinking water. To get as much fluoride as those rats did, human beings would have to drink more than 380 eight-ounce glasses of fluoridated water a day.

Today, more than half the people living in the United States have access to adequately fluoridated public water supplies. The result? A lifelong 50 to 70 percent reduction in cavities among the residents of these communities.

- ✔ Send electrical messages between cells so that your muscles will move, your eyes can see, your brain can think, and so on

- ✔ Regulate body temperature — cooling your body with moisture (perspiration) that evaporates on your skin

- ✔ Lubricate your moving parts

Maintaining the Right Amount of Water in Your Body

As much as three-quarters of the water in your body is in *intracellular fluid,* the liquid inside body cells. The rest is in *extracellular fluid,* all the other body liquids, such as

- ✔ Interstitial fluid (the fluid between cells)

- ✔ Blood plasma (the clear liquid in blood)

- ✔ Lymph (a clear, slightly yellow fluid collected from body tissues that flows through your lymph nodes and eventually into your blood vessels)

- ✔ Bodily secretions

- ✔ Urine

A healthy body has just the right amount of fluid inside and outside each cell, a situation medical folk call *fluid balance.* Maintaining your fluid balance is essential to life. If too little water is inside a cell, it will shrivel and die. If there is too much water, the cell will burst.

A balancing act: The role of electrolytes

Your body maintains its fluid balance through the action of substances called *electrolytes,* mineral compounds that dissolve into electrically charged particles called ions.

Many minerals, including calcium, phosphorus, and magnesium, form compounds that dissolve into charged particles. But nutritionists generally use the term electrolyte to describe sodium, potassium, and chlorine. The most familiar electrolyte is the one found on every dinner table: sodium chloride, plain old table salt. (In water, its molecules dissolve into two ions: one sodium ion and one chloride ion.)

Under normal circumstances, the fluid inside your cells has more potassium than sodium and chloride. The fluid outside is just the opposite: more sodium and chloride than potassium. The cell wall is a *semi-permeable membrane;* some things pass through, but others do not. Water molecules and small mineral molecules flow through freely, but larger molecules such as proteins do not.

The process by which sodium flows out and potassium flows in to keep things on an even keel is called the *sodium pump.* If this process were to cease, sodium ions would build up inside your cells. Sodium attracts water; the more sodium there is inside the cell, the more water will flow in. Eventually, the cell would burst and die. The sodium pump, regular as a clock, prevents this from happening so you can move along, blissfully unaware of those efficient, electric ions.

What happens if you don't get enough water and electrolytes

Drink more water than you need, and your healthy body will simply shrug its shoulders, so to speak, urinate more copiously, and readjust the water level. It's hard for a healthy person on a normal diet to drink himself or herself to death on water.

But if you do not get enough water, your body will let you know pretty quickly.

The first sign is thirst, that unpleasant dryness in your mouth caused by the loss of water from cells in your gums, tongue, and cheeks.

What else do those electrolytes do?

In addition to keeping fluid levels balanced, sodium, potassium, and chloride (the form of chlorine found in food) ions create electrical impulses that allow cells to send messages back and forth among themselves so that you can think, see, move, and perform all the bio-electrical functions that you take for granted.

Sodium, potassium, and chloride are also major minerals (see Chapter 11) and essential nutrients. Like other nutrients, they are useful in bodily processes:

✔ Sodium helps digest proteins and carbohydrates and keeps your blood from becoming too acidic or too alkaline.

✔ Potassium is used in digestion, to synthesize proteins and starch, and as a major constituent of muscle tissue.

✔ Chloride is a constituent of hydrochloric acid, which breaks down food in your stomach. It is also used by white blood cells to make *hypochlorite,* a natural antiseptic.

The second sign is reduced urination. This is a protective mechanism triggered by _ADH,_ a hormone secreted by the hypothalamus, a gland at the base of your brain. The initials are short for antidiuretic hormone. Remember, a diuretic is a substance such as caffeine, which increases urine production. ADH does just the opposite, helping your body conserve water rather than eliminate it.

If you do not pay heed to these signals, your tissues will begin to dry out. You are dehydrating, and if you don't — or can't — get water, you will not survive.

How to Get the Water You Need

Because you don't store water, you need to take in a new supply every day, enough to replace what you lose when you breathe, perspire, urinate, and defecate. On average, this adds up to 1,500 – 3,000 milliliters (50 – 100 ounces; 6 – 12.5 cups) a day. Here's where the water goes:

- 850 – 1,200 milliliters (28 – 40 ounces) is lost in breath and perspiration.
- 600 – 1,600 milliliters (20 – 53 ounces) is lost in urine.
- 50 – 200 milliliters (1.6 – 6.6 ounces) is lost in feces.

About 15 percent of the water you need is created by digesting and metabolizing food. The end products of digestion and metabolism are carbon dioxide (a waste product you breathe out of your body) and water composed of hydrogen from food and oxygen from the air that you breathe. The rest of your daily water comes directly from what you eat and drink.

Fruits and vegetables are full of water; lettuce, for example, is 90 percent water. And you get water from foods that you'd never think of as water sources: hamburger (more than 50 percent), cheese (the softer the cheese, the higher the water content — Swiss cheese is 38 percent water; skim milk ricotta, 74 percent), a plain, hard bagel (29 percent water), milk powder (2 percent), and even butter and margarine (10 percent). Only oils have no water.

You can get water from, well, plain water. Eight 10-ounce glasses give you 2,400 milliliters, approximately enough to replace what your body loses every day. You also get water from liquids, such as milk, coffee, tea, soft drinks, and fruit juices.

But here's an interesting fact: Not all liquids are equally liquefying. The caffeine in coffee and tea and the alcohol in beer, wine, and spirits are diuretics, chemicals that makes you urinate more copiously. While caffeinated and alcohol beverages provide water, they also increase its elimination from your body.

Excuse me for a minute. I'm getting a drink of water.

How does water know where to go?

Osmosis is the principle that governs how water flows through a semi-permeable membrane such as the one surrounding a body cell.

Here's the principle: Water flows through a semi-permeable membrane from the side where the liquid solution is least dense to the side where it is more dense. In other words, the water, acting as if it has a mind of its own, tries to equalize the density of the liquid on both sides of the membrane.

How does the water know which side is more dense? Now that one's easy: Wherever the sodium content is higher. When there is more sodium inside the cell, more water flows in to dilute it. When there is more sodium in the fluid outside the cell, water flows out to dilute that.

Osmosis explains why drinking sea water does not hydrate your body. When you drink sea water, liquid flows out of your cells to dilute the salty solution in your intestinal tract. The more you drink, the more water you lose. You are literally drinking yourself into dehydration.

Of course, the same thing happens — though certainly to a lesser degree — when you eat salted pretzels or nuts. The salt in your mouth makes your saliva more salty. This draws liquid out of the cells in your cheeks and tongue, which feel uncomfortably dry. You need . . . a drink of water!

Who Needs Extra Water and Electrolytes?

In the United States, most people regularly consume much more sodium than they need. In fact, some people who are sodium-sensitive may end up with high blood pressure that can be lowered if they reduce their sodium intake.

Potassium and chloride are found in so many foods that, here, too, a dietary deficiency is a rarity. In fact, the only recorded case of chloride deficiency was among infants given a formula liquid from which the chloride was inadvertently omitted.

The estimated minimum daily requirements for sodium, potassium, and chloride are one-size-fits-all averages.

✔ **Sodium:** 500 milligrams for a healthy adult weighing 70 kilograms (154 pounds)

✔ **Potassium:** 2,000 milligrams for a healthy adult weighing 70 kilograms (154 pounds)

✔ **Chloride:** 750 milligrams for a healthy adult weighing 70 kilograms (154 pounds)

Most Americans get much more as a matter of course. And there are times when you actually need extra water and electrolytes.

You're sick to your stomach

Repeated vomiting or diarrhea drains your body of water and electrolytes. You also need extra water to replace the liquid lost in perspiration when you have a high fever.

When you lose enough water to be dangerously dehydrated, you also lose the electrolytes you need to maintain fluid balance, regulate body temperature, and trigger dozens of biochemical reactions. Plain water won't replace those electrolytes. Check with your doctor for a drink that will hydrate your body without upsetting your tummy.

Death by dehydration: Not a pretty sight

Every day, you lose an amount of water equal to about four percent of your total weight. If you do not take in enough water to replace what you lose naturally by breathing, perspiring, urinating, and defecating, warning signals go off loud and clear.

Early on, when you have lost just a little water, equal to about one percent of your body weight, you feel thirsty. If you ignore thirst, it gets more intense.

When water loss rises to about two percent of your weight, your appetite fades. Your circulation slows as water seeps out of blood cells and blood plasma. And you experience a sense of emotional discomfort, a perception that things are, well, not right.

By the time your water loss equals four percent of your body weight (5 pounds for a 130-pound woman; 7 pounds for a 170-pound man), you are slightly nauseated, your skin is flushed, and you are very, very tired. With less water circulating through your tissues, your hands and feet tingle, your head aches, your temperature rises, you breathe faster and your pulse quickens.

After this, things begin to spiral downhill. When your water loss reaches 10 percent of your body weight, your tongue swells, your kidneys start to fail, and you are so dizzy that you cannot stand on one foot with your eyes closed. In fact, you probably can't even try: Your muscles are in spasm.

When you lose enough water to equal 15 percent of your body weight, you are deaf and pretty much unable to see out of eyes that are sunken and covered with stiffened lids. Your skin has shrunk, and your tongue has shriveled.

When you have lost water equal to 20 percent of your body weight, you've had it. You are at the limit of your endurance. Deprived of life-giving liquid, your skin cracks, and your organs grind to a halt. And — sorry about this — so do you. *Ave atque vale.*

You're exercising or working hard in a hot environment

When you are warm, your body perspires. The moisture evaporates and cools your skin so that blood circulating up from the center of your body to the surface is cooled. The cooled blood returns to the center of your body, lowering the temperature (your "core temperature") there, too.

If you do not cool your body down, you will continue to lose water. If you do not replace the lost water, things can get dicey because you're not just losing water, you're also losing electrolytes. The most common cause of temporary sodium, potassium, and chloride depletion is heavy, uncontrolled perspiration.

Deprived of water and electrolytes, your muscles cramp, you are dizzy and weak, and perspiration, now uncontrolled, no longer cools you. Your core body temperature begins to rise, and without relief — air conditioning, a cool shower, plus water, ginger ale, fruit juice — you may progress from heat cramps to heat exhaustion to heat stroke, the last potentially fatal.

You're on a high-protein diet

You need extra water to eliminate the nitrogen compounds in protein. This is true of infants on high-protein formulas as well as adults on high-protein reducing diets. See Chapter 6 to find out why too much protein may be so harmful.

You're taking certain medications

Because some medications interact with water and electrolytes, ask your doctor whether you need extra water and electrolytes if she prescribes:

- ✔ **Diuretics:** They increase the loss of sodium, potassium, and chloride.
- ✔ **Neomycin (an antibiotic):** It binds sodium into insoluble compounds, making it less available to your body.
- ✔ **Colchicine (an antigout drug):** It lowers your absorption of sodium.

You have high blood pressure

In 1997, when researchers at Johns Hopkins analyzed the results of more than 30 studies dealing with high blood pressure, they found that people taking daily supplements of 2,500 mg (2.5 grams) of potassium were likely to have blood pressure several points lower than those not taking the supplements. Ask your doctor about this one, and remember: Food is also a good source of potassium. One whole banana has 594 milligrams of potassium; one cup of dates – 1,160 milligrams; and one cup of raisins – 1,239 milligrams.

When ginger ale won't cut it

Serious dehydration calls for serious medicine such as the World Health Organization's handy-dandy, two-tumbler electrolyte replacement formula.

WAIT!!! STOP!!!! If you are reading this while lying in bed exhausted by some variety of *turista,* the traveler's diarrhea acquired from impure drinking water, do not make the formula without absolutely clean glasses, washed in bottled water. Better yet, get paper cups.

Now, here's what you need:

Glass #1

8 ounces orange juice

A pinch of salt

½ teaspoon sweetener (honey, corn syrup)

Glass #2

8 ounces boiled or bottled or distilled water

¼ teaspoon baking soda

Take a sip from one glass, then the other, and continue until finished. If diarrhea continues, contact your doctor.

Water is water. Or is it?

Chemically speaking, water's an odd duck. It is the only substance on earth than can exist as a liquid (water) and a solid (ice) — but not a bendable "plastic." No, snow is not plastic water. It's a grouping of solids (ice crystals).

Water may be "hard" or "soft." These terms have nothing to do with how the water feels on your hand. They describe the liquid's mineral content.

✔ Hard water is water that rises to the earth's surface from underground springs. It has lots of minerals (usually calcium carbonate), which it picks up as it moves up through the ground.

✔ Soft water is "surface water," the run-off from rain-swollen streams or rainwater that falls directly into reservoirs. It has fewer minerals.

Hard water may contain as many as 100 particles of calcium, magnesium, iron, and sodium for every 1 million parts of water (shorthand: 100 ppm). Hard water is not high in sodium. The mineral particles can make it taste salty and feel slightly gritty on your skin, and when you wash with hard water, it can leave a mineral "scum" on your skin, hair, and clothes.

Soft water has no salty taste and it leaves your skin, hair, and clothes clean. Is your drinking water hard or soft? The answer may depend on where you live. In the northeastern United States and other places where the major part of the water supply comes from reservoirs, the water that flows from your tap is likely to be soft. In the southwestern United States and other places where the water supply comes mostly from wells and springs, the water is likely to be hard.

What you get at the supermarket is another thing altogether.

Many Americans either do not like the flavor of their tap water or they believe that it is not as pure as it should be. So they buy bottled water. Here's what they get:

Distilled water is tap water that has been distilled: boiled until it turns to steam, which is then collected and condensed back into a liquid free of impurities, chemicals, and minerals. (The name may also be used to describe a liquid produced by ultrafiltration, a process that removes everything from the water except water molecules.) Distilled water is very important in chemical and pharmaceutical processing. You will appreciate the fact that it doesn't clog your iron, makes "clean" ice cubes, and serves as a flavor-free mixer or base for tea and coffee.

Mineral water is spring water. It is naturally alkaline, which makes it a natural antacid and a mild diuretic (a substance that increases urination).

Spring water is also a mineral water, but the term is used to describe water from springs nearer to the earth's surface so it has fewer mineral particles and what some people describe as a "cleaner" taste than mineral water.

Spring-like or spring fresh are terms designed to make something sound more highfalutin' than it really is. These products aren't spring water; they are probably filtered tap water.

Still water is spring water that flows up to the surface on its own. **Sparkling water** is pushed to the top by naturally-occurring gases in the underground spring. The big difference? Sparkling water has bubbles; still water doesn't.

Part III
Healthy Eating

The 5th Wave   By Rich Tennant

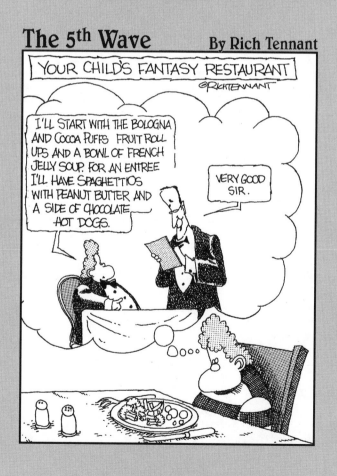

In this part . . .

You can find out how to put foods together to build a healthy diet right here. The chapters in this part are chock-full of rules and guidelines and strategies for making selections that enhance your body while pleasing your palate. And, oh, yes, there's an explanation of why you get hungry and why you find some foods more appetizing than others — an important factor in creating a nutritious diet. (Hey, if it doesn't taste good, why would you want to eat it?)

Chapter 14

Why You Eat When You Eat

. . . .

In This Chapter

▶ The difference between appetite and hunger

▶ Body signals that say, "Feed me"

▶ Why you feel full after eating

▶ What happens when your appetite goes wild

. . . .

*B*ecause you need food to live, your body is no slouch at letting you know that it's ready for breakfast, lunch, dinner, and maybe a few snacks in between. This chapter explains the signals your body uses to get you to the table, to the drive-thru of your favorite restaurant, or to the vending machine down the hall.

The Difference between Hunger and Appetite

People eat for two reasons. The first reason is hunger; the second is appetite. Hunger and appetite are *not* synonyms. In fact, hunger and appetite are entirely different processes.

Hunger is the need for food. It is

> ✔ A physical reaction (chemical changes in your body related to a naturally low level of glucose in your blood several hours after eating)
>
> ✔ An instinctive, protective mechanism that makes sure that your body gets the fuel it requires to function reasonably well

Appetite is the desire for food. It is

> ✔ A sensory or psychological reaction (looks good! smells good!) that stimulates an involuntary physiological response (salivation, stomach contractions)
>
> ✔ A conditioned response to food (see the sidebar on Pavlov's dogs)

Pavlov's performing puppies

Ivan Petrovich Pavlov (1849-1936) was a Russian physiologist who won the Nobel Prize in physiology/medicine in 1904 for his research on the digestive glands. Pavlov's Big Bang, though, was his identification of respondent conditioning — a fancy way of saying that you can train people to respond physically (or emotionally) to an object or stimulus that simply reminds them of something that they love or hate.

Pavlov tested respondent conditioning on dogs. He began by ringing a bell each time he offered food to his laboratory dogs so that the dogs learned to associate the sound of the bell with the sight and smell of food.

Then he rang the bell without offering the food, and the dogs responded as though food was on tap — salivating madly, even though the dish was empty.

Respondent conditioning applies to many things other than food. For example, it can make a winning Olympic athlete teary at the sight of the flag that represents his country. Food companies are great at using respondent conditioning to encourage you to buy their products: When you see a picture of a deep, dark, rich chocolate bar, doesn't your mouth start to water, and. . . . Hey, come back! Where are you going?

The practical difference between hunger and appetite is this: When you are hungry, you eat one hot dog. After that, your appetite may lead you to eat two more hot dogs just because they look appealing or taste good.

In other words, appetite is the basis for the familiar saying: "Your eyes are bigger than your stomach." Not to mention the well-known advertising slogan: "Bet you can't eat just one." Hey, these guys know their customers.

How You Know You're Hungry

The clearest signals that your body wants food, right now, are the physical reactions from your stomach and your blood that let you know it is definitely time to put more food in your mouth and — eat!

The noisy stomach

An empty belly has no manners. If you do not fill it right away, your stomach will issue an audible — sometimes embarrassing — call for food. This rumbling signal is called a *hunger pang*.

Hunger pangs are actually plain old muscle contractions. When your stomach's full, these contractions and their continued waves "down" the entire length of the intestine — known as *peristalsis* — move food through your digestive tract (see Chapter 2 for more about digestion). When your stomach's empty, the contractions just squeeze air, and that makes noise.

This phenomenon was first observed in 1912 by an American physiologist named Walter B. Cannon. (Cannon? Rumble? Could I make this up?) Cannon convinced a fellow researcher to swallow a small balloon attached to a thin tube connected to a pressure-sensitive machine. Then Cannon inflated and deflated the balloon to simulate the sensation of a full or empty stomach. Measuring the pressure and frequency of his volunteer's stomach contractions, Cannon discovered that the contractions were strongest and occurred most frequently when the balloon was deflated and the stomach "empty." Cannon drew the obvious conclusion: When your stomach is empty, you feel hungry.

The blood knows

Every time you eat, your pancreas secretes *insulin,* a hormone that enables you to move blood sugar (glucose) out of the blood and into cells where it is needed for various chores. *Glucose* is the basic fuel your body uses for energy. (See Chapter 8.) As a result, the level of glucose circulating in your blood rises and then declines naturally, producing a vague feeling of emptiness, perhaps weakness, that prompts you to eat.

What meal is this, anyway?

There's no doubt about breakfast and lunch. The first comes right after you wake up in the morning; the second, in the middle of the day, sometime around noon.

But when do you eat dinner? And what about supper?

According to my Webster's New International Dictionary of the English Language (2nd edition, 1941 — 15 pounds, including the new binding I put on when the old one crumbled after I dropped the darned thing on its spine once too often), dinner is the main meal of the day, usually eaten around mid-day, although (get this) some people, "especially in cities," have their dinner between 6 p.m. and 8 p.m. — which probably makes it their supper, because Webster's calls that a meal you eat at the end of the day.

In other words, dinner is lunch except when it's supper. Help!

Most people experience this natural rise and fall as a relatively smooth cycle that lasts about four hours. Throughout the world, the cycle prompts a feeding schedule that generally provides four meals during the day: breakfast, lunch, "tea" (a mid-afternoon meal), and supper.

In the United States, a three-meals-a-day culture forces you to fight your natural rhythm by going without food from lunch at noon to supper at 6 p.m. or later. The unpleasant result is that when glucose levels decline around 4 p.m., and people in many countries are enjoying afternoon tea, lots of Americans get really testy and try to satisfy their natural hunger by grabbing the nearest food, usually a high-fat, high-calorie snack.

Beating the four-hour hungries

In 1989, David Jenkins, M.D., Ph.D., and Tom Wolever, M.D., Ph.D., of the University of Toronto, set up a "nibbling study" designed to test the idea that if you even out digestion — by eating several small meals rather than three big ones — you could spread out insulin secretion and keep the amount of glucose in your blood on an even keel all day long.

The theory turned out to be right. People who ate five or six small meals rather than three big ones felt better and experienced an extra bonus: lower cholesterol levels. After two weeks of nibbling, the people in the Jenkins-Wolever study showed a 13.5 percent lower level of low-density lipoproteins than people who ate exactly the same amount of food divided into three big meals.

How You Know You're Full

The satisfying feeling of fullness after eating is called *satiety,* the signal that says, okay, hold the hot dogs, I've had plenty, and I need to push back from the table.

As nutrition research and the understanding of brain functions have become more sophisticated, scientists have discovered that your *hypothalamus,* a small gland in the middle and toward the back of the brain on top of the *brain stem* (the part of the brain that connects to the top of the spinal cord), seems to house your appetite controls in an area of the brain where hormones and other chemicals that control hunger and appetite are made (see Figure 14-1). For example, the hypothalamus releases neuropeptide Y (NPY) and peptide YY, two chemicals that latch onto brain cells and then send out a signal: More food!

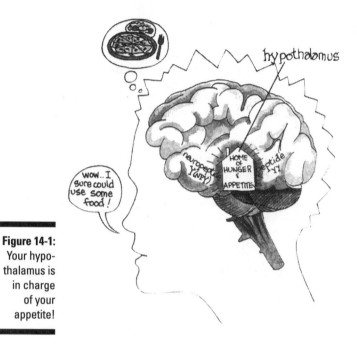

Figure 14-1:
Your hypo-
thalamus is
in charge
of your
appetite!

Other body cells also play a role in making your body say, "I'm full." In 1995, researchers at Rockefeller University discovered a gene in *fat cells* (the body cells where fat is stored) that directs the production of a hormone called *leptin* (from the Greek word for *thin*). Leptin appears to tell your body how much fat you have stored, thus regulating your hunger (need for food to provide fuel). Leptin also reduces the hypothalamus's secretion of NPY, the hormone that signals hunger. When the Rockefeller folks injected leptin into specially bred "fat mice," the mice ate less, burned food faster, and lost significant amounts of weight.

Eventually, researchers hope that this kind of information can lead to the creation of safe and effective drugs to combat obesity.

Environment, Appetite, and Hunger

Your environment, physical as well as psychological, definitely affects both appetite and hunger, sometimes leading you to eat more than normal, sometimes less.

Baby, it's cold outside

You are more likely to feel hungry in cool places rather than in warm ones. And you are more likely to want high-calorie dishes in cold weather than in hot weather. Just think about the foods that tempt you in winter — stews, roasts, thick soups — versus those you find pleasing on a simmering summer day — salads, chilled fruit, simple sandwiches.

This difference is no accident. Food gives you calories. Calories keep you warm. To make sure that you get what you need, your body even processes food faster when it's cold out. Your stomach empties more quickly as food speeds along through the digestive tract, which means those old hunger pangs show up sooner than expected, which means you eat more and stay warmer and . . . well, you get the picture.

Stretch, lift, move, exercise

Everybody knows that working out gives you a big appetite, right? Not necessarily. True, people who exercise regularly are likely to have a healthy (read: normal) appetite, but they're rarely hungry immediately after exercising because

 ✔ Exercise pulls stored energy — glucose and fat — out of body tissues, so your glucose levels stay steady and you don't feel hungry.

 ✔ Exercise slows the passage of food through the digestive tract. Your stomach empties more slowly and you feel fuller longer.

   Caution: If you eat a heavy meal right before heading for the gym or the stationary bike in your bedroom, the food sitting in your stomach may make you feel stuffed. Sometimes, you may develop cramps.

 ✔ Exercise (including mental exertion) reduces anxiety. For some people, that means less desire to reach for a snack.

When you hurt, who wants food?

Severe physical stress or trauma — a broken bone, surgery, a burn, a high fever — reduces appetite and slows the natural contractions of the intestinal tract. If you eat at times like this, the food may back up in your gut or even stretch your bowel enough to tear it. In situations like this, intravenous feeding — fluids with nutrients sent through a needle directly into a vein — give you nutrition without irritation.

Medicine and appetite

When you take medicine, you may be more (or less) likely to eat. Some drugs used to treat common conditions affect your appetite. When you use these medicines, you may find yourself eating more (or less) than usual.

This side effect is rarely mentioned when doctors hand out prescriptions, perhaps because it is not life-threatening and usually disappears when you stop taking the drug. Here is a list of some medicines from *The Essential Guide to Prescription Drugs* (New York: Harper Collins, 1995) by James W. Long and James J. Rybacki that may increase your appetite:

✔ Antidepressants (mood elevators)

✔ Antihistamines ("allergy pills")

✔ Diuretics (chemicals that make your kidneys work harder and cause you to urinate more)

✔ Tranquilizers (calming drugs)

As a general rule, drugs in the following groups may decrease your appetite:

✔ Antibiotics

✔ Anticancer agents

✔ Anticholesterol products

✔ Antifungal agents

✔ Anti-Parkinson drugs

✔ Antiseizure medication

✔ Blood pressure medication

✔ Diet pills

Not every drug in a particular class of drugs (that is, antibiotics or antidepressants) has the same effect on appetite. For example, the antidepressant drug amitriptyline (Elavil) increases your appetite and may cause weight gain; another antidepressant drug, fluoxetine (Prozac) does not.

The fact that a drug affects appetite is almost never a reason to avoid using it. But knowing that a relationship exists between the drug and your desire for food can be helpful. Plain common sense dictates that you ask your doctor about possible drug/appetite interactions whenever she prescribes a drug for you. If the drug package the pharmacist gives you doesn't come with an "insert," ask for it. Read the fine print about side effects and other interesting details — such as the direction to avoid alcohol or driving or using heavy machinery.

When Your Appetite Goes Haywire: Eating Disorders

An eating disorder is a psychological illness that leads you to eat either too much or too little. Indulging in a hot fudge sundae once in a while is not an eating disorder. Neither is dieting for three weeks so that you can fit into last year's dress this New Year's Eve.

The difference between normal indulgence and dieting versus an eating disorder is that the first is acceptable, healthy behavior while an eating disorder is a potentially life-threatening illness that requires immediate medical attention.

People who eat too much

Not everyone who is larger or heavier than the current American ideal has an eating disorder. Human bodies come in lots of different sizes and some people are just naturally larger or heavier than others. An eating disorder may be present, though, when

- ✔ A person continually confuses the desire for food (appetite) with the need for food (hunger)
- ✔ A person who has access to a normal diet experiences psychological distress when denied food
- ✔ A person uses food to relieve anxiety provoked by what he or she considers a scary situation — a new job, a party, ordinary criticism, a deadline

Traditionally, doctors have found treating obesity (see Chapter 3) very difficult. However, recent research suggests that some people overeat in response to irregularities in the production of chemicals that regulate satiety (your feeling of fullness). This research opens the path to new kinds of drugs that can control extreme appetite.

People who eat too little

Some people relieve their anxiety not by eating but by refusing to eat or by regurgitating food after they've eaten it. The first kind of behavior is called anorexia nervosa; the second, bulimia.

Anorexia nervosa (voluntary starvation) is virtually unknown in places where food is hard to come by. It seems to be an affliction of affluence, most likely to strike the young and well-to-do. It is nine times more common among women than among men.

Many doctors who specialize in treating people with eating disorders suggest that anorexia nervosa may be an attempt to control one's life by rejecting a developing body. In other words, by starving themselves, anorexics avoid developing breasts and hips. By not growing wide, they avoid growing up.

If left untreated, anorexia nervosa can end in death by starvation.

Bulimia (voluntary vomiting), like anorexia nervosa, occurs chiefly among the young and more commonly among young women than young men.

Unlike anorexics, bulimics do not refuse to eat. In fact, they may often binge (consume enormous amounts of food in one sitting: a whole chicken, several pints of ice cream, a loaf of bread).

But bulimics do not want to keep the food they eat in their bodies. They may use laxatives to increase defecation but their most characteristic method for getting rid of food is regurgitation. Bulimics may simply retire to the bathroom after eating and stick their fingers into their throats to make themselves throw up. Or they may use emetics (drugs that induce vomiting). Either way, danger looms.

The human body is not designed for repeated stuffing followed by regurgitation. Bingeing may dilate the stomach to the point of rupture; constant vomiting may severely irritate or even tear through the lining of the esophagus (throat). In addition, the continued use of large quantities of emetics may result in a life-threatening loss of potassium that triggers irregular heartbeat or heart failure, factors that supposedly contributed to the 1983 death of singer Karen Carpenter, an anorexic/bulimic who — at one point in her disease — weighed only 80 pounds, but still saw herself as overweight. (One symptom of anorexia and/or bulimia is the inability to look in a mirror and see yourself as you really are. Even at their most skeletal, people with these eating disorders perceive themselves as grossly fat.)

As you can see, eating disorders are life-threatening conditions. But they can be treated. If you (or someone you know) experiences any of the signs and symptoms just described, the safest course is to seek immediate medical advice and treatment.

If you have Internet access, you can get more information from the Web site of The American Anorexia/Bulimia Association, Inc. (www.aabainc.org).

Maintaining a Healthy Appetite

The best way to deal with hunger and appetite is to learn to recognize and follow your body's natural cues.

If you are hungry, eat — in reasonable amounts that make maintaining a realistic weight possible for you. (Confused about how much you should weigh? Check out the weight table in Chapter 3.)

Perhaps the greatest secret about controlling appetite is to remember that nobody's perfect. Make one day's indulgence guilt-free by reducing your calorie intake proportionately over the next few days. A little give here, a little take there, and you will stay on target overall.

Chapter 15

Why You Like the Foods You Like

*T*aste is the ability to perceive flavors in food and beverages. *Preference* is the appreciation of one food and distaste for another. Decisions about taste are physical reactions dependent on specialized body organs called *taste buds*. Decisions about food preferences may depend on your genes, your medical history, and your personal reactions to specific foods, like former President George Bush's loathing for broccoli, described in detail later in this chapter.

Tasting Food

Your taste buds are sensory organs that enable you to perceive different flavors in food — in other words, to taste the food you eat.

Taste buds ("taste papillae") are not flowers. They are tiny bumps on the surface of your tongue (see Figure 15-1). Each one contains groups of receptor cells that anchor an antenna-like structure called a microvillus, which projects up through a gap ("pore") in the center of the taste bud, sort of like a thread sticking through the hole in Life Savers candy. (For more on the microvilli — plural, more than one microvillus — and how they behave in your digestive tract, see Chapter 2.)

The microvilli in your taste buds transmit "messages" from flavor chemicals in the food along nerve fibers to your brain, which translates the messages into perceptions: "Oh, wow, that's good," or "Man, that's awful."

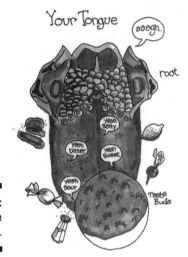

Figure 15-1:
Your tongue
up close.

The four basic flavors

Your taste buds recognize four basic flavors: sweet, sour, bitter, and salt.

Early on, scientists thought that everyone had specific taste buds for specific flavors: sweet taste buds for sweets, sour taste buds for sour, and so on. However, the prevailing theory today is that groups of taste buds work together so that flavor chemicals in food link up with chemical bonds in taste buds to create patterns that you recognize as *sweet, sour, bitter,* and *salt.* The technical term for this process is "across fiber pattern theory of gustatory ciding."

The nose knows

Your nose is very important to your sense of taste. Like the taste of food, the aroma of food also stimulates sensory messages. Think about how you sniff your brandy before drinking and how the wonderful aroma of baking bread warms the heart and stirs the soul — not to mention the salivary glands. When you can't smell, you can't really taste. As anyone who's ever had a cold knows, when your nose is stuffed and your sense of smell is deadened, almost everything tastes like plain old cotton.

Your health and your taste buds

Some illnesses and medicines alter your ability to taste foods. The result may be partial or total *ageusia* (the medical term for "loss of taste"). Or you may experience *flavor confusion* — meaning that you mix up flavors, translating sour as bitter, or sweet as salt, or vice versa.

Table 15-1 lists some medical conditions that affect your sense of taste.

Table 15-1	These Things Make Tasting Food Difficult
This Condition	*May Lead to This Problem*
A bacterial or viral infection of the tongue	Secretions that block your taste buds
Injury to your mouth, nose, or throat	Damage to the nerves that transmit flavor signals
Radiation therapy to mouth and throat	Damage to the nerves that transmit flavor signals

Here are some medical drugs that make it difficult to taste food. Good news: Your sense of taste usually returns to normal when you stop taking the drug.

- Captopril (Capoten), a drug to lower blood pressure
- Griseofulvin (Fulvicin, Grifulvin, Grisactin, Gris-PEG), an anti-fungus drug
- Lithium (Cibalith-S, Eskalith, Lithobid, Lithonate, Lithotabs), an antidepressant/antimanic drug
- Metronidazole (Flagyl), an anti-infective drug
- Penicillamine (Cuprimine, Depen), an antirheumatic
- Rifampin (Rifadin, Rimactane), an antituberculosis drug

Source: James W. Long and James J. Rybacki, *Essential Guide to Prescription Drugs* (New York: HarperPerennial, 1995).

Fooling your taste buds

Combining foods can short-circuit your taste buds' ability to identify flavors correctly. For example, when you sip wine (even an apparently smooth and silky one), your taste buds say, "Hey, that alcohol's sharp." Take a bite of cheese first, and the wine will taste smoother (less acidic) because the cheese's fat and protein molecules coat your receptor cells so that acidic wine molecules cannot connect.

A similar phenomenon occurs in serial wine tastings (tasting many wines, one after another). Try two equally dry, acidic wines, and the second will seem mellower because acid molecules from the first one fill up space on the chemical bonds that perceive acidity. Drink a sweet wine after a dry one, and the sweetness will be even more pronounced.

Here's another way to fool your taste buds: Eat an artichoke. The "meat" at the base of the artichoke leaves contains *cynarin,* a sweet-tasting chemical that makes any food you taste after the artichoke taste sweeter.

What Tastes Good

When it comes to deciding what tastes good, all human beings and most animals have four things in common: They like sweets, crave salt, go for the fat, and avoid the bitter (at least at first).

These choices are rooted deep in biology and evolution. In fact, you could say that whenever you reach for something that you consider good to eat, the entire human race — especially your own individual ancestors — reaches with you.

Foods your body needs

Here's something to chew on: The foods that taste good — sweet foods, salty foods, fatty foods — are essential for a healthy body.

✔ Sweet foods are a source of quick energy because their sugars can be converted quickly to glucose, the molecule your body burns for energy. (Check out Chapter 8 for an explanation of how your body uses sugars.)

Better yet, sweet foods make you feel good. Eating them seems to tell your brain to release natural pain killers called *endorphins.* Sweet foods may also stimulate an increase in blood levels of *adrenaline,* a hormone secreted by the adrenal glands. (Adrenaline is sometimes labeled the "fight-or-flight" hormone because it is secreted most heavily when you feel threatened and must decide whether to stand your ground — "fight" — or hurry away — "flight.")

✔ Salt is vital to life. As Chapter 13 explains, salt enables your body to maintain its fluid balance and to regulate chemicals called electrolytes that give your nerve cells the power needed to fire electrical charges that energize your muscles, power up your organs, and transmit messages from your brain.

- Fatty foods are even richer in calories (energy) than sugars. So it is no surprise that you want them most when you are very hungry. (Chapter 2 and Chapter 7 explain how you use fats for energy.)

- Which fatty food you want may depend on your gender. Several studies suggest that women like their fats with sugar — Hey, where's the chocolate? Men seem to prefer their fat with salt — Bring on the fries!

Foods that are easy to find

Marvin Harris is an anthropologist whose special interest is the history of food. In a perfectly delightful book called *Good To Eat: Riddles of Food and Culture* (Simon & Schuster, 1986), Harris poses this interesting situation:

Suppose you live in a forest where someone has pinned $20 and $1 bills to the upper branches of the trees. Which will you reach for? The $20 bills, of course. But wait. Suppose there are only a couple of $20 bills, but millions and millions of $1 bills. Does that change the picture? You betcha.

Searching for food is hard work. You don't want to spend so much time trying to find food that you use up more calories than the food can provide. Substitute "chickens" for $20 bills and "large insects" for $1 bills, and you can see why people who live in places where insects far outnumber the chickens will spend their time and energy on picking off the plentiful high-protein bugs rather than chasing after the occasional chicken — although they wouldn't turn it down if it fell into the pot.

So, you may say that Harris' "first rule of food choice" is that people tend to eat and enjoy what is easily available, which explains the differences in cuisines in different parts of the world.

Here's a second rule: In order for a food to be appealing ("good to eat"), it has to be both nutritious and relatively easy or economical to produce.

A food that meets one test but not the other is likely to be off the list. For example:

- The human stomach cannot extract nutrients from grass. So even though grass grows here, there, and everywhere, under ordinary circumstances, grass never ends up in your salad.

- Cows are harder to raise than plants, especially under the hot South Asian sun; pigs eat what people do, so they compete for your food supply. In other words, although they are highly nutritious, sometimes neither the cow nor the pig is economical to produce. This is a reasonable anthropological explanation for why some cultures have prohibited their use as food.

Stirring the stew: The culinary benefits of immigration

If you are lucky enough to live in a place that draws lots of immigrants, your dining experience is flavored with other people's (meaning: other cultures') favorite foods. In the United States, for example, the "melting pot" is not an idle phrase. "American" cooking literally bubbles with contributions from every group that stepped ashore on what former President Lyndon Baines Johnson used to call the "good ole U. S. of A."

Table 15-2 lists some of the foods and food combinations characteristic of specific ethnic/regional cuisines. Imagine how few you might sample living in a place where everybody shares exactly the same ethnic, racial, or religious background. Just thinking about it is enough to make me want to stand up and shout, "Hooray for diversity at the dinner table!" (Check out Figure 15-2 for the visuals!)

Table 15-2	Geography and Food Preference
If Your Ancestors Came from Here	*You Are Likely to Be Familiar with This Flavor Combination*
Central & Eastern Europe	Sour cream and dill or paprika
China	Soy sauce plus wine and ginger
Germany	Meat roasted in vinegar and sugar
Greece	Olive oil and lemon
India	Cumin and curry
Italy	Tomatoes, cheese, and olive oil
Japan	Soy sauce plus rice wine and sugar
Korea	Soy sauce plus brown sugar, sesame, and chili
Mexico	Tomatoes and chili peppers
Middle Europe	Milk and vegetables
Puerto Rico	Rice and fish
West Africa	Peanuts and chili peppers

Source: A. W. Logue, *The Psychology of Eating and Drinking* (New York: W. H. Freeman and Company, 1986).

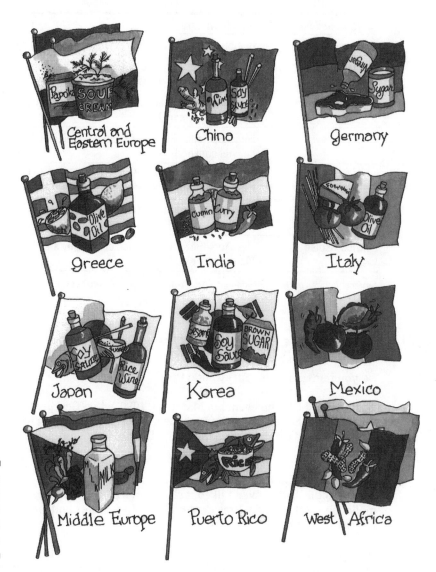

Figure 15-2:
Ethnic and regional cuisines abound.

Of course, enjoying other peoples' food doesn't mean you don't have your own special treats. Table 15-3 is a flag-waver: A list of made-in-America taste sensations, many created here by immigrant chefs whose talents flowered in American kitchens.

Table 15-3	Born in the USA
This Food Item	*Was Born Here*
Baked beans	Boston (Pilgrim adaptation of Native American dish)
Clam chowder	Boston (named for "la chaudière," a large copper soup pot, used by fishermen to make a communal soup)
Hamburger	Everywhere (originally called a Hamburg steak, except in Hamburg, Germany)
Jambalaya	Louisiana (combination of French Canadian with native coastal cookery)
Potato chips	Saratoga Springs, New York (credited to a chef at Moon's Lake House Hotel)
"Spoon bread"	Southern United States (adapted from Native American corn pudding)
Vichyssoise	New York (Ritz Carlton Hotel; created by a chef born near Vichy, France)

Source: James Trager, *The Foodbook* (New York: Grossman Publishers, 1970).

When Food Is Offensive

Do you remember the Yucky Food Press Conference?

That's what I call the events of March 23, 1990, when George Bush, President of the United States, interrupted a question on foreign policy to explain why he had banned broccoli from the White House dining room and the galley of Air Force One.

The President's actual words (I have the clipping right here) were: "I do not like broccoli. And I haven't liked it since I was a little kid and my mother made me eat it. And I'm President of the United States and I'm not going to eat any more broccoli."

Why some of us should loathe broccoli but love — as Mr. Bush reputedly does — refried beans and beef jerky (or vice versa) is still something of a mystery to the sensory experts. They suggest, but cannot prove, that your food preferences depend on your genes, your culture, and your personal experience.

If you are allergic to a food or have a metabolic problem that makes digesting it hard for you, you may eat the food less frequently but you'll enjoy it as much as everyone else does. For example, people who cannot digest lactose, the sugar in milk, may end up gassy every time they eat ice cream but they still like the way the ice cream tastes.

Genetics at the dinner table

Virtually everyone instinctively dislikes bitter foods, at least at first tasting. This dislike is a protective mechanism. Bitter foods are often poisonous, so disliking stuff that tastes bitter is a primitive but effective way to eliminate potentially toxic food.

According to Linda Bartoshuk, Ph.D., Professor of Surgery (Otolaryngology) at the Yale University School of Medicine, about two-thirds of all human beings carry a gene that makes them more sensitive than usual to bitter flavors. This gene may have given their ancestors a leg up in surviving their evolutionary food trials.

People with this gene can taste very small concentrations of a chemical called phenylthiocarbamide (PTC). Because PTC is potentially toxic, Dr. Bartoshuk tests for the trait by having people taste a piece of paper impregnated with 6-N-propylthiouracil, a thyroid medication whose flavor and chemical structure are similar to PTCs. People who say the paper tastes bitter are called "PTC tasters." People who taste only paper are called "PTC non-tasters."

If you are a PTC taster, you are likely to find the taste of saccharin, caffeine, the salt substitute potassium chloride, and the food preservatives sodium benzoate and potassium benzoate really nasty. Ditto for the flavor chemicals common to cruciferous vegetables — members of the mustard family, including radishes, cabbage, brussels sprouts, cauliflower, and George Bush's broccoli.

No such ambivalence exists among people who have gotten truly sick, we're talking nausea and vomiting here, after eating a specific food. If this happens to you, you probably will come to like its flavor less. Sometimes, your revulsion may be so strong that you will never try the food again — even if you know that what actually made you sick was something else entirely, like riding a roller coaster just before eating, or having the flu, or taking a drug whose side effects upset your stomach.

Does it matter if you like your food? Yes. It does. The simple act of putting food into your mouth should stimulate the flow of saliva and the secretion of enzymes that you need to digest the food. Some studies suggest that if you really like your food, your pancreas may release as much as 30 times its normal amount of digestive enzymes.

But if you truly loathe what you are eating, your body may refuse to take it in. No saliva flows; your mouth becomes so dry that you may not even be able to swallow the food. If you do manage to choke it down, your stomach muscles and your digestive tract may convulse in an effort to be rid of the awful stuff.

Beyond Instinct: Learning to Like Unusual Foods

Exposure to different people and cultures often expands your taste horizons. Some taboos — horse meat, snake, dog — may simply be too emotion-laden to be overcome. Others with no emotional baggage fall to experience. Most people hate very salty, very bitter, very acidic, or very slippery foods such as caviar, coffee, Scotch whisky, and oysters on first taste, but later learn to enjoy them.

Coming to terms with these foods can be both physically and psychologically rewarding.

- Many bitter foods, such as coffee and unsweetened chocolate, are relatively mild stimulants that temporarily improve mood and physical performance.

- Strongly flavored foods, such as salty caviar, offer a challenge to the taste buds.

- Foods such as oysters, which may seem totally disgusting the first time you see or taste them, are symbols of wealth or worldliness. Trying them implies a certain sophistication in the way you face life.

Happily, an educated, adventurous sense of taste can be a pleasure that lasts as long as you live. Professional tea tasters, wine tasters, and others (maybe you?) who have developed the ability to recognize even the smallest differences among flavors continue to enjoy their gift well into old age. Although your sense of taste does decline as you grow older, you can keep it perking as long as you supply the stimuli in the form of tasty, well-seasoned food.

In other words, as they say about adult life's other major sensory delight, "Use it or lose it."

Chapter 16

What Is a Healthful Diet?

•••

In This Chapter

▶ The Dietary Guidelines for Americans

▶ How to measure your fat intake

▶ Safe limits on salt and sugar

▶ A definition of moderate drinking

•••

he American Heart Association says to limit your consumption of fats and cholesterol. The American Cancer Society says to eat more fiber. The National Research Council says to watch out for fats, sugar, and salt. The American Diabetes Association says to eat regular meals so that your blood sugar stays even. The Food Police say if it tastes good, forget it!

The U.S. Departments of Agriculture and Health and Human Services have incorporated some of these rules into the Dietary Guidelines for Americans and even added some more of their own. The Dietary Guidelines are to punitive food rules what Häagen-Dazs no-fat chocolate sorbet is to ordinary ice cream: a delicious, reasonable, and totally guilt-free alternative.

Before you begin to read this chapter, make sure that you have a couple of bookmarks or some paper clips or maybe even a few pencils on hand. The material you'll find here often refers back to information in other chapters, so you'll have to skip back and forth and you'll need to have a way to keep your place while you're moving around the book.

What Are Dietary Guidelines for Americans?

The Dietary Guidelines for Americans are seven sensible suggestions first published by the Departments of Agriculture and Health and Human Services in 1980, with three revised editions since then (1985, 1990, and 1995). The guidelines are meant for people who want to maintain a healthy lifestyle.

They describe food choices that promote good health, provide the energy for an active life, and may reduce the risk or severity of chronic illnesses, such as diabetes and heart disease.

The best thing about these guidelines is that they seem to have been written by real people who actually like food. You can tell right up front by the second paragraph, which is headlined "Eating is one of life's greatest pleasures."

The guidelines work best in conjunction with a "food pyramid" that groups foods into categories and tells you how many servings of each you should consume each day, and with the new food labels that show nutrient content for all the foods you buy. You can read more about the pyramid and the labels in Chapter 17. Right now, the job is to spell out the guidelines themselves. Here they are, numbers 1 through 7.

#1: Eat a Variety of Foods

Think of food as little packages of nutrients. For example, an orange is vitamin C, vitamin A, calcium, phosphorus, potassium, thiamin, riboflavin, niacin, some simple carbohydrates (sugar), complex carbohydrates (fiber), and a little protein. Sounds great, but there's a catch.

Oranges don't have either vitamin B12 or iron. To get the first you need food from animals — poultry, fish, beef, milk, cheese, or eggs. To get the second, you need either the animal foods or whole grains, raisins, nuts, seeds, potato skins, and enriched grain products. The situation is the same in reverse, of course. If all you eat is foods from animals, your diet will be missing fiber, vitamin E, and vitamin C.

In short, no one food or class of foods, regardless of its benefits, can give you all the nutrients you need. A healthful diet always means variety.

Table 16-1 lists the different groups of foods you need each day (and Figure 16-1 illustrates them). You can find out how to use these foods in specific combinations in Chapter 17.

Table 16-1	Five Food Groups = One Healthful Diet	
Food Group	*Foods in This Group*	*Recommended Servings per Day**
Grain products	Bread, cereal, pasta, rice	6 – 11
Vegetables	Whole vegetables, vegetable juices	3 – 5

Food Group	Foods in This Group	Recommended Servings per Day*
Fruits	Whole fruits, fruit juices	2 – 4
Milk products	Milk, yogurt, cheese	2 – 3
Meat group	Meat, poultry, fish, dry beans, eggs, nuts	2 – 3

* The number of servings is given in ranges. The lower end of the range applies to people consuming fewer calories (that is, 1,500 calories a day); the higher end, to people consuming more calories (that is, 2,500 to 3,000 calories a day).

Source: *Dietary Guidelines for Americans,* 4th ed. (Washington D.C.: U.S. Department of Agriculture, U.S. Department of Health and Human Services, 1995).

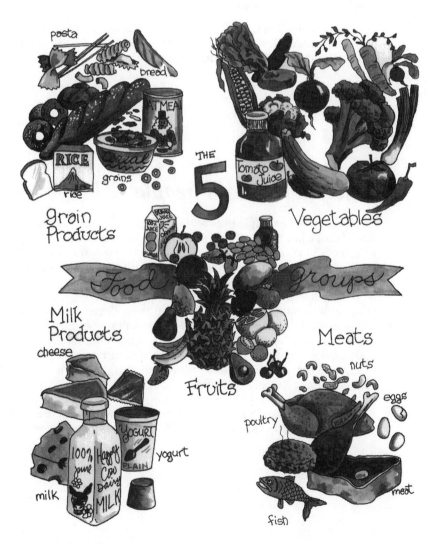

Figure 16-1:
The five food groups.

#2: Balance the Food You Eat with Physical Activity — Maintain or Improve Your Weight

If you take in more calories from food than you use up running your body systems (heart, lungs, brain, and so forth) and doing a day's physical work, you will store the extra calories as body fat. In other words, you will gain weight. The reverse is also true. If you spend more energy in a day than you take in as food, you will pull the extra energy you need out of stored fat. You will lose weight.

I'm no mathematician, but I can reduce this principle to two simple equations in which E stands for energy (calories), > stands for "greater than", < stands for "less than", and W stands for weight:

E (in) > E (out) = +W

E (in) < E (out) = –W

It ain't the Theory of Relativity, but you get the picture!

Calories and real people

Here's a real-life example of how the energy in, energy out theory works. Stick one of those bookmarks I told you to keep on hand right here, and flip back to Table 3-1 in Chapter 3. Table 3-1 shows you how to calculate the number of calories a person can consume each day without pushing up the poundage. Even being mildly active increases the number of calories you can wolf down without gaining weight. The more strenuous the activity, the more plentiful the calorie allowance. Suppose that you are a 25-year-old man who weighs 140 pounds. The formula in Table 3-1 shows that you require 1,652 calories a day to run your body systems. Clearly, you need more calories to do your daily physical work — simply moving around or exercising. Different levels of physical activity require different levels of energy (calorie) intake. According to the National Research Council:

- ✔ Mild activity such as carpentry or housecleaning increases the number of calories you can consume each day without gaining weight to 2,645.

- ✔ Moderate activity such as walking briskly at up to 4 miles per hour raises the total number of calories you can consume each day without gaining weight to 2,810.

✔ Working your little butt off at a heavy activity such as playing a football game or digging ditches pushes the amount of calories you can consume each day without gaining weight up to 3,471.

In other words, a 140-pound man who steps up his physical activity from "mild" to "heavy" can consume 826 extra calories without gaining weight. That happens to be just about the amount of calories in 4 cups of al dente spaghetti plus 1 cup of fat-free tomato sauce. Neat.

Not everybody can — or should — run right out and start chopping down trees or throwing touchdown passes to control his or her weight. In fact, if you have gained a lot of weight recently or have been overweight for a long time or haven't exercised in a while or have a chronic medical condition, you should check with your doctor before starting any new regimen. (**Caution:** Check out of any health club that puts you right on the floor without checking your vital signs — heartbeat, respiration, and so forth.)

Table 16-2 is a list of some forms of moderate activity for healthy adults.

Table 16-2	Exercise for Recovering Couch Potatoes
Activity	
Walking (at the rate of 3 to 4 miles per hour)	
General stretching and calisthenics	
Table tennis	
Lawn mowing	
Golf (pulling a cart or carrying your clubs)	
Home repair, painting the walls	
Jogging	
Swimming	
Bicycling (at the rate of less than 10 miles per hour)	
Gardening	
Dancing	

Source: *Dietary Guidelines for Americans,* 4th ed. (Washington D.C.: U.S. Department of Agriculture, U.S. Department of Health & Human Services, 1995).

Other reasons to exercise

Weight control is a good reason to step up your exercise level, but it's not the only one. Here are four more:

✔ **Exercise increases muscles.** If you exercise regularly, you will end up with more muscle tissue than the average bear. Because muscle tissue weighs more than fat tissue, athletes (even weekend warrior types) may end up weighing more than they did before they started exercising to lose weight. But a recent study from the U.S. Department of Agriculture Grand Forks (North Dakota) Human Nutritional Research Center says that a higher muscle-to-fat ratio is healthier and more important in the long run than actual weight in pounds. Exercise that changes your body's ratio of muscle to fat gives you a leg up in the longevity race.

✔ **Exercise reduces the amount of fat stored in your body.** People who are fat around the middle as opposed to the hips (an "apple" shape versus a "pear") are at higher risk of weight-related illness. Exercise helps to reduce abdominal fat and thus lower your risk of these weight-related diseases. To identify your own body type, use a tape measure to compare your waist line to your hips (around the buttocks). If your waist (abdomen) is bigger, you're an apple. If your hips are bigger, you're a pear.

✔ **Exercise strengthens your bones.** Osteoporosis (thinning of the bones leading to repeated fractures) doesn't happen only to little old ladies. True, on average, a woman's bones thin faster and more dramatically than a man's, but after the mid-30s, everybody — male as well as female — begins to lose bone density. Exercise can slow, halt, or even, in some cases, reverse the process. In addition, being physically active develops the muscles that help support bones. Stronger bones equals less risk of fracture equals less risk of potentially fatal complications.

✔ **Exercise increases brain power.** You know that aerobic exercise increases the flow of oxygen to the heart. But did you also know that it increases oxygen to the brain?

When a rush job (or a rush of anxiety) keeps you up all night, a judicious exercise break can keep you bright until dawn. According to Judith J. Wurtman, Ph.D., nutrition research scientist at Massachusetts Institute of Technology (M.I.T.) and author of *Managing Your Mind and Mood Through Food,* when you are awake and working during the hours you would normally be asleep, your internal body rhythms tell your body to cool down, even though your brain is racing along. Simply standing up and stretching, walking around the room, or doing a couple of sit-ups every hour or so will speed up your metabolism, warm up your muscles, increase your ability to stay awake and, in Dr. Wurtman's words, "prolong your ability to work smart into the night."

#3: Choose a Diet with Plenty of Grain Products, Vegetables, and Fruits

A group of foods packed with vitamins, minerals, lots of complex carbohydrates (starch and fiber), and very little fat — what are these wonder workers? Plants. Only plant foods give you this sterling combination of vitamins and minerals plus complex carbohydrates. Plant foods are low in calories and high in fiber. And they contain chemicals called antioxidants that prevent free radicals (incomplete pieces of molecules) from hooking up with each other to form potentially toxic substances. As a result, the list of benefits associated with a diet based largely on plants seems to grow longer every day.

Plant foods

✔ Add lots of bulk but few calories to your diet so you feel full without adding weight

✔ Are low in fat and have no cholesterol, which means they reduce your risk of heart disease

✔ Are high in fiber, which reduces the risk of heart disease; prevents constipation; reduces the risk of developing hemorrhoids or makes existing ones less painful; moves food quickly through your digestive tract, thus reducing the risk of diverticular disease (inflammation caused by food's getting caught in the folds of your intestines and causing tiny out-pouchings of the weakened gut wall); and lowers your risk of cancer of the mouth, throat (esophagus and larynx), and stomach

Note: Whether eating lots of fiber also lowers the risk of colon cancer is in question. A final judgment awaits the results of several studies currently underway.

✔ Are rich in beneficial substances called phytochemicals also believed to reduce your risk of heart disease and cancer (for more about these wonder-workers, see Chapter 12).

For all these reasons, the guidelines recommend that most of the calories in your diet should come from grains, fruits, and vegetables — including dry beans, which are listed in the meat category in Table 16-1 but are (as you undoubtedly know) vegetables.

#4: Choose a Diet Low in Fat, Saturated Fat, and Cholesterol

Fat is an essential nutrient. Even the dreaded cholesterol is vital to life. In fact, a 1996 study in the journal *Science* shows that cholesterol, which may increase an adult's risk of heart disease, is vital to an embryo's healthy development. Cholesterol triggers the action of genes that tell cells to become specialized body structures — arms, legs, backbone, and so forth. Approximately one in every 9,000 babies is born with a birth defect linked to a failure to make the cholesterol needed to perform this vital function.

Adults, though, should control fat intake so as to control calories and reduce the risk of obesity-related illnesses such as heart disease, diabetes, and some forms of cancer.

The magic 30 percent

Overall, the guidelines suggest a diet that derives no more than 30 percent of its calories from fat.

The question is, how do you figure out the 30 percent? Eating's supposed to be fun — not math at every meal. Not to worry. The chart in the Appendix lists the amount of calories and other nutrients in real-life portions of hundreds of foods: a cup of milk, or a slice of bread, one piece of fruit, or a chicken leg (roasted, no skin).

You can use this chart to figure out the percentage of fat in practically anything you want to eat. Take, for example, one wedge of Camembert cheese in the 3-wedge box on every supermarket shelf. As you can plainly see, it has about 115 calories and 9 grams of fat. Remember that one gram of fat has nine calories. To find out the percentage of calories that come from fat:

1. **Multiply the grams of fat by 9 (the number of calories in one gram of fat).**

   For our cheese example, 9 grams multiplied by 9 gives you the number of calories from fat: 81.

2. **Divide the result from Step 1 by the total number of calories. The result is the percent of calories from fat.**

   Continuing our cheese example, divide 81 (the number of calories from fat) by 115 (the total number of calories in the wedge). The result — 70 percent — is the percent of calories from fat in one wedge of Camembert cheese.

The super 10 percent

The guidelines also suggest that you get no more than 10 percent of your total daily calories from saturated fat (for a definition of the different kinds of fat in foods, see Chapter 7).

Once again, it's the Appendix to the rescue. The chart you find there shows the grams of saturated fat, monounsaturated fat, and polyunsaturated fat for each item. You can use the 9-calories-a-gram formula from the previous section to figure out how many calories you get from the saturated fat in a food.

Or, hey, you could read the package label. Since May 1994, all packaged food sold in the United States has been required to carry nutritional information, including the fat content. Milk, peas, soup, chocolate cake — you name it, and you can find the saturated fat content per serving right there on the side of the package. We'll talk more about these savvy new labels in Chapter 17.

Right now, check out Table 16-3. It tells you how many grams of fat equal the recommended daily intake for diets providing 1,500; 2,000; 2,500; and 3,300 calories a day. This table shows you how many grams of fat make up 10 percent and 30 percent of the total calories in four different diet regimens. For example, if you consume 1,500 calories a day, 30 percent of the total equals 450 calories. Divide that by 9 (the number of calories in one gram of fat) to get 50 grams of fat, the total amount suggested by the Dietary Guidelines for Americans.

Table 16-3	How Much Fat Do the Guidelines Allow?	
Calories (Total Per Day)	*30 Percent of Total Daily Calories =This Many Grams of Fat**	*10 Percent of Total Daily Calories = This Many Grams of Fat**
1,500	450 calories = 50 grams	150 calories = 17 grams
2,000	600 calories = 67 grams	200 calories = 22 grams
2,500	750 calories = 83 grams	250 calories = 28 grams
3,300	990 calories = 110 grams	330 calories = 37 grams

* numbers rounded

Source: *Nutritive Value of Foods* (Washington D.C.: U.S. Department of Agriculture, 1991).

The basic 300-or-less

The Dietary Guidelines recommend that a person consuming 2,000 calories a day get no more than 300 milligrams of cholesterol from food. If your diet provides fewer calories, your cholesterol intake should also drop.

#5: Choose a Diet Moderate in Sugars

Sugars are energy foods. That's good. But they add calories, and if you use them carelessly, they nourish those bacteria that rot your choppers. The solution to the first problem is moderation. The solution to the second is boring but valid: Brush your teeth and floss after every meal.

Question: Which is worse for your teeth, a piece of chocolate or a couple of raisins? Yes, this is a trick question. Yes, the answer is raisins.

The explanation's simple. Both foods have lots of sugar, but the chocolate is less detrimental because it dissolves quickly and is washed out of your mouth (and off your teeth) by your saliva. Raisins are sticky. Unless you brush and floss after eating, they will cling to your teeth, providing a long-lasting banquet for those pesky tooth decay bacteria.

Although sugars occur naturally in fruits and vegetables, it's a safe bet that most of the sugar in your diet is added to other foods. Here are the sugars that you are likely to find on food labels. You can assume the food is high in sugar if the sugar word shows up in first or second place on the ingredient list.

- Brown sugar
- Corn sweetener
- Corn syrup
- Fructose
- Fruit juice concentrate
- Glucose (dextrose)
- High-fructose corn syrup
- Honey
- Invert sugar (50:50 fructose-glucose)
- Lactose
- Maltose
- Molasses
- Raw sugar
- Sugar (sucrose)
- Syrup

#6: Choose a Diet Moderate in Salt and Sodium

Sodium is a mineral that helps regulate your body's fluid balance, the flow of water into and out of every cell (see Chapter 13). The aim is to keep enough water inside the cell so that it can perform its daily jobs, but not so much that the cell — packed to bursting — explodes.

Most people have no problems with sodium. They eat a lot one day, a little less the next, and their bodies adjust. Others, however, do not react so evenly. For them, a high-sodium diet appears to increase the risk of high blood pressure. If you already have high blood pressure, you can tell fairly quickly whether lowering the amount of salt in your diet lowers your blood pressure. But no test is available right now to tell whether someone who does not have high blood pressure will develop it by consuming a diet high in sodium.

Because limiting sodium intake to a moderate level won't harm anyone, the guidelines advocate avoiding excessive amounts of salt. This helps reduce blood pressure levels for people who are salt-sensitive.

Reducing salt intake has another, unadvertised benefit. It may lower your weight a bit. Why? Because sodium is *hydrophilic* (hydro = water; philic = loving). Sodium attracts and holds water. When you eat less salt, you retain less water, you are less bloated, and you feel thinner.

Do not reduce salt intake drastically without checking with your doctor first. Remember, sodium is an essential nutrient, and the guidelines advocate moderate use, not no use at all.

The obvious question: What's moderate? One answer is found on the new Nutrition Facts food labels, which list a Daily Value (that is, a recommended amount) of 2,400 milligrams of sodium per day. How much is that? Slightly more sodium than you would get in one level teaspoon of table salt (sodium chloride).

Like sugar, sodium occurs naturally in foods. The foods with the highest amounts of naturally occurring sodium are natural cheeses, sea fish, and shellfish. Some foods are low in sodium but pick up lots of salt when they are processed. For example, one cup of cooked fresh green peas that I checked has 2 milligrams of sodium but one cup of canned peas may have 493 milligrams of sodium. To be fair, most canned and processed vegetables are now available in low-sodium versions as well. The difference is notable: One cup of low-sodium canned peas has 8 milligrams of sodium, 485 milligrams less than regular canned peas.

You also get added sodium in the salt on snack foods such as potato chips and peanuts, not to mention the salt you add yourself from the shaker on virtually every American table. Not all the sodium you swallow is sodium chloride. Sodium compounds are also used as preservatives, thickeners, and buffers (chemicals that smooth down acidity).

Table 16-4 lists several different kinds of sodium compounds in food. Table 16-5 lists sodium compounds in over-the-counter (OTC) drug products.

Table 16-4	The Sodium Compounds Found in Food
Compound	*What It Is or Does*
Monosodium glutamate (MSG)	Flavor enhancer
Sodium benzoate	Keeps food from spoiling
Sodium caseinate	Thickens foods and provides protein
Sodium chloride	Table salt (flavoring agent)
Sodium citrate	Holds carbonation in soft drinks
Sodium hydroxide	Makes it easy to peel the skin off tomatoes and fruits before they are canned
Sodium nitrate/nitrite	Keeps food (cured meats) from spoiling
Sodium phosphates	Mineral supplement
Sodium saccharin	No-calorie sweetener

Sources: "The Sodium Content of Your Food," *Home and Garden Bulletin,* No. 233 (Washington, D.C.: U.S. Department of Agriculture, August 1980); Ruth Winter, *A Consumer's Dictionary of Food Additives* (New York: Cleown, 1978).

Table 16-5	Some Sodium Compounds in OTC Drug Products
Sodium Compound	*What It Is*
Sodium ascorbate	A form of vitamin C used in nutritional supplements
Sodium bicarbonate	Antacid
Sodium biphosphate	Laxative
Sodium citrate	Antacid
Sodium fluoride	Mineral used in nutritional supplements and as a decay preventive in tooth powders
Sodium phosphates	Laxative
Sodium saccharin	Sweetener
Sodium salicylate	Analgesic (similar to aspirin)

Sources: Handbook of Nonprescription Drugs, 9th ed. (Washington, D.C.: American Pharmaceutical Association, 1990); *Physicians' Desk Reference,* 48th ed. (Montvale, N.J.: Medical Economics Data Production, 1994).

#7: If You Drink Alcohol Beverages, Do So in Moderation

Sounds like Mom-and-apple-pie advice, right? Right. But — and you've heard this song before — what's *moderation,* anyway? Laymen (you and me, babe) might define moderate in terms of the effects alcohol has on the ability to perform simple tasks such as speaking and thinking clearly or moving in a straight line. Obviously, if the amount of alcohol you drink makes you slur your words or bump into the furniture, that's not moderate.

Nutrition scientists use a more precise standard, defining moderate as the amount of alcohol your body can metabolize without increasing your risk of serious illness such as cancer or liver damage. To metabolize alcohol, you need an enzyme called *alcohol dehydrogenase* (ADH), which is secreted by glands in your stomach (gastric alcohol dehydrogenase), your intestinal wall (intestinal alcohol dehydrogenase), and your liver (liver alcohol dehydrogenase).

For unknown reasons, women secrete smaller amounts of alcohol dehydroge-nase than men do. As a result, women metabolize alcohol more slowly and feel its effects faster and more intensely. The old wives' tale that He can drink Her "under the table" is no myth. It's physiology.

The Dietary Guidelines define moderate drinking as one drink a day for a woman, two drinks a day for a man. Aha, you say, but what's one drink? Good question. Here's the answer:

- 12 ounces of regular beer (150 calories)
- 5 ounces of wine (100 calories)
- ⅕ ounce of 80-proof distilled spirits (100 calories)

Source: Dietary Guidelines for Americans, 4th ed. (Washington, D.C.: U.S. Department of Agriculture, 1995).

Some people should not drink at all, not even in moderation. This includes alcoholics, people who plan to drive a car or take part in other activities that require attention to detail or real physical skill, and people using medication (prescription drugs or over-the-counter products). For information about who should and should not drink, as well as a list of drugs that interact with alcohol, see Chapter 9.

Okay: Now Relax

Life is not a Scout test. You don't have to follow the Dietary Guidelines for Americans every single day of your life. Nobody's perfect, and the guidelines are meant to be broken — once in a while. For example, the ideal rule is that no more than 30 percent of your daily calories should come from fat. But you can bet that you'll exceed your 30 percent this Saturday, when you dance by the buffet table at your best friend's wedding and see

- ✔ Camembert cheese (70 percent of the calories from fat)
- ✔ Sirloin steak (56 percent of the calories from fat) and salad with Thousand Island dressing (90 percent of the calories from fat)
- ✔ Whipped cream cake (I can't count that high.)

Is this a crisis? Should you stay home? Must you keep your mouth shut tight all night? Are you kidding? Here's the Real Rule: Let the good times roll every once in a while. After the party's over, compensate. For the rest of the week, emphasize lots of the nutritious, delicious low- or no-fat foods that should make up most of your regular diet:

- ✔ Fresh fruit (virtually no calories from fat)
- ✔ Vegetable salads (ditto — but watch the dressing!)
- ✔ Roast white meat turkey, no skin (20 percent of its calories from fat)
- ✔ Pasta (5 percent) with fat-free cheese (zip, zero, zilch)

By the end of the week, you're likely to have averaged out to that desirable 30 percent with no fuss and no muss, and right in line with that headline from the first page of the guidelines that I mention in the beginning of this chapter: "Eating is one of life's greatest pleasures." Amen to that.

Chapter 17

Making Wise Food Choices

• •

In This Chapter

▶ The Food Guide Pyramid

▶ The features of the new food labels

▶ Using the pyramid and food labels to choose nutritious meals

▶ Some commonsense rules for successful snacking

• •

*T*his is a very important chapter because it describes two valuable nutrition aids — the Food Pyramid and the new food package label — and tells you how to use them to create a healthful diet.

This is a difficult chapter because it's bursting with numbers and details. Health writers love this kind of material, but health editors hate it, mostly because they often have to spend hours turning it into warm and fuzzy reader-friendly sentences.

But don't let the multiple factoids and statistics turn you off. The information you'll find here really is vital for making good food choices. Take a deep breath, keep your highlighter handy, and jump right in.

The Food Pyramid

The food pyramid is building blocks for grown-ups. Instead of the letters of the alphabet, these blocks represent food groups you can put together to form (what else?) a pyramid, broad at the bottom, narrowing to a point on top.

> ✔ The broad base represents the foods you should eat every day, the ones that should account for most of the calories you consume.
>
> ✔ The pointy top — a much smaller space — represents the foods that you should eat only once in a while.
>
> ✔ The middle blocks — larger than the top, smaller than the bottom — stand for foods that you should eat in moderate amounts every day.

What the food pyramid says to you

The essential message of all good guides to healthy food choices is that no one food is either good or bad — it's how much and how often you eat it that counts.

With that in mind, the food pyramid delivers three important messages:

- ✔ **Balance.** You can't build a pyramid with a set of identical blocks. You need blocks of different sizes, including the one with a point on the top. The variously sized blocks in the food pyramids show that a healthful diet is balanced: A little more of this, a little less of that.

- ✔ **Variety.** The fact that the pyramid contains so many building blocks tells you that no single food will give you all the nutrients you need.

- ✔ **Moderation.** Having some foods up at the small, pointy top tells you that while every food is valuable, some — such as fats and sweets — are best used in very small amounts.

Clearly, the virtue of the food pyramid is that it allows you to eat practically everything you like — as long as you follow the recommendations on how much and how frequently (or infrequently) to eat it.

The USDA Food Guide Pyramid

The first food pyramid was created by the U.S. Department of Agriculture (USDA) in 1992 in response to criticism that the original government guide to food choices — the Four Food Group Plan (vegetables and fruits, breads and cereals, milk and milk products, meat and meat alternatives) — was too heavily weighted toward high-fat, high-cholesterol foods from animals.

Figure 17-1 is a picture of the USDA Food Guide Pyramid. As you can see, this pyramid is based on daily food choices. It shows you which foods are in what groups — unlike the Four Food Group Plan, the pyramid separates fruits and vegetables into two distinct groups — and lists the number of servings from each food group that you should have each day.

The number of servings is given in ranges. The lower end is for people consuming about 1,600 calories a day; the upper end, for people whose daily diet nears 3,000 calories.

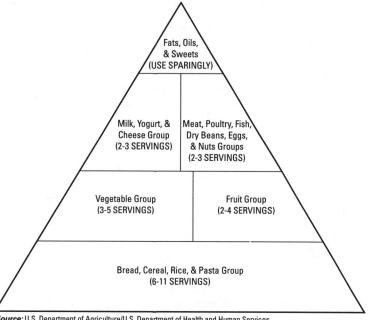

Source: U.S. Department of Agriculture/U.S. Department of Health and Human Services

Figure 17-1:
The USDA
Food Guide
Pyramid.

What's a serving? Not to worry. That's spelled out in Table 17-1.

Table 17-1	What's a Serving?
Food Group	**Serving Size**
Bread	1 slice bread
Cereal	1 ounce ready-to-eat cereal ½ cup cooked cereal
Rice, pasta	½ cup cooked rice or pasta 5-6 small crackers
Vegetables	1 cup raw leafy vegetables ½ cup chopped raw vegetables ½ cup cooked chopped vegetables ¼ cup vegetable juice
Fruits	1 medium piece of fresh fruit (apple, banana, orange, peach) ½ cup cooked or canned chopped fruit ½ cup fruit juice

(continued)

Table 17-1 *(continued)*

Food Group	Serving Size
Milk products	1 cup milk 1 cup yogurt ½ ounce natural cheese 2 ounces processed cheese
Meat	2 to 3 ounces cooked lean meat
Fish	2 to 3 ounces cooked fish
Poultry	2 to 3 ounces cooked lean poultry
Dry beans	½ cup cooked dry beans
Eggs	1 egg
Nuts, seeds	2 tablespoons peanut butter ⅓ cup nuts or seeds
Fats, oils, sweets	no specific amount; very little

Source: The Food Guide Pyramid (Washington, D.C.: International Food Information Council Foundation, U.S. Department of Agriculture, Food Marketing Institute, 1995).

One useful aspect of the USDA Food Guide Pyramid is that it recommends different numbers of daily servings for people consuming different amounts of calories each day. For example, consider the different recommendations of servings from the bread group at different levels of calorie consumption:

✔ At the 1,600 calorie-a-day level sufficient for women who do not exercise and for many older adults, the USDA recommends 6 servings a day from the bread group.

✔ At the 2,200 calorie-a-day level that meets the needs of most children and active women and many sedentary men, the USDA recommends 9 servings a day from the bread group.

✔ At the 2,800 calorie-a-day level that provides the energy required by most teenage boys, many active men, and some very active women, the USDA recommends 11 servings a day from the bread group.

You may want to check out the International Food Information Council's Web page on the Food Pyramid at ificinfo.health.org/brochure/ pyramid.htm

Table 17-2 lists the USDA serving recommendations for three levels of calorie consumption.

Table 17-2	How Many Servings: Daily Choices Based on the USDA Food Guide Pyramid		
Food Group	*1,600 Calories*	*2,200 Calories*	*2,800 Calories*
Bread group	6	9	11
Fruit group	2	3	4
Vegetable group	3	4	5
Milk group*	2-3	2-3	2-3
Meat group	5 ounces	6 ounces	7 ounces

* Requirements higher for women who are pregnant or nursing.

Source: *The Food Guide Pyramid* (Washington, D.C.: International Food Information Council Foundation, U.S. Department of Agriculture, Food Marketing Institute, 1995).

The Mediterranean Diet Food Pyramid

A second valuable food pyramid is the one based on the Mediterranean Diet. The Mediterranean Diet food pyramid (shown in Figure 17-2) was developed in 1993 by the World Health Organization, Harvard School of Public Health, and Oldways Preservation and Exchange Trust, a nonprofit organization based in Cambridge, Massachusetts. It describes food choices that match the traditional diet of countries such as Italy and Greece, which border on the Mediterranean Sea. In this part of the world, people share a number of dietary practices. For example, they

- ✔ Eat lots of grains
- ✔ Eat plenty of fresh fruits and vegetables
- ✔ Use olive oil as their primary fat
- ✔ Consume only moderate amounts of milk products (primarily cheese and yogurt, rather than milk and butter)
- ✔ Use fish and poultry rather than red meat as their main source of high-protein foods from animals
- ✔ Drink wine with meals

Over the past decade, a number of studies have confirmed that people who follow this diet are likely to have a lower risk of heart disease and a lower risk of some kinds of cancer (notably colon cancer). People who follow this diet also seem to live longer than most.

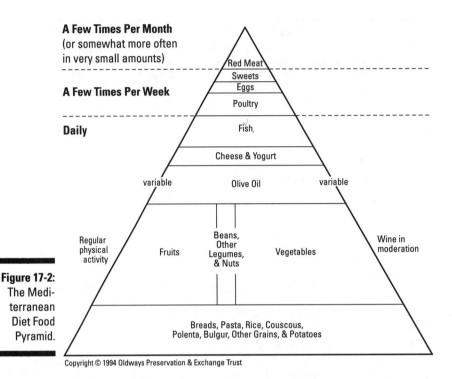

A Few Times Per Month
(or somewhat more often
in very small amounts)

A Few Times Per Week

Daily

Red Meat

Sweets

Eggs

Poultry

Fish

Cheese & Yogurt

variable   Olive Oil   variable

Regular
physical
activity

Fruits

Beans,
Other
Legumes,
& Nuts

Vegetables

Wine in
moderation

Breads, Pasta, Rice, Couscous,
Polenta, Bulgur, Other Grains, & Potatoes

Figure 17-2:
The Medi-
terranean
Diet Food
Pyramid.

Unlike the USDA Food Guide Pyramid, the Mediterranean Diet Pyramid is not
a guide to daily food choices. It has no recommended number of daily servings. Instead, this pyramid concentrates on an overall eating pattern, showing
how frequently you should use a given group of foods — daily, a few times a
week, or a few times a month — and asks you to use your own sense of pro-
portion to figure out how much of each food you should include in your diet.

And there's more. Oldways and the Harvard School of Public Health, with
Baylor University, have also created diet pyramids specifically for two popular
ethnic cuisines. The Traditional Healthy Asian Diet Pyramid (see Figure 17-3)
and the Healthy Traditional Latin American Diet Pyramid (see Figure 17-4)
reflect differences in eating patterns (and the foods generally available) in
other parts of the world.

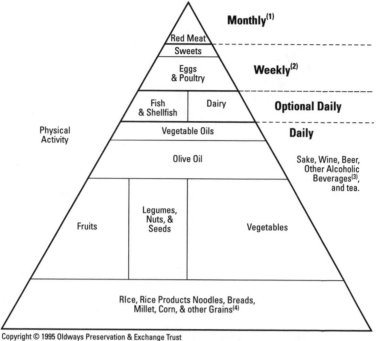

Figure 17-3:
The
Traditional
Healthy
Asian Diet
Pyramid.

Copyright © 1995 Oldways Preservation & Exchange Trust

(1) Or more often in very small amounts.

(2) Dairy foods are generally not part of the healthy, traditional diets of Asia, with the notable exception of India. In light of the current nutrition research, if dairy foods are consumed on a daily basis, they should be used in low to moderate amounts, and preferably low in fat.

(3) Wine, beer, and other alcoholic beverages should be consumed in moderation and primarily with meals and avoided whenever consumption would put an individual or others at risk.

(4) Minimally refined whenever possible.

For example, the Asian pyramid features rice and noodles in the grain group and puts fish, shellfish, and dairy products in the same block. Milk almost never appears in an Asian diet because many Asians lack sufficient amounts of lactase, the enzyme required to digest lactose, the sugar in milk. The Latin American diet pyramid makes similar adjustments, featuring tortillas, beans, and rice.

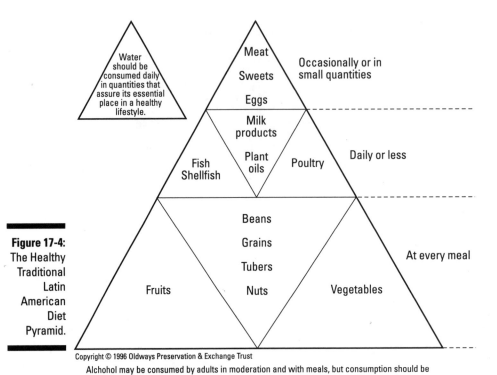

Alchohol may be consumed by adults in moderation and with meals, but consumption should be avoided during pregnancy and whenever it would put the individual or others at risk.

Figure 17-4:
The Healthy Traditional Latin American Diet Pyramid.

Comparing the Food Pyramids

The USDA Food Guide Pyramid, the Mediterranean Diet pyramid, the Asian Diet Pyramid, and the Latin American Diet Pyramid are all meant to help you make healthy food choices. But like painters looking at the same sunset, one emphasizing detail, the other, color, these pyramids interpret a "healthy diet" in different ways.

Overall approach: Give me the lowdown

The USDA Food Guide Pyramid puts more emphasis on meat, poultry, and seafood. The Mediterranean, Asian, and Latin American pyramids rely more heavily on fiber-rich complex carbohydrates (grains and other starchy foods). As a result, using the latter pyramids can tilt you toward a diet that is lower in calories than one assembled from the USDA food pyramid.

Servings: Tell me when

Here's a thorny proposition: Do you spell out servings in detail and spare folks from complicated computing — or do you simply say, hey, here's what you should be eating: Go to it!

The USDA pyramid goes the first route. Unfortunately, the authoritative recommended servings are sometimes hard to reconcile with equally authoritative practical advice. For example, the recommended serving size for meat, fish, or poultry is 3 ounces, but the suggested servings shown in Table 17-2, based on how many calories you get from your daily diet, are not multiples of three. Holy calculator, Batman!

The Mediterranean pyramid avoids the problem by omitting serving sizes entirely. Instead, it appeals to your common sense. You're supposed to look at a dinner plate and say something like this: I should get more of my calories from grains and fruit than from meat and milk, so that's how I'll fill up my plate.

Are you this disciplined? Then the Mediterranean pyramid's laid-back approach will work out fine. But if you're a person who likes everything just so, you may actually enjoy the challenge of trying to figure out exactly how many shreds of beef make up a one-and-one-half-serving portion.

Watch those proteins

Critics contend that, like the Four Food Group Plan, the USDA pyramid puts too much emphasis on foods from animals. Worse yet, it does not distinguish between good protein choices (lean beef, chicken without the skin) and bad protein choices (hot dogs, roast duck with skin) — which means that you can follow all the "good advice" and still end up loading your plate (and your body) with fat, saturated fat, and cholesterol.

More troubling, the recommended daily servings of protein foods may raise your fat consumption into the nutritional stratosphere.

For example, the USDA pyramid suggests two to three servings from the meat category and an equal number of servings of dairy products. In theory, this permits you to down 9 ounces of red meat plus 3 cups of whole milk a day. How much fat, saturated fat, and cholesterol is that? Check out the appropriate entries in the chart in the Appendix, which shows the nutrient content of hundreds of real-life food servings. I'm telling you to do this yourself, rather than doing the addition for you, because I suspect that the total would make my heart skip a beat.

By contrast, the protein choices in the Mediterranean diet include plant foods (nuts, seeds, beans) that are naturally cholesterol-free and low in saturated fats. And this pyramid translates "dairy" to mean mostly yogurt and cheese — foods that have less artery-clogging fat than plain, whole milk.

Using fats wisely

The USDA pyramid recommends using fats only sparingly, but it does not differentiate between animal fats (butter, lard) and vegetable fats (oils and margarine).

The Mediterranean pyramid actually recommends a fat: olive oil. Recent research shows that olive oil, which is rich in oleic acid, a monounsaturated fatty acid, does not raise the level of the "bad" cholesterol linked to heart disease. In addition, olive oil — like other vegetable oils — has plenty of vitamin E, which may protect heart health by preventing cholesterol from blocking your arteries. (Fazed by fats? Flip to Chapter 7.)

Where did my drink go?

The USDA pyramid does not include alcohol beverages. Sometimes the pyramid comes with an explanation that alcohol belongs in the food group at the tiny, tippy top — the one for foods such as sweets and oils ("use sparingly").

By contrast, the Mediterranean pyramid puts wine right on the diagram, off to the side at the "in moderation" section of the design. According to the Dietary Guidelines for Americans (see Chapter 16), that means one drink a day for a healthy woman, two drinks a day for a healthy man.

Chapter 9 spells out the health benefits of moderate alcohol consumption, so I won't bore you by repeating it here. But I will explain the rationale for saying "wine" rather than "alcohol beverages" (that is, beer, wine, and spirits).

Unlike distilled spirits — whiskey, gin, tequila, rum, vodka — wine contains small amounts of beneficial phytochemicals (phyto = plants), including some vitamins and minerals. Of course, beer also has some vitamins and minerals, so simple deductive logic suggests that the wine is simply an integral part of the ethnic eating patterns of the Mediterranean diet.

Creating Your Own Food Pyramid

Why not put together your own food pyramid based on your personal preferences? For example, if you are a vegetarian, your pyramid would still be based on grains plus vegetables and fruits, but you would eliminate the meat group and substitute combinations of "complementary" protein foods such as milk products with grain foods or beans with grains as described in Chapter 6.

In making your pyramid, you also want to take into account any medical conditions such as allergies or a chronic illness that require you to emphasize or avoid specific foods. For example, if corn products give you hives and milk makes you wheeze, you'd eliminate the first from the grain group and substitute nondairy foods such as soy "milk" for the dairy products category.

Figure 17-5 gives you an empty pyramid for the USDA regimen, and Figure 17-6 is an empty pyramid for the Mediterranean diet. You can fill these in at your pleasure. Wait: Make some copies first (and don't forget to enlarge!), so you'll have extras if you mess up the first one. The only rules are the general ones outlined in Chapter 16: Control fat and cholesterol; moderate the sweets; and build with a base of high-fiber, nutrient-rich plants.

And neatness counts. Just kidding.

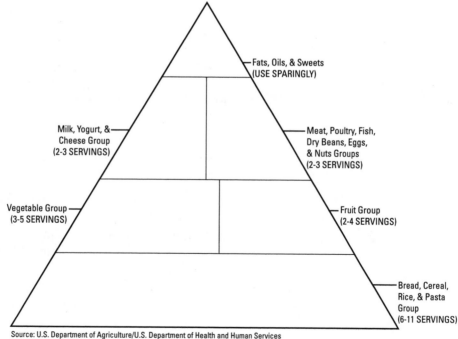

Figure 17-5:
Make your own USDA food pyramid.

Fats, Oils, & Sweets
(USE SPARINGLY)

Milk, Yogurt, & Cheese Group
(2-3 SERVINGS)

Meat, Poultry, Fish, Dry Beans, Eggs, & Nuts Groups
(2-3 SERVINGS)

Vegetable Group
(3-5 SERVINGS)

Fruit Group
(2-4 SERVINGS)

Bread, Cereal, Rice, & Pasta Group
(6-11 SERVINGS)

Source: U.S. Department of Agriculture/U.S. Department of Health and Human Services

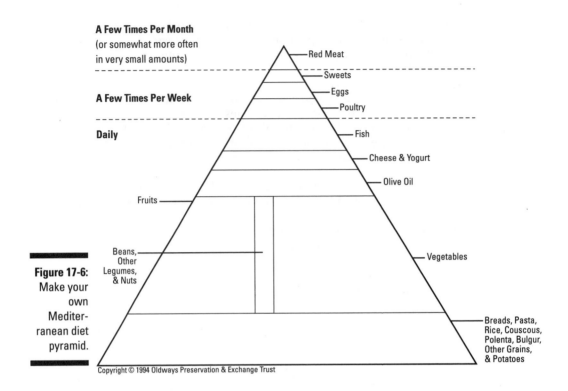

A Few Times Per Month
(or somewhat more often
in very small amounts)

A Few Times Per Week

Daily

Red Meat
Sweets
Eggs
Poultry
Fish
Cheese & Yogurt
Olive Oil
Fruits
Beans, Other Legumes, & Nuts
Vegetables
Breads, Pasta, Rice, Couscous, Polenta, Bulgur, Other Grains, & Potatoes

Figure 17-6:
Make your own Mediterranean diet pyramid.

Copyright © 1994 Oldways Preservation & Exchange Trust

The New, Improved Food Labels

Once upon a time, the only reliable consumer information on a food label was the name of the food inside. The 1990 Nutrition Labeling and Education Act changed that forever with a spiffy new set of consumer-friendly food labels that include

- A mini-nutrition guide showing the food's nutrient content and evaluating its place in a balanced diet

- Accurate ingredient listings, with all ingredients listed in order of their prominence in the food and clear identification of ingredients previously listed simply as *colorings* and *sweeteners*

- Scientifically-reliable information about the relationship between specific foods and specific chronic health conditions such as heart disease and cancer

These new labels are *de rigueur* for more than 90 percent of all processed, packaged foods, everything from canned soup to "fresh" pasteurized orange juice. Food sold in really small packages — a pack of gum, for example — can omit the nutrition label but must carry a telephone number or address so that an inquisitive consumer (you) can call or write for the information.

Just about the only processed foods exempted from the nutrition labeling regulations are those with no appreciable amounts of nutrients or those whose content varies from batch to batch:

✔ Plain (unflavored) coffee and tea

✔ Some spices and flavorings

✔ Deli and bakery items prepared fresh in the store where they are sold directly to the consumer and food produced by small companies

✔ Food sold in restaurants, unless it makes a nutrition content or health claim (How do you eat well when eating out? Check out Chapter 18.)

Labels are voluntary for fresh raw meat, fish, or poultry, and fresh fruits and vegetables, but many markets — perhaps under pressure from customers (Hint! Hint!) — do put posters or brochures with generic nutrition information near the meat counter or produce bins.

Just the facts, ma'am

The star of the new food labels is the Nutrition Facts chart on the back (or side) of the package. This chart has three important elements: serving sizes, amounts of nutrients per serving, and percent Daily Value. (See Figure 17-7.)

Nutrition Facts
Serving Size 1/2 cup (122 g)
Servings Per Container about 3.5

Amount Per Serving

Calories 40	Fat Cal. 5
	% Daily Value*
Total Fat 0.5 g	**1%**
Sodium 5 mg	**0%**
Total Carb. 9 g	**3%**
Fiber 5 g	**21%**
Sugars 4 g	
Protein 2 g	

Vitamin A 300% (80% as beta-carotene)	
Calcium 2%	Iron 4%

Not a significant source of saturated fat, cholesterol, and vitamin C.
*Percent Daily Values are based on a 2,000 calorie diet.

Figure 17-7: A typical Nutrition Facts chart.

Serving size: This varies from package to package. Serving sizes don't always reflect the typical amount that an adult may eat. In some cases, the serving size may be a very small amount.

Calories: The calories contained in a single serving.

% daily values: The percentage of nutrients that one serving contributes to a 2,000-calorie diet. Parents or children may need more or less than 2,000 calories per day.

Nutrient amounts: The nutritional values of the most important, but not all, vitamins and other nutrients in the product.

Serving size

No need to stretch your brain trying to translate gram-servings or ounce-servings into real servings. This label does it for you, listing the servings in comprehensible kitchen terms such as one cup or one waffle or two pieces or one teaspoon. It also tells you how many servings are in the package.

The serving size is exactly the same for all products in a category. In other words, the Nutrition Facts chart allows you to compare at a glance the nutrient content for two different brands of yogurt, Cheddar cheese, string beans, soft drinks, and so on.

When you check the labels, the suggested serving sizes may seem small (especially with so-called lowfat items). Think of these serving sizes as useful guides.

Amount per serving

The Nutrition Facts chart tells you the amount (per serving) for several important nutrients:

- ✔ Calories
- ✔ Calories from fat
- ✔ Total fat (in grams)
- ✔ Saturated fat (in grams)
- ✔ Cholesterol (in milligrams)
- ✔ Total carbohydrate (in grams)
- ✔ Dietary fiber (in grams)
- ✔ Sugars (in grams)
- ✔ Protein (in grams)

Percent Daily Value

The "percent Daily Value" enables you to judge whether a specific food is high, medium or low in fat, cholesterol, sodium, carbohydrates, dietary fiber, sugars, protein, vitamin A, vitamin C, calcium, and iron.

The percent Daily Value for vitamins and minerals is based on a set of recommendations called the *reference daily intakes (RDI),* which are similar, but not identical, to the recommended dietary allowances (RDAs) for vitamins and minerals in Chapter 10 and Chapter 11.

RDIs are based on allowances set in 1973, so some RDIs are now out of date. For example, the Daily Value for calcium is 1,000 milligrams, but many studies — and two National Institutes of Health Conferences — suggest that post-menopausal women who are not using hormone replacement therapy should consume 1,500 milligrams calcium a day to reduce their risk of osteoporosis.

The percent Daily Value for fats, carbohydrates, protein, sodium, and potassium is based on the *daily reference values (DRV)*. DRVs are standards for nutrients such as fat and fiber known to raise or lower the risk of certain health conditions such as heart disease and cancer. For example, the Dietary Guidelines for Americans suggest that no more than 30 percent of your daily calories should come from fat. That means a 2,000-calorie-a-day diet should have no more than 600 calories from fat. To translate fat calories to grams of fat (the units used in the DRVs), divide the number of calories (600) by 9 (the number of calories in one gram of fat). The answer: 67, slightly higher than the actual DRV. But close enough.

Nutritionists use similar calculations to set the DRVs for

- Saturated fat (10 percent of your calories/9 calories a gram)

- Carbohydrates (60 percent of your calories/4 calories a gram)

- Dietary fiber (11.5 percent of your calories/4 calories a gram)

- Protein (10 percent of your calories/4 calories a gram)

Health claims

Ever since man (and woman) came out of the caves, people have been making health claims for certain foods. These folk remedies are comforting, but the evidence to support them is mostly anecdotal: "I had a cold. My mom gave me chicken soup, and here I am, all bright and bushy-tailed. Of course, it did take a week to really feel better. . . ."

The health claims approved by the USDA and the Food and Drug Administration (FDA) for inclusion on the new food labels are another matter entirely. If you see one of these statements suggesting that a particular food or nutrient plays a role in reducing your risk of a specific medical condition, you can be absolutely 100-percent sure that a real relationship exists between the food and the medical condition. You can also be sure that scientific evidence from well-designed studies support the claim.

In other words, the USDA/FDA-approved health claims are medically sound and scientifically specific. They highlight the known relationships between

- **Calcium and bone density:** A label describing a food as "high in calcium" may truthfully say: "A diet high in calcium helps women maintain healthy bones and may reduce the risk of osteoporosis later in life."

✔ **A high-fat diet and a higher risk of cancer:** A label describing a food as "low in fat" may truthfully say: "A diet low in fat reduces the risk of coronary heart disease."

✔ **A diet high in fat, saturated fat, and cholesterol and a higher risk of heart disease:** A label describing a food as "lowfat, low cholesterol" or "no fat, no cholesterol" may truthfully say: "This food follows the recommendations of the American Heart Association's diet to lower the risk of heart disease."

✔ **A high-fiber diet and a lower risk of some kinds of cancer:** A label describing a food as "high-fiber" may truthfully say: "Foods high in dietary fiber may reduce the risk of certain types of cancer."

✔ **A high-fiber diet and a lower risk of heart attack:** A label describing a food as "high-fiber" may truthfully say: "Foods high in dietary fiber may help reduce the risk of coronary heart disease."

✔ **Sodium and hypertension (high blood pressure):** A label describing a food as "low-sodium" may truthfully say: "A diet low in sodium may reduce the risk of high blood pressure."

✔ **A fruit-and-vegetable-rich diet and a low risk of some kinds of cancer:** Labels on fruits and vegetables may truthfully say: "A diet high in fruits and vegetables may lower your risk of some kinds of cancer."

✔ **Folic acid (folate) and a lower risk of neural tube (spinal cord) birth defects such as spina bifida:** Labels on folate-rich foods may truthfully say, "A diet rich in folates during pregnancy lowers the risk of neural tube defects in the fetus."

Which leaves you with only two questions: What's "high"? What's "low"? See the next section.

How high is high? How low is low?

Today, savvy consumers reach almost automatically for packages labeled "Low Fat" or "High Fiber." But it's a dollars-to-doughnuts sure bet that hardly one shopper in a thousand actually knows what "low" and "high" mean.

Because these are potent terms that promise real health benefits, the new labeling law has created strict, science-based definitions:

✔ *High* means that one serving provides 20 percent or more of the Daily Value for a particular nutrient. Other ways to say "high" are "rich in" or "excellent source," as in "milk is an excellent source of calcium."

✔ *Good source* means one serving gives you 10 to 19 percent of the Daily Value for a particular nutrient.

✔ *Light* (sometimes written *lite*) is used in connection with calories, fat, or sodium. It means the product has one-third fewer calories, or 50 percent less fat, or 50 percent less sodium than usually found in this type of product.

✔ *Low* means that the food contains an amount of a nutrient that allows you to eat several servings without going over the Daily Value for that nutrient.

- *Low calorie* means 40 calories or less per serving

- *Lowfat* means 3 grams of fat or less

- *Low saturated fat* means 1 gram or less

- *Low cholesterol* means 20 milligrams or less

✔ *Free* means "negligible" — not "none."

- *Calorie-free* means fewer than 5 calories per serving

- *Fat free* means less than 0.5 grams of fat

- *Cholesterol-free* means less than 2 milligrams of cholesterol or 2 grams or less saturated fat

- *Sodium-free* or *salt-free* means less than 5 milligrams of sodium

- *Sugar-free* means less than 0.5 grams of sugar

Bonus! Bonus! Bonus!

The extra added attraction on the new food label is the totally complete ingredient listing, with every single ingredient listed in order of its weight: heaviest first, lightest last. In addition, the label must spell out the true identity of some classes of ingredients known to cause allergic reactions:

✔ Vegetable proteins (*hydrolyzed corn protein* rather than the old-fashioned *hydrolyzed vegetable protein*)

✔ Milk products (*nondairy* products such as coffee whiteners may contain the milk protein caseinate, which comes from milk)

✔ F D & C yellow No. 5, a full, formal chemical name instead of *coloring*

Naming the precise source of sweeteners (*corn sugar monohydrate* rather than just *sugar monohydrate*) is still voluntary. But — as with information about raw meat, fish, and poultry — manufacturers and stores just may respond to consumer pressure. (Repeat advice: Hint! Hint!)

"Organic" and "health": Two label terms in search of a meaning

Two highly-charged food words are "organic" (as in "organic food") and "health" (as in "health food"). Do you know what they mean? Don't be embarrassed to say no. Neither do most health professionals.

To a chemist, "organic" means a substance that contains carbon, hydrogen, and oxygen. By this chemical standard, all foods — and all human beings — are organic.

Yet some people use organic to describe plant foods grown without pesticides or synthetic chemicals, or to describe the poultry, fish, beef, and lamb from animals raised on a diet with no antibiotics or other medicating chemicals to assure healthy and efficiently-producing animals.

But these descriptions are not standards regulated by any federal agency. So USDA is currently attempting to create regulations that will legally define the term organic.

✔ In December 1997, USDA released its first proposal on new standards for "organic foods."

✔ In May 1998, after receiving more than 280,000 comments from the public, food growers, and food marketers, the agency announced that although bio-engineered and irradiated foods are safe, they may not carry the "organic" label.

✔ In October 1998, USDA issued three more proposals on how animals yielding organic food are to be treated and how the agency will certify producers of organic foods.

Final rules are now expected sometime late in 1999 or early in the year 2000. As for "health food," an imprecise term applied indiscriminately to yummy good stuff such as high protein, lowfat pasta made from artichoke flour and yummy are-you-kidding-stuff such as high-fat carob candy bars, that remains a term used at the manufacturers' discretion.

Until someone proposes a more concrete definition for "health food" or USDA regulations on which foods can be labeled "organic" are finalized, organic foods and health foods may still be satisfying and delicious.

But the label terms are apt to leave you hungry — for more information.

How to Use the Food Guide Pyramid and New Food Labels

The food pyramids and the new food labels are easy to use. Compulsive list-makers may even think they're fun. Here are some possibilities: The food pyramid is a dandy shopper's helper. You can use the food guide pyramids to set up shopping lists.

Copy the two empty pyramids in Figures 17-5 and 17-6 and stick them on your fridge. During the week, make a shopping list by filling in the blanks on the pyramid of your choice. For example, pasta goes into the box for grains at the bottom of either pyramid. Margarine goes in the "fats and sweets" box at the top of the USDA pyramid. Parmesan cheese for your pasta goes in the "cheese and yogurt" box on the Mediterranean pyramid. And so on.

When it's time to zip out to the supermarket, check the shopping-list pyramid. Add or subtract items as required to bring your shopping list into line with the nutritional guidelines of the pyramid you've chosen. Too heavy on meat? Eliminate one meat purchase and add dry beans to your Mediterranean pyramid, or swap beans for meat in the meat section of the USDA pyramid. When the whole thing looks about right, it's time to shop. Neat, isn't it?

The Nutrition Facts label allows you to eat your cake — nutritiously. At the supermarket, use the Nutrition Facts chart to compare products and choose the best alternatives.

Here's a good example. You find yourself irresistibly drawn to double dark chocolate ice cream (lots of fat, saturated fat, cholesterol, and a whopping 230 calories per ½ cup serving). But then, just as your hand is opening the freezer door, ready to reach for the ice cream, suddenly . . . out of the corner of your eye, you see the Nutrition Facts chart on the label on the no-fat but equally irresistible chocolate sorbet. It says, "No fat, no saturated fat, no cholesterol, and only 90 to 130 calories per serving." When you put the labels side-by-side, do you need to ask which one comes out the winner?

The food pyramid helps balance meals and individual dishes. Back home in the kitchen, when you start to prepare meals, you increase the nutritional value by thinking of individual dishes as mini-food pyramids.

For example, you can improve the nutritional status of that low-fat, high-sugar irresistible chocolate sorbet by adding high-fiber complex carbohydrate cereal flakes and raisins (lowfat, plus C and B vitamins). Now your reasonable sweet dessert is a three-food-group hit: grains, fruit, and sweets.

Or you may serve up a nutritional home run with a combination food such as burritos, newly popular among citizens who have never been closer to Mexico than a lunch at Taco Bell.

The following shows two versions of the burrito, one based on the USDA Food Guide Pyramid, the other based on the Mediterranean Diet Pyramid. Both are lowfat, high-fiber, and packed with plenty of vitamins, minerals, and other nutrients. And both satisfy virtually anyone's personal standards of good-to-eat. With no-fat, virtually-nothing-but-flavor hot sauce, of course.

The USDA Food Guide Pyramid Burrito:

> 2 ounces of chicken = one meat group serving
>
> one tortilla = one grain group serving
>
> 3 tablespoons cheese = ½ milk group serving
>
> ⅓ cup chopped tomato = ½ vegetable group serving
>
> ½ cup shredded lettuce = ½ vegetable group serving

The Mediterranean Diet Pyramid Burrito:

> ½ cup cooked red beans
>
> one tortilla
>
> 3 tablespoons lowfat cheese
>
> ⅓ cup chopped tomato
>
> ½ cup shredded lettuce
>
> ¼ cup shredded onions

Strategies for smart snacking

Do you get really hungry every afternoon around 4 p.m.? So hungry that your stomach growls?

Does this make you so testy that you consider emigrating to some place like Great Britain, where everyone knows that a normal human being needs an extra meal between lunch and dinner? Does your desperation trip you into a snack of the food uglies — stuff that adds calories without contributing nutrients?

Will you be even the teensiest bit surprised to hear that the food pyramids and the food labels can help you avoid this dilemma?

Here's how:

- ✔ Use the food pyramid to choose munchies that are a valuable part of your overall daily diet.
- ✔ Use the Nutrition Chart on food labels to pick foods that satisfy hunger while conforming to nutritional guidelines.

As for actual choices, although you know that fruits and veggies are good snacks, that doesn't mean that you're stuck with boring carrot sticks or an apple.

The food pyramid says "fruits and vegetables," not raw fruits and raw vegetables. Yes, a fresh apple's fine. But so is a baked apple (100 calories), fragrant with cinnamon and decorated with no-fat sour cream (30-45 calories for two tablespoons). Carrot strips are okay. So are vegetarian baked beans — yes, baked beans (140 calories plus 26 grams of carbohydrates, 7 grams of protein, 7 grams of dietary fiber, and 2 grams of fat per ½ cup serving).

Given the prevalence of the microwave in offices as well as home kitchens, taming the 4 p.m. hungries without sacrificing your diet principles is easy.

The Final Word on Diagrams and Stats

At the beginning of this chapter, I warned you that keeping track of all the facts might be difficult. But now I think that you can pretty much boil them all down to one nutritional Golden Rule exemplified by the food pyramids and the Nutrition Facts food label:

> *Keep things in proportion.*

Come to think of it, that's not a bad philosophy for life.

Chapter 18

Eating Smart When Eating Out

● ●

In This Chapter

▶ Adapting a restaurant menu to your nutritional needs

▶ Evaluating menu health claims

▶ Understanding the nutrition value of fast food

▶ Getting the lowdown on brand name fast food items

● ●

*E*ating out is in. You don't have to cook, and somebody else washes the dishes. The challenge is to avoid letting luxury lull you into ceding responsibility for your food choices to some chef whose heart belongs to butter. This chapter lays out strategies for making your excellent adventure nutritionally sound. You find out how to edit a menu in a *white-tablecloth* restaurant (the food professional's description of an upscale eatery) to balance gustatory pleasure with commonsense nutrition. And you figure out how to juggle fast food so as to fill out a nutrient-rich food guide pyramid (described in Chapter 17).

No cooking, no dishes, no guilt. Who could ask for anything more?

How to Edit a Posh Restaurant Menu

From a nutritional point of view, restaurant dining *de luxe* has three basic pitfalls:

✔ The serving sizes are too big.

✔ The garnishes and side dishes are too rich.

✔ The meal has too many courses.

Not to worry. Exercise a little care and caution, and you can order from any menu, secure in the knowledge that pleasing your palate doesn't mean tossing away all nutritional common sense. The following list of strategies can make any restaurant experience a joy.

Keep the first course simple

Set the nutritional tone of dinner right off the bat with your choice of appetizer. You have two possible alternatives. The first alternative is to opt for a really rich, high-density food such as pâté de foie gras (literally: fat liver paste) and then coast downward, calorie-fat-and-cholesterol-wise, for the rest of the meal. A second alternative is to choose a tasty but low-calorie, lowfat appetizer such as clear soup, a salad with lemon juice dressing, or shellfish such as shrimp cocktail (10 to 30 calories a shrimp) with no-fat (catsup/horseradish) sauce. This choice allows you more food later on.

Order an appetizer as a main dish

My favorite New York City restaurant, a bistro on Second Avenue, serves an appetizer consisting of a really big (and I mean huge) bowl of maybe 25 steamed mussels in their shells in a tomato-based sauce with one crusty piece of French bread underneath to sop it up with. When I add a glass of cold, dry white wine and one more piece of bread, this appetizer becomes a meal in itself. With a lot fewer calories and less fat than most any entry on the menu. Cheaper, too.

Don't butter the bread

Don't oil it, either. Many chic and trendy restaurants now serve up a dish of flavored olive oil in place of butter. True, the olive oil has less saturated fat than butter, and it has no cholesterol. But the calorie count is exactly the same. All fats and oils (butter, margarine, vegetable oils) give you about 100 calories a tablespoon. Don't take my word for it: Check it out in the Appendix, which has the complete list of nutrients in hundreds of different foods. *Note:* You may get even more calories from the oil if you do a lot of dipping.

Consumer alert: Don't assume that your bread is lowfat just because you didn't butter it. Many different types of bread come already buttered (or oiled). One example is foccacia, the newly-popular, thick squares of savory Italian bread. Others are popovers and muffins.

To test the fat content of your bread, pick up a piece or put it on your napkin. If your hand feels sticky or the bread leaves an oily spot on your napkin, you have your answer.

Call for naked vegetables

Victorians boiled vegetables into a yucky muck — no color, no texture, no taste. Then came butter, cheese, and cream sauces, often burnished under the broiler to a browned crust. Now, smart restaurant cooks rely on herbs and spices, reduced (boiled down and thickened) fat-free bouillons, unusual salad combinations, and imaginative treatments such as purees and kabobs to make their vegetables tasty but trim. The result? Food heaven and nutrition joy. The vegetable flavors come through, and the calories stay very, very, very low.

To reap the low-calorie rewards, avoid veggie dishes labeled

- ✔ Au beurre (with butter)
- ✔ Au gratin (with cheese sauce)
- ✔ Batter-dipped
- ✔ Breaded
- ✔ Fritters (fried)
- ✔ Fritto (fried)
- ✔ Hollandaise (sauce with butter and egg yolks)
- ✔ Tempura (battered and fried)

Minimize the main dish

I won't insult you by telling you to avoid fried foods. If you're reading this book, you already know that the best choice is something broiled, baked, or roasted — without added fat, and with the drippings siphoned off. But I can't avoid noting that you can lower the fat content of any main dish simply by wielding a mean knife and fork to cut away the vestiges of fat.

Another approach is to order a main course meat dish without the main part. That is, have your meat, fish, or poultry in your small-serving appetizer, and then ask your waiter to assemble a dish of veggies as an entree. It may be pricey to have a special dish assembled, and you may have to beg a bit, but most reputable restaurants will work with you. Especially if you point out that your strategy is allowing you to order three dishes — appetizer, main dish, and dessert (well, at least something sweet; more about that later) — instead of one.

What you want are all the nifty little extras that come with the meat course. Not that boring steamed stuff. And definitely not veggies so raw they have no taste. The difference between raw cauliflower and cauliflower that's been steamed for 30 minutes, then dusted with dill, is so vast that people who insist on passing out the stuff cold should be charged with vegetable abuse.

Demand tiny boiled onions. Baby peas with mint. Pickled beets and red cabbage. Sugared carrots. Sautéed spinach. Darling little boiled or baked potatoes with a crust of paprika or cumin. The more, the merrier. The result may not be entirely fat-free, but it will almost certainly have fewer calories, more fiber, less fat, and a wider variety of vitamins than plain meat or poultry.

Control the portions

Restaurants do not make friends by serving up teensy little portions. In fact, tiny servings probably sank "nouvelle cuisine," the late '80s fad that put one string bean, three garden peas, one half artichoke heart, and one sliced cherry tomato on three lettuce leaves and called it the salad course.

Reality dictates that the portions on restaurant plates will rarely come within hailing distance of the official serving sizes issued by the U.S. Department of Agriculture. To protect yourself against humongous portions, you need to store real-life versions of the "recommended" portions in your memory banks. To do that, use an 8-ounce measuring cup and a kitchen scale to run through some basic practice drills at home:

- ✔ Broil a small steak or roast a chicken breast. Use the kitchen scale to weigh a 3-ounce portion. Does the steak look like a deck of cards? How about a small calculator? That's one serving.

- ✔ Boil some rice. After the rice is done, fill the measuring cup to the half mark. Take out the rice and roll it into a tennis ball or a billiard ball. Hey, whatever. That's one serving.

- ✔ Shred some greens. Fill the measuring cup to the 8-ounce mark. Turn the greens out onto a salad plate. That's one serving.

- ✔ Open one can of beets or one can of fruit cocktail. Fill the measuring cup to the halfway mark with one or the other. Spoon the beets or fruit onto a plate. That's one serving.

- ✔ Open a can of soda. Pour it into the measuring cup, right up to the 8-ounce mark. Pour that into a glass. Add some ice. It's probably more than you get in an upscale restaurant, less than you get at the burger barn. No matter: It's still one certified USDA serving.

Now that you have a picture of a serving in your mind, you can slice away the extra from your restaurant plate — and take it home for lunch or dinner the next day. That's what "doggie bags" are for.

Sideline the sauces

Dining out is a treat, so treat yourself — within reason. You can have your béarnaise (egg yolks, butter), béchamel (butter, flour, heavy cream), brown sauce (beef drippings, flour), and hollandaise (butter, egg yolks), as long as you have them in reasonable amounts.

Ask the waiter to bring the sauce on the side, take one tablespoonful (about a soup spoonful), and hand the rest back to the waiter. When ordering from an Italian menu, the general rule is to avoid the olive-oil-based white sauces and choose the tomato-based red sauce. Many restaurants now make their red sauces skinny — all tomato, little or no oil. If the chef where you're eating fattens up the tomato sauce with olive oil, forget this rule.

Share dessert — or substitute espresso

After a heavy meal, your body often craves something sweet. Lower your calories, fat, and so on by splitting a dessert with your dinner partner. Or opt for rich but fat-free sweetened coffees: Espresso, Greek, and Turkish brews seem most satisfying. Hate coffee? Have a cola.

Ask for proof

When the menu says, "Eat me. I'm healthy!" — ask for proof. The people who make and market processed foods are required by law to provide detailed ingredient labels on their packages. Restaurants are ordinarily exempt. They don't have to tell you exactly what's in the beef Stroganoff or vegetable stir-fry. The exception is a dish for which the restaurant makes a health claim.

The restaurant may write "lowfat" or "heart-healthy" next to the item on the menu or mark the entry with a little red heart to signify the same thing. When a restaurant does this, the Nutrition Education and Labeling Act says it has to back it up. The law is flexible; it does not require an ingredient listing on the menu, but it says that the restaurant can comply by making a notebook available that accomplishes at least one of the two following tasks:

✔ The notebook can list the nutrient content of each labeled dish or show that the dish was made according to a recipe from an authoritative professional association or dietary group, such as the American Heart Association.

✔ The notebook can show that the nutritional values for the dish are based on a reliable nutrition guide such as USDA's voluminous Handbook #8, several volumes with perhaps a thousand pages of nutritional analysis for all kinds of food. As with the new improved labels on food packages, this policy is designed to make sure that any food that claims to be "healthy" really is.

Surviving on Fast Food

Fast food can be good food. Choose carefully, and you can enjoy burgers while still meeting the recommended daily dietary allowances for all important vitamins and minerals. A fast-food burger on a bun, plus a salad, and a small, lowfat milk shake or a cup (8-ounce) milk or a small Coke may not sound like great nutrition, but the version served up in fast-food restaurants can actually be relatively low in fat and relatively high in valuable nutrients.

Table 18-1 compares the nutrient values of three basic McDonald's meals. All three meals meet current USDA recommendations that no more than 30 percent of your calories should come from fat (although Meal #1 is high in saturated fat). They meet cholesterol guidelines and provide lots of vitamin A and vitamin C. Meal #1 and Meal #2 are also calcium-rich.

✔ The "burger" is the basic, small, no-frills hamburger.

✔ The "garden salad" includes one packet of fat-free herb vinaigrette dressing.

✔ The shake is a small (414 milliliters or about 14 ounces) vanilla shake.

✔ The milk is an 8-ounce container of lowfat (1 percent) milk.

✔ The cola is a 16-ounce cup (small).

The initials DV stand for Daily Value, a nutritional guideline suggesting how much of each nutrient you should get each day on a 2,000-calorie diet. For the complete skinny on the DV and how it is used on food labels, check out Chapter 17.

Stop! Before you bite into that burger, remember that the following chart is only a guide. Menus and ingredients may change, so check the nutrition brochure at your local burger haven.

Table 18-1	Nutritious Fast-Food Meals? Yes, Nutritious Fast-Food Meals.		
Nutrient Values	*Meal*		
	Burger, Garden Salad, Small Lowfat Vanilla Shake	*Burger, Garden Salad, Milk*	*Burger, Garden Salad, Small Coke*
Calories	710	450	490
% calories from fat	24%	24%	16%
% DV saturated fat	47%	26%	17%
% DV cholesterol	23%	13%	10%
% DV dietary fiber	22%	21%	21%
% DV vitamin A	130%	130%	120%
% DV vitamin C	50%	50%	45%
% DV calcium	50%	45%	15%

Source: The McDonald's Corporation

The fast-food pyramid

Talk about smart marketing — the folks at Wendy's have come up with a real doozy — a diagram showing how to fit Wendy's menu items into the USDA Food Guide Pyramid, the good-for-you guide I describe in Chapter 17.

Trans fat: The Boooo! factor

Once upon a time, fast-food restaurants — indeed, most restaurants — fried up their foods in butter, which is loaded with saturated fat and cholesterol that gum up your arteries and increase your risk of heart disease. Then, prodded by the Food Police, restaurants switched to vegetable fats, which are low in saturated fat and have no cholesterol. Hooray? Well, not exactly. Instead of using heart-healthy vegetable oils, fast-food restaurants use solid vegetable shortenings, a crucial difference. The shortenings are solid because they contain "hydrogenated" vegetable oils. Chapter 7 explains the chemistry of hydrogenation (adding hydrogen atoms to fats).

Hydrogenated vegetable oils are high in trans fatty acids, a form of fat that may clog your arteries as efficiently as saturated fats and cholesterol. An order of fries may have as much artery-hostile fat as a 4-ounce burger. Boooo!

You don't have to be Albert Einstein to realize how valuable this promotional tool can be to customers. If you're a vegetarian or if you prefer the Mediterranean Diet (which relies less heavily on meat than does the USDA Pyramid), you can easily adapt the Wendy's pyramid, eliminating the meat and substituting — ruffles and flourishes please! — Wendy's broccoli and cheese baked potato (for less fat, leave off the cheese). Figure 18-1 shows Wendy's smart adaptation.

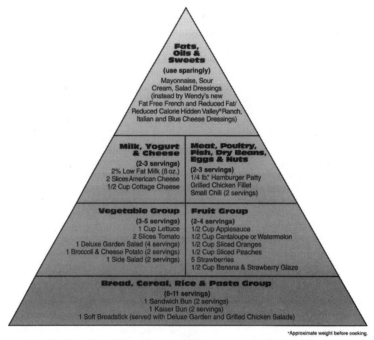

Figure 18-1:
Morphing
the USDA
Food Guide
Pyramid into
Wendy's
Food
Pyramid.

Source: Wendy's International, Inc.

Fast food ingredient guides

The reason it was so easy to put together the information in Figure 18-1 is that, like their more expensive cousins, fast-food restaurants that make health claims for their food must also make nutrition information available. If brochures aren't available at your local store, don't be shy: Write or call for a copy or check out the restaurant's Web site.

Burger King Corporation
Consumer Relations
17777 Old Cutler Road
Miami, Florida 33157
Phone: 305-378-7011
www.burgerking.com

KFC (Kentucky Fried Chicken)
Public Affairs Department
KFC Corporation
P.O. Box 32070
Louisville, Kentucky 40232
www.kentuckyfriedchicken.com

McDonald's Nutrition Information Center
McDonald's Corporation
Oak Brook, Illinois 60521
Phone: 630-623-FOOD
www.mcdonalds.com/food/nutrition

Wendy's International Inc.
Customer Service Department
4288 W. Dublin-Granville Rd.
Dublin, Ohio 43017
Phone: 614-764-3100
www.wendys.com/the_menu/nut_frame.html

Part IV
Food Processing

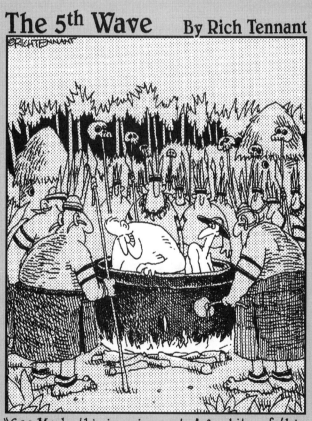

The 5th Wave   By Rich Tennant

"Gee, Mark - this is an iron pot. A few bites of this stew should help you shake that anemia."

In this part . . .

*H*ave you ever wondered why canned green beans aren't as green as fresh ones? Or why an originally translucent egg white turns white when you cook it? Or why frozen carrots are mushy when you defrost them? Or — modern technology at its most mysterious — why exposing food to radiation keeps it fresh longer? Wonder no more. Just shift your eyes to the right to find out what happens when you cook, freeze, dry, or zap food.

Chapter 19

What Is Food Processing?

In This Chapter

▶ A definition of food processing

▶ The four goals of food processing

▶ The advantages of food processing

▶ Nutritional benefits of processed food

This chapter is not the liveliest one in this book. In fact, it is sort of like a study guide for the next three chapters, written to bring you up to speed on the goals and techniques of food processing. The information here is pretty rudimentary: A catalog of the basic food-processing techniques, a direct explanation of how these techniques make food more (or less) palatable, a nifty home experiment to demonstrate the results of bacterial action on ordinary food (a raw chicken leg/a piece of cheese), and a very short guide to the potential health benefits of enriched, altered, or fake foods.

Can you safely pass this by? Sure. Will you profit by stopping to browse? Definitely. The choice, as they say, is yours.

By the way, my personal nomination for liveliest chapter is Chapter 3. I like it because it explains how (and why) to be sensible about your weight, rather than spending precious time and energy trying to fit your body into someone else's one-size-fits-all scheme. Try it. You'll like it.

What Food Processing Is

Say "processed food" and most people think "cheese spread." They're right, of course. Cheese spread is a processed food. But so are baked potatoes, canned tuna, frozen peas, skim milk, pasteurized orange juice, and scrambled eggs. In broad terms, food processing is any technique that alters the natural state of food — everything from cooking to freezing to pickling to drying and more and more and more.

Each form of processing changes food from a living thing (animal or vegetable) into an integral component of your healthful diet. Overall, food processing aims to

- Lengthen shelf life
- Reduce the risk of food-borne illnesses
- Maintain or improve texture and flavor
- Upgrade the nutritional value of foods

How Processing Preserves Food

"Natural" does not necessarily translate as "safe" or "good to eat." Food spoils (naturally) when microbes living (naturally) on the surface of the meat, carrot, peach, or whatever reproduce (naturally) to a population level that overwhelms the food.

Sometimes you can see, feel, or smell this happening. Mold grows on cheese. Meat or chicken begin to feel slippery. Milk smells sour. The mold on the cheese, the slippery slickness on the surface of the meat or chicken, and the odor of the milk are caused by microbes growing out of control. Don't even argue with them; throw out the food.

All food processing is designed to prevent what happens to the chicken (or the cheese). It aims to preserve food and extend its shelf life (the period of time when it is safe and nutritious) by stemming the natural tide of biological destruction. This section discusses how food processing works.

Wait! Not all microbes are bad guys. We use "good" ones to ferment milk to yogurt and to make wines and beers.

Preservative method #1: Temperature control

Exposing food to high heat for a sufficiently long period of time reduces the natural population of bacterial spoilers, killing microbes that may otherwise make you sick. For example, pasteurization (heating milk or other liquids such as fruit juice to 145–154.4°F for 30 minutes) kills all disease-causing and most other bacteria, as does high-temperature, short-time pasteurization (161°F for 15 seconds).

Chilling also protects food. It works by slowing the rate of microbial reproduction. For example:

- ✔ Milk refrigerated at 50°F or lower may stay fresh for almost a week because the cold prevents organisms that survived pasteurization or are present in the fridge from developing or reproducing.

- ✔ Fresh chicken frozen to 0°F or lower may remain safe for up to 12 months (whole) or 9 months (cut up).

Preservative method #2: Removing the water

Like all living things, microbes on food need water. Dehydrate the food and the bugs won't reproduce so that the food stays fresher longer. That's the rationale behind raisins, prunes, and pemmican, a dried mix of meat, fat, and berries adapted from East Coast Native Americans and served to 18th- and 19th-century sailors of every national stripe. Dehydration (loss of water) occurs when food is

- ✔ Exposed to air and sunlight
- ✔ Heated for several hours in a very low (250°F) oven or smoked (the smokehouse acts as a very low oven)

Preservative method #3: Controlling the air flow

Just as microbes need water, they also need air. Reducing the air supply almost always reduces the bacterial population. The exception is *anaerobic* (meaning "without air") bacteria, such as botulinum organisms, that thrive in the absence of air. Go figure!

Foods are protected from air by vacuum-packaging. A vacuum — from *vacuus,* the Latin word for *empty* — is a space with virtually no air. Vacuum-packaging is done on a container (generally a plastic bag or a glass jar) from which the air is removed before sealing. When you open a vacuum-packed container, you hear a sudden little pop as the vacuum is broken.

If there's no pop, the seal has already been broken, allowing air inside. This means the food inside may be spoiled or may have been tampered with. Do not taste-test: Throw out the entire package, food and all.

Preservative method #4: Chemical warfare

About two dozen chemicals are used as "food additives" or "food preservatives" to prevent spoilage. (If the mere mention of chemicals or food additives makes the hair on the back of your neck rise, chill out with Chapter 22.) Here are the most common chemical preservatives:

✔ **Acidifiers.** Most microbes do not thrive in highly acid settings, so a chemical that makes a food more acidic prevents spoilage. Wine and vinegar are acidifying chemicals; so is citric acid, the natural preservative in citrus fruits, and lactic acid, the naturally produced acid in yogurt.

✔ **Mold inhibitors.** Sodium benzoate, sodium propionate, and calcium propionate slow (but do not entirely stop) the growth of mold on bread. Sodium benzoate is also used to prevent the growth of molds in cheese, margarine, and syrups.

✔ **Bacteria-busters.** Salt is hydrophilic (hydro = water; phil = loving). When you cover fresh meat with salt, the salt draws water up and out of the meat — and up and out of the cells of bacteria living on the meat. Presto: The bacteria die; the meat dries. And you get to eat corned beef (large grains of salt were once known as corns).

Preservation method #5: Irradiation

Irradiation is a technique that exposes food to gamma radiation, a high-energy light stronger than the X rays your doctor uses to make a picture of your insides. Gamma rays (also known as pico rays) are ionizing radiation, the kind of radiation that kills living cells. As a result, irradiation prolongs the shelf life of food by

✔ Killing microbes and insects on plants (wheat, wheat powder, spices, dry vegetable seasonings)

✔ Preventing potatoes and onions from producing new sprouts at the eyes

✔ Slowing the rate at which some fruits ripen

✔ Killing disease-causing organisms such as Trichinella, Salmonella, E. coli, and Listeria (the organism responsible for a recent outbreak of food poisoning due to packaged meats and cold cuts) on meat and poultry

In 1998, the FDA (which had already approved the use of radiation for plant foods, pork, and poultry) put its stamp of approval on irradiating fresh red meat products as a way to enhance, but not replace, the safe handling and storage of meat in the processing plant, in the supermarket, and in your kitchen.

Here is a basic list of the methods used to extend the shelf life of food. Each method is explained in detail in Chapter 20, Chapter 21, or Chapter 22.

✔ **Temperature methods**

- Cooking

- Canning

- Refrigeration

- Freezing

✔ **Air control**

- Canning

- Vacuum packaging

✔ **Moisture control**

- Dehydration

✔ **Chemical methods**

- Acidification

- Mold inhibition

- Salting (dry salt or brine)

✔ **Irradiation**

How Processing Makes Food Safer

This section is short but sweet: Reducing or limiting the growth of food's natural microbe population not only lengthens shelf life, it also lowers the risk of food-borne illness. Increased food safety is a natural consequence of most processing that keep foods usable longer. Next.

Can the Concorde tenderize your steak?

Tough cuts of meat, such as chuck, are less expensive than tender cuts, such as sirloin, so a pot of gold awaits the person who comes up with an efficient way to tenderize beef in large batches right at the packing plant.

One contender for the gold ring may have emerged at the USDA's Beltsville Agriculture Research Center outside Washington, D.C., where food scientists have been experimenting with immersing meat in water and bombarding it with shock waves.

The process, called *Hydrodyning,* also appears to knock microbes off the meat.

Will the process tenderize meat without turning it to mush? Is it cost effective? Can you do the same thing by running outdoors to catch the sonic boom when the supersonic Concorde passes by? Only time will tell.

How Processing Makes Food Taste Better

One advantage of commercial food processing is that it allows you to enjoy things never seen in Nature — like the ever-popular cheese spread. A more prosaic benefit of food processing is that it intensifies aroma and flavor, almost always for the better. For example:

- **Drying concentrates flavor.** A prune has a different, darker, more intensely sweet flavor than a fresh plum. On the other hand, dried food can be hard and tough to chew. (Think beef jerky.)

- **Heating heightens aroma by quickening the movement of aroma molecules.** In fact, your first tantalizing hint of dinner is usually the scent of cooking food. Chilling has the opposite effect: It slows the movement of the molecules. To sense the difference, sniff a plate of cold roast beef versus hot roast beef straight from the oven. Or sniff two glasses of vodka, one warm, one icy from the freezer. One comes up scent-free. The other has the olfactory allure of pure gasoline. Guess which is which?

- **Warming foods also intensifies flavors.** This development is sometimes beneficial (warm roast beef is somehow more savory than cold roast beef), sometimes not (warm milk is definitely not as popular as the icy-cold version).

- **Finally, changing the temperature also changes texture.** Heating softens some foods (butternut squash is a good example) and solidifies others. (Think eggs.) Chilling keeps the fats in pâté firm so the stuff doesn't melt down into a puddle on the plate. Ditto for the gelatin that keeps dessert molds and dinner aspics standing upright.

How Processing Makes Food More Nutritious

Food processing not only makes a wide variety of seasonal foods (mostly fruits and vegetables) available all year long, it also enables food producers to improve the nutritional status of lots of basic foods by enriching or altering them to meet the needs of modern consumers. And last, but definitely not least, food processing gives us some totally fake but widely appreciated substitute fats and sweeteners.

Added nutrients

The addition of vitamins and minerals to basic foods has helped eliminate many once-common nutritional deficiency diseases. The practice is so common that you take the following for granted:

- Bread, cereals, and grains are given extra B vitamins to replace the vitamins lost when whole grains are stripped of their nutrient-rich covering to make white flour or white rice or de-germed cornmeal. This reduces the risk of the B vitamin deficiency diseases beriberi and pellagra.

- Bread, cereals, and grains are also given iron to replace what's lost in milling and make it possible for American women to reach the RDA (recommended daily dietary allowance) for this important mineral.

- All milk sold in the U.S. has added vitamin D to reduce the risk of the bone-deforming vitamin D deficiency diseases rickets (among children) and osteomalacia (among adults).

Altered foods

Dairy products are a good example of altered foods with lower natural fat, saturated fat, and cholesterol content. Skim milk — milk from which the fat has been removed — becomes a higher-calcium product when fat-free milk proteins are added to make a creamier liquid with less fat and cholesterol than whole milk.

Modern food chemistry can also make milk more digestible. Many people of Asian, middle Eastern, or African ancestry do not produce sufficient amounts of lactase, the enzyme needed to digest lactose, the sugar in milk. These people have no problems with yogurt, whose lactose has been partially predigested by lactase from the bacteria that thicken the milk and convert it to yogurt. Now grocers also carry lactose-free cheese and milk with added lactase.

Alternative fats

Fat carries desirable flavors and makes food "rich." But it is also high in calories and some fats (the saturated kind described in Chapter 7) can clog your arteries. One way to deal with this is to eliminate the fat from food (see milk, in the previous section). Another is to head for the food lab and create a no-or-low calorie, non-clogging substitute, such as Olestra/Olean or Simplesse.

Olestra/Olean

Olestra/Olean, approved by the FDA in 1996, is a no-calorie chemical from sugar and vegetable oils used in snack foods such as potato chips. Olestra is indigestible, which means it adds no calories, fat, or cholesterol to food. Unfortunately, as it speeds through your intestinal tract, it is likely to pick up and swoosh along some fat-soluble nutrients such as vitamin A, vitamin D, vitamin E, and cancer-fighting carotenoids (see Chapter 10).

One Harvard study suggests that eating three small servings of snack foods made with Olestra in one week can lower your blood concentrations of carotenoids 10 percent. Because carotenoids seem to protect against *macular degeneration,* an age-related loss of vision, the Boston data estimate that widespread use of Olestra might lead to as many as 600 extra cases of macular degeneration a year in the United States. Did I mention Olestra may also cause diarrhea when eaten in excess?

However, in the spring of 1998, an 18-member FDA Food Advisory Committee reaffirmed the agency's original decision that Olestra is safe for use in snack foods. The committee concluded that the fat alternative's gastrointestinal effects and its effects on carotenoid absorption do not significantly affect public health.

For more information about the activities of the FDA's Center for Food Safety and Applied Nutrition, which ran the tests evaluating Olestra, visit the Web site at vm.cfsan.fda.gov/list.HTML.

Simplesse

Simplesse is a low-calorie fat substitute made by heating and blending proteins from egg whites and/or milk into extremely tiny round balls that taste like fat. Simplesse has 1 to 2 calories a gram versus 9 calories a gram for real fats or oils. Simplesse is not recommended for young children, because they need the essential fatty acids in real fats, and it may be problematic for

- ✔ People sensitive to milk
- ✔ People sensitive to eggs
- ✔ People on low-protein diets (for example, kidney disease patients)

Substitute sweeteners

Here's a scientific tidbit. Most substitute sweeteners were discovered by accident in laboratories where researchers touched a paper or a pencil, then stuck their fingers in their mouths to discover, Eureka! It's sweet. As Harold McGee, author of *On Food and Cooking* (Collier Books, 1988), says: Fingers in the mouth? It makes you wonder what goes on in all those labs!

The best-known substitute sweeteners (in order of their discovery) are:

- **Saccharin:** This synthetic sweetener was discovered by accident (the fingers-in-the-mouth-syndrome) at Johns Hopkins in 1879. Proposed to be banned in 1977 after it was linked to bladder cancer in rats, it is still on the market, and diabetics who have used saccharin for years show no excess levels of bladder cancer. However, a warning label may appear with saccharin indicating that it is a mild rodent carcinogen. In December 1998, the executive committee of the National Toxicology Program (NTP) recommended that saccharin be taken off the list of suspected human carcinogens. (*Note:* Most people think saccharin is very sweet, but if you hate broccoli, you are likely to think saccharin is bitter. Check out Chapter 15 to see why.)

- **Cyclamates** *(cy-cla-mates)***:** These surfaced (on somebody's finger, of course) in 1937 at the University of Illinois. They were tied to cancer in laboratory animals and banned (1969) in the U.S., but not in Canada and many other countries. But there has never been any evidence of ill effects in human beings. Cyclamates are available for use as a table-top sweetener in Canada; in the U.S., the FDA is currently reconsidering its ban.

- **Aspartame:** Another accidental discovery (1965), this is a combination of two amino acids, aspartic acid and phenylalanine. The problem with aspartame is that, during digestion, it breaks down into its constituent ingredients. The same thing happens when aspartame is exposed to heat. That's trouble for people born with a phenylketonuria (PKU), a metabolic defect characterized by a lack of the enzyme needed to digest phenylalanine. The excess amino acid can pile up in brain and nervous tissue, leading to mental retardation in young children.

- **Sucralose:** Sucralose, which was discovered in 1976, is the only no-calorie sweetener made from sugar. Your body does not recognize it as a carbohydrate or a sugar, so it zips through your intestinal tract unchanged. More than 100 scientific studies conducted over a 20-year period attest to its safety, and the FDA has recently approved its use in a variety of foods, including baked goods, candies, substitute dairy products, and frozen desserts.

- **Acesulfame-K** (*a-see-sul-fame;* the *K* is the chemical symbol for potassium)**:** This artificial sweetener, with a chemical structure similar to saccharin, is found in baked goods, chewing gum, and other food products. In 1998, the FDA approved its use in soft drinks, whose shelf life it seems to prolong.

Table 19-1 compares the calorie content and sweetening power of sugar versus substitute sweeteners. For comparison, sugar has 4 calories a gram.

Table 19-1	Comparing Substitute Sweeteners	
Sweetener	*Calories Per Gram*	*Sweetness Relative to Sugar**
Sugar (sucrose)	4	
Acesulfame-K	0	150 – 200 times sweeter than sugar
Aspartame	4**	160 – 200 times sweeter than sugar
Cyclamates	0	30 – 60 times sweeter than sugar
Saccharin	0	200 – 700 times sweeter than sugar
Sucralose	0	600 times sweeter than sugar

*The range of sweetness reflects estimates from several sources.

**Aspartame has 4 calories per gram, but you need so little to get a sweet flavor that you can count it as 0 calories per serving.

A Last Word: Follow That Bird!

You can sum up the essence of food processing by following the trail of one chicken from the farm to your table. (Vegetarians are excused from this section.)

A chicken's first brush with processing comes right after slaughtering. It's plucked, cut into pieces, and packed off to the food processor or the supermarket. Either way, it travels on ice to slow the natural bacterial decomposition. In the food factory, your chicken may be boiled and canned whole, or boiled and cut up and canned in small portions like tuna fish, or boiled into chicken soup to be canned or dehydrated into bouillon cubes, or cooked with veggies and canned as chicken à la king, or fried and frozen in whole pieces, or roasted, sliced, and frozen into a chicken dinner, or . . . you get the picture (and if you don't, check out Figure 19-1).

If you buy a "fresh" (raw) chicken instead of a cooked one, you perform similar rituals in your own kitchen. First it goes to the refrigerator (or freezer), then to the stove for thorough cooking to make sure that no stray bacteria contaminates your dinner table (or you), then back to the fridge for the leftovers. In the end, the chicken's been processed. And you have eaten. That is the point of this story.

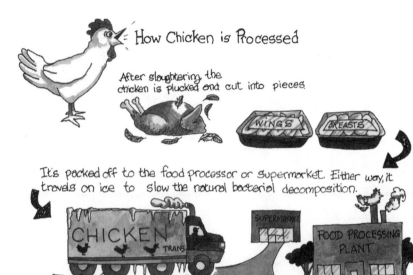

How Chicken is Processed

After slaughtering, the chicken is plucked and cut into pieces.

It's packed off to the food processor or supermarket. Either way, it travels on ice to slow the natural bacterial decomposition.

In the food factory, your chicken may be boiled and canned whole, or boiled and canned in small portions, or boiled into chicken soup, or dehydrated into bouillon cubes, fried or frozen into whole pieces, or.... you get the picture......

Figure 19-1:
From the farm to your table: chicken processing.

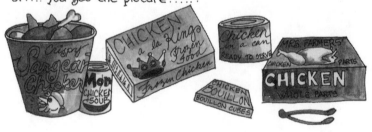

Chapter 20

Cooking and Nutrition

*Y*ou can bet that the first cooked dinner was an accident involving some poor wandering animal and a bolt of lightning that — zap! — charred the beast into medium sirloin. Then a caveman attracted by the aroma tore off a sizzled hunk, and forthwith offered up the first restaurant rating: "Yum."

After that, it was but a hop, a skip, and a jump, anthropologically speaking, to gas ranges, electric broilers, and microwave ovens. This chapter explains how these handy technologies affect the safety, nutritional value, appearance, flavor, and aroma of the foods that you heat.

What's Cooking?

Ever since man discovered fire and learned how to control cooking rather than having to wait for a passing thunderbolt, the human race has generally relied on three simple ways to heat food:

  ✔ **An open flame:** You hold the food directly over — or under — the flame or put the food on a griddle on top of the flame. The electric heating coil is a 20th-century variation on the open flame.

  ✔ **A closed box:** You put the food in a closed box (an oven) and heat the air in the oven to create high-temperature dry heat.

  ✔ **Hot liquid:** You submerge the food in hot liquid or suspend the food over the liquid so that it cooks in the steam escaping from the surface.

Cooking food in a wrapper such as aluminum foil combines two methods: open fire (the grill) or a closed box (the oven) plus the steam from the food's own juices (hot liquid).

Here are the basic methods used to cook food with heat generated by fire or an electric coil:

Open Flame	Hot Air	Hot Liquid
Broiling	Baking	Boiling
Grilling	Roasting	Deep-frying
Toasting		Poaching
		Simmering
		Steaming
		Stewing

How hot is boiling water?

Water is a molecule (H_2O) composed of three atoms: two hydrogens and one oxygen. When water is exposed to energy (heat), some of the water molecules vaporize (separate into their gaseous components). The vapors collect in tiny pockets at the bottom of the vessel (pot). Continued heating energizes the vapors; they begin to push up against the water.

To break through the water's surface, the vapors must acquire enough energy to equal the force (pressure) of the atmosphere (air) pushing down on the water. The temperature at which this happens is called the boiling point.

At sea level (elevation: 0 feet), the atmosphere is heavier (has more oxygen) than at higher elevations. That's why you breathe more easily in Miami (elevation: 10 feet) than atop Mt. McKinley in Alaska (elevation: 20,320 feet).

The heavier air at sea level exerts more pressure against the surface of the water in your pot, so making the water boil takes more energy (higher heat).

At sea level, the boiling point of water is 212°F (100° on the Centigrade — "C" — scale). As a general rule, the boiling point of water drops one degree Fahrenheit for every 500-foot increase in altitude over sea level. In other words, at an altitude 500 feet above sea level, the boiling point for water is 211°F (99.4°C); at 1,000 feet, it is 210°F (98.9°C).

The following chart shows the approximate boiling points for water in specific American cities.

Altitude	Place	Boiling Point F	Boiling Point C
Sea level	Atlantic City, NJ	212	100
500 feet	Austin, TX	211	99.4
5,000	Denver, CO	202	94.4
6,000	Cheyenne, WY	200	93.3
7,000	Santa Fe, NM	198	92.2

Source: The World Almanac and Book of Facts 1994 (Mahwah, NJ: World Almanac, 1993).

Note: How fast the water is boiling does not affect the temperature — a slow boil (few bubbles) is as hot as a fast one (lots of bubbles).

Converting between Fahrenheit and Centigrade

Pssst! Here's how to convert temperatures from Fahrenheit (F) to Centigrade (C) and back again:

1. degrees Centigrade = $\dfrac{(\text{degrees F} - 32)}{9} \times 5$

   For example, to convert the Fahrenheit boiling point of water (212°F) to the Centigrade boiling point of water (100°C):

   $$\dfrac{212 - 32 \times 5 = 100}{9}$$

2. degrees Fahrenheit = $\dfrac{(\text{degrees C}) \times 9}{5} + 32$

   For example, to convert the Centigrade boiling point of water (100°C) to the Fahrenheit boiling point of water (212° F):

   $$\dfrac{100 \times 9 + 32 = 212}{5}$$

Cooking with Electromagnetic Waves

A gas or electric stove generates thermal energy (heat) that warms and cooks food. A microwave oven generates electromagnetic energy (microwaves) produced by a device called a magnetron (see Figure 20-1).

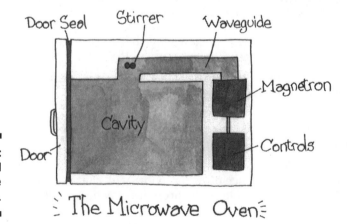

Figure 20-1: Your typical microwave oven.

Microwaves sail through glass, paper, and plastic right into food where they agitate water molecules so that they vibrate against each other. The vibration of the water molecules generates more energy (heat) that warms and cooks the food. The dish holding food in a microwave oven generally stays cool because it has so few water molecules.

Cooking and Food Safety

Many microbes living naturally in food are harmless or even beneficial. For example:

- Lactobacilli (lacto = milk; bacilli = rod-shaped bacteria) are used to digest sugars in milk and convert the milk to yogurt.

- Nontoxic molds convert milk to blue cheese (the blue ribbons in the cheese are — mold!).

Some organisms, however, carry the risk of food poisoning. Are you surprised to learn that every year, as many as 81 million Americans experience diarrhea — a common symptom of food poisoning — after eating food contaminated with such an organism?

Some forms of food poisoning are far more serious. The United States is not immune to their effects:

- In the winter of 1998–99, illness and deaths were reported due to consumption of packaged meats contaminated with Listeria monocytogenes.

  This incident was particularly troublesome because the contaminated products (packaged meats) were made to be served cold. The only way to reduce the risk would have been to reheat the "cold cuts" — unlikely except with hot dogs, which must be boiled or broiled, not microwaved, to reach a safe internal temperature of 165°F.

  Note: Pregnant women who consume Listeria-contaminated food may have an increased risk of injury to the fetus.

- Both children and adults have died in this country following consumption of undercooked chopped meat containing Escherichia coli 0157:H7 (sometimes abbreviated *E. coli*).

- The toxin produced by Clostridium botulinum (C. botulinum), which thrives in the absence of air (as in low-acid, canned food), is potentially fatal. Your only warning of its presence may be a swollen can — which should be discarded without being opened.

- Raw meat and poultry or unpasteurized milk contaminated with Campylobacterium jejuni (C. jejuni) have been linked to Guillain-Barré syndrome, a paralytic illness that sometimes follows flu infection.

Although these organisms are equal-opportunity bad guys — anyone who eats food carrying them may get sick — they are most dangerous for the very young, the very old, and those whose immune systems have been weakened by illness or medication.

Cooking food thoroughly and keeping it hot (or chilling quickly) once it has been cooked destroys many dangerous bugs or slows the rate at which they reproduce, thus reducing the risk of food poisoning. Table 20-1 lists some common *pathogens* (disease-causing organisms) linked to food-borne illness, shows where you're likely to find them, and tells how to keep them under control.

Table 20-1 lists some disease-causing organisms in foods. Table 20-2 lists the recommended safe cooking temperatures for various foods.

Table 20-1	Disease-Causing Organisms in Food
The Bug	*Where You Find It*
Campylobacterjejuni	Raw meat and poultry, unpasteurized milk
Clostridium botulinum	Canned low-acid foods, smoked fish
Clostridium perfringens	Foods made from poultry or meat
E. coli	Raw beef
Listeria monocytogenes	Raw meat and seafood, raw milk, some raw cheeses
Salmonella bacteria	Poultry, meat, eggs, dried foods, dairy products
Staphyloccus aureaus	Custards, salads (that is, egg, chicken, and tuna salad)

Source: USDA Meat and Poultry Hotline.

Two hours — and you're out!

Micro-organisms thrive on food at temperatures between 40°F (the temperature inside a well-tuned refrigerator should be several degrees lower) and 140°F (the cooking temperature that inactivates many — though not all — bad guys). For maximum safety, follow the USDA/FDA "Two-Hour Rule": Never allow food to sit at temperatures between 40°F and 140°F for more than two hours.

More questions about food safety? Call

✔ USDA Meat and Poultry Hotline: 800-535-4555

✔ FDA Seafood Hotline: 800-332-4010

Table 20-2	How Hot Is Safe?
This Food . . .	*Is Done (Generally Safe to Eat) when Cooked to This Internal Temperature*
Eggs and Egg Dishes	
Eggs	Cook until yolk and white are firm
Egg dishes	160°F
Ground Meat and Meat Mixtures	
Turkey, chicken	165°F
Veal, beef, lamb, pork*	160°F
Fresh Beef*	
Medium rare	145°F
Medium	160°F
Well-done	170°F
Fresh Pork	
Medium	160°F
Well-done	170°F
Poultry	
Chicken, whole	180°F
Turkey, whole	180°F
Poultry breasts, roasts	170°F
Poultry thighs, wings	Cook until juices run clear
Stuffing (cooked alone or in bird)	165°F
Duck and goose	180°F
Ham	
Fresh (raw)	160°F
Precooked (to reheat)	140°F

*Undercooked hamburger is a major source of the potentially lethal organism E. coli. To be safe, the internal temperature must read 165°F.

Source: USDA Food Safety and Inspection Service, "A Quick Consumer Guide to Safe Food Handling," *Home and Garden Bulletin,* No. 248 (August 1995).

How Cooking Changes the Texture of Food

Exposure to heat alters the structure of proteins, fats, and carbohydrates, so it changes food's *texture* (the way food particles are linked to make the food feel hard or soft). In other words, cooking can turn crisp carrots mushy and can turn soft steak to tough.

Protein

Proteins are made of very long molecules that sometimes fold over into accordion-like structures (see Chapter 6 for details on proteins). Heating food does not lower its protein value, but it does

✔ Break protein molecules into smaller fragments

✔ Cause protein molecules to unfold and form new bonds to other protein molecules

✔ Make proteins clump together

Need an example? Think of the egg. When you cook one, the long protein molecules in the white unfold, form new connections to other protein molecules, and link up in a network that tightens to squeeze out moisture so that the egg white hardens and turns opaque. The same unfold-link-squeeze reaction turns translucent poultry firm and white and makes gelatin set. The longer you heat proteins, the stronger the network becomes, and the tougher, or more solid, the food will be.

Grains: Split personality performers

In cooking, grains, such as corn, exhibit split personalities — part protein, part complex carbohydrates. When you boil an ear of corn, the protein molecules inside the kernels do the break-unfold-network dance. At the same time, carbohydrate starch granules begin to absorb moisture and soften.

The trick to boiling perfect corn is to control this process, removing the corn from the water when the starch granules have absorbed enough moisture to soften the kernels but before the protein network has tightened.

That's why cookbooks advise a short stay in the pot. But if you're a person who likes corn chewy, just let it boil away, 15 minutes, 30 minutes — you be the judge.

A hot story

When you heat fats, their molecules break apart into chemicals known as "free radicals" which may hook up with other molecule fragments to form potentially carcinogenic (cancer-causing) compounds. These compounds are produced in higher numbers at higher heats; the usual safe cutoff is around 500°F (right before "broiling" on the oven dial). Burned fat or smoking oil, for example, has more nasties than plain melted fat or oil that is warm but not smoking.

As a result, many nutritionists warn against eating the crisp, crinkly, absolutely yummy browned top layer of foods, especially burned meats which, in 1998, were tentatively linked to a higher risk of breast cancer in women. Of course, the theory has yet to be proven, and as with so much in modern nutrition, the story may be more complicated than it seems at first glance.

Why? Because in 1996, Martha Belury, of Purdue University, discovered that cheeseburgers — yes, cheeseburgers, grilled, fried, broiled, whatever — are rich in CLA (short for conjugated dienole linoleic acid, a form of an essential fatty acid — a topic covered in Chapter 7.

In Belury's lab, CLA slowed or reversed skin, breast, and stomach cancers in mice at the three stages of tumor development: early, when the cell is first damaged; midway in the process, when pre-cancerous cells multiply to form tumors; and late, when tumors begin to enlarge and spread to other organs.

Does this happen in people? Nobody knows. But it sure reminds me of the Woody Allen movie *Sleeper,* in which the hero wakes up sometime in the future to discover that corned beef sandwiches are health food. Hey, you can't make this stuff up!

To see this work, scramble two eggs — one beaten and cooked plain and one beaten with milk and then cooked. Adding liquid (milk) makes it more difficult for the protein-network to squeeze out all the moisture. So the egg with the added milk cooks up softer than the plain egg.

Fat

Heat melts fat, which can run off food, lowering the calorie count. In addition, cooking breaks down connective tissue — the supporting framework of the body, which includes some adipose (fatty) tissue — thus making the food softer and more pliable. You can see this most clearly when you cook fish. The fish "flakes" when it's done because its connective tissue has been destroyed.

When meat and poultry are stored after cooking, their fats continue to change, this time by picking up oxygen from the air. Oxidized fats have a slightly rancid taste more politely known as *warmed-over flavor.* You can slow — but not entirely prevent — this reaction by cooking and storing meat, fish, and poultry under a blanket of food rich in *antioxidants,* chemicals that prevent other chemicals from reacting with oxygen. Vitamin C is a natural antioxidant, so gravies and marinades made with tomatoes and citrus fruits slow the natural oxidation of fats.

Carbohydrates

Cooking has different effects on simple carbohydrates and complex ones (if you are confused about carbohydrates, see Chapter 8). When heated

- ✔ Simple sugars — such as sucrose or the sugars on the surface of meat and poultry — caramelize, or melt and turn brown. (Think of crème caramel.)

- ✔ Starch, a complex carbohydrate, becomes more absorbent, which is why pasta expands and softens in boiling water.

- ✔ Some dietary fibers (gums, pectins, hemicellulose) dissolve, so vegetables and fruits soften when cooked.

The last two reactions — absorption and dissolved cell walls — can improve the nutritional value of foods by making the nutrients inside previously fiber-stiffened cells more available to your body.

How Cooking Changes Food Flavors and Aroma

Heat degrades (breaks apart) flavor and aroma chemicals. As a result, most cooked food has a more intense flavor and aroma than raw food.

A good example is the mustard oils that give cruciferous vegetables, such as cabbage and cauliflower, their distinctive (some may say offensive) odor. The longer you cook these vegetables, the worse they smell. On the other hand, heat destroys *diallyl disulfide,* the chemical that gives raw garlic its bite and bark, so cooked garlic tastes and smells milder than the raw version.

How Cooking Changes Food Color

Carotenoids — the natural red and yellow pigments that make carrots yellow, sweet potatoes orange, and tomatoes red — are practically impervious to heat and the acidity or alkalinity of cooking liquids. No matter how you cook them or how long, carotenoids stay bright and sunny.

You can't say the same for the other pigments in food. The ones that make food naturally red, green, or white react to heat, acids (such as wine, vinegar, or tomato juice), and basic (alkaline) chemicals (such as mineral water or baking soda and water), usually for the worse. Here's a brief run-down on the color changes that you can expect when you cook food.

✔ Red beets and cabbage get their color from pigments called *anytho-cyanins*. Acids make these pigments redder. Alkaline solutions fade anythocyanins from red to bluish purple.

✔ Potatoes, cauliflower, rice, and white onions are white because they contain white pigments called *anthoxanthins*. When anthoxanthins are exposed to alkaline chemicals (mineralized water or baking soda), they turn yellow or brownish. Acids prevent this reaction. Boil cauliflower florets in tomato juice, rinse off the juice, and you'll see — white cauliflower!

✔ Green veggies are colored by *chlorophyll,* a pigment that reacts with acids in cooking water (or in the vegetable itself) to form *pheophytin,* a brown pigment. The only way to short-circuit this reaction is to protect the vegetables from acids. Old-time cooks added alkaline baking soda, but that increases the loss of certain vitamins (see "Protecting the Nutrients in Cooked Foods," later in this chapter). Fast cooking at high heat or cooking in lots of water (which dilutes acids) lessens these color changes.

✔ The natural red color of fresh meat comes from *myoglobin* and *hemoglobin* in blood. When meat is heated, the pigment molecules are *denatured,* broken into fragments. They lose oxygen and turn brown or — after long cooking — turn the really unappetizing gray characteristic of "steam table" meats. This inevitable change is more noticeable in beef than in pork or veal because beef starts out naturally redder.

Red to blue and back again

The following recipe lets you see colors change right before your very eyes.

1 small can sliced beets

1 saucepan

3 small glass bowls

1 cup water

1 teaspoon baking soda

3 tablespoons white vinegar

Line up the glass bowls on your kitchen counter. Open the can. Remove 6 slices of beets. Put 2 slices in the first glass bowl and 4 slices into the saucepan. Put the rest in a small container and refrigerate for dinner. No sense wasting good beets!

Mix the baking soda into the water and add this alkaline solution to the saucepan. Heat for 4 minutes; don't heat too high — the solution foams. Turn off the heat. Remove the beets from the pan. Put 2 slices each in the second and third glass bowls.

Ignore the second bowl. Add the vinegar (an acid) to the third bowl. Wait 2 minutes. Now look: The beets in the first bowl (straight from the can) should still be bright red; the beets in the second bowl, faded by the baking soda, should be darker, almost navy blue; the beets in the third bowl, restored by the vinegar, should be heading back to bright red. Not yet? Add another tablespoon of vinegar.

Ain't chemistry grand?

How Pots and Pans Affect Food

A pot is a pot is a pot, right? No way! In fact, your choice of pot can affect the nutrient value of food by

✔ Adding nutrients to the food, or

✔ Slowing the natural loss of nutrients during cooking, or

✔ Actively increasing the loss of nutrients during cooking

In addition, some pots make the food's natural flavors and aromas more intense, which can make the food more — or less — appetizing. Read on to find out how your pot can change your food. And vice versa.

Aluminum

Aluminum is lightweight and conducts heat well. That's good. But the metal

✔ Makes some aroma chemicals smellier (particularly those in the cruciferous vegetables — cabbage, broccoli, brussels sprouts, and so on)

✔ Flakes off, turning white foods (such as cauliflower or potatoes) yellow or brownish

 Early speculation aside, aluminum flaking is not hazardous to your health: Cooking with aluminum pots does not increase your risk of developing Alzheimer's disease. True, salty or acidic foods (wine, tomatoes) in aluminum pots increase the flaking, but even then, the amount of aluminum you get from the pot is less than you get naturally every day from food and water (see Chapter 11 for the lowdown on aluminum as a natural nutrient).

Copper

Copper pots heat steadily and evenly. To take advantage of this property, many aluminum or stainless steel pots are made with a layer of copper sandwiched into the bottom. But naked copper is a potentially poisonous metal. That's why copper pots are lined with tin or stainless steel. If you cook with copper, check the lining of the pot periodically. If it's damaged — meaning that you can see the orange copper peeking through the silvery lining — have the pot relined or throw it out.

Copper and egg whites: A chemical team

When you whip an egg white, its proteins unfold, form new bonds, and create a network that holds air in. That's why the runny white turns into stable foam.

You can certainly whip egg whites successfully in a glass or ceramic bowl — chilled, and absolutely free of any fat, including egg yolk, that would prevent the proteins from linking tightly. But the best choice is copper: the ions (particles) flaking off the surface bind with and stabilize the foam. (Aluminum ions stabilize but darken the whites.)

But wait. Isn't copper toxic? (See Chapter 11.) Yes, but the amount you get in an occasional batch of whites is so small it's insignificant, safety-wise.

Ceramics

The chief virtue of plain terra cotta (the orangy clay that looks like red bricks) is its *porosity,* a fancy way of saying that terra cotta roasting and baking pans allow excess steam to escape while holding in just enough moisture to make bread so moist and chicken such tender pickings.

Decorated ceramic vessels are another matter. For one thing, the glaze makes the pot much less porous, so that meat or poultry cooked in a covered painted ceramic pan steams instead of roasts. The practical result: a soggy surface rather than a crisp one.

More important, some pigments used to paint or glaze the pots contain lead. To seal the decoration and prevent lead from leaching into food, the painted pots are *fired* (baked in an oven). If the oven is too cool or the baking time too short, lead leaches — most heavily when in contact with acidic foods such as fruit juices or foods marinated in wine or vinegar.

Ceramics made in the United States, Japan, and Great Britain are generally considered safe, but for maximum protection, hedge your bets. Unless the pot comes with a tag or brochure that specifically says it's acid-safe, don't use it for cooking or storing foods. And always wash decorated ceramics by hand; repeated passes through the dishwasher can wear down the surface.

Enamelware

Enameled pots are made of metal covered with *porcelain,* a fine translucent china. Enamelware heats more slowly and less evenly than plain metal. A good quality enameled surface resists discoloration and does not react with food. But it can chip and it is easily marked or scratched by cooking utensils other than wood or hard plastic. If the surface chips and you can see the metal underneath, discard the pot lest metals flake into your food.

Glass

Glass is a neutral material that does not react with food. Two cautions with glass:

✔ Do not use a glass-and-metal pot in the microwave oven. The metal blocks microwaves. More important, it can cause *arcing* — a sudden electrical flare that may damage the oven and scare you out of your wits.

✔ Remember that glass breaks. Sometimes all over the floor. Are you a person who often drops things? Pass on the glass.

Iron cookware

Like aluminum, iron pots are a good news/bad news item. Iron conducts heat well and stays hot significantly longer than other pots. It is easy to clean. It lasts forever, and it releases iron ions into food, which may improve the nutritional value of dinner.

In 1985, nutrition researchers at Texas Tech University in Lubbock set out to measure the iron content of foods cooked in iron pots. Among their discoveries: beef stew (0.7 milligrams of iron per 100 grams/3.5 ounces, raw) can end up with as much as 3.4 milligrams of iron per 100 grams after cooking slightly longer than an hour in an iron pot.

Alas! There's a downside. The iron that flakes off the pot may be a form of the mineral that your body cannot absorb. Also, more iron is not necessarily better. It encourages oxidation (bad for your body) and can contribute to excess iron storage in people who have *hemochromatosis* (a condition that leads to iron buildup that may damage internal organs).

By the way, did I mention that pumping iron is not a bad way to describe the experience of cooking with iron pots? They are really, really heavy.

Nonstick

Nonstick surfaces are made of plastic (polytetrafluoroethylene to be exact; PTFE for short) plus hardeners — chemicals that make the surface, well, hard. So long as the surface is unscratched and intact, the nonstick surface does not react with food.

Nonstick pots are a dieter's delight. They let you cook without added fat, but using them may also lighten your wallet. They scratch easily. Unless you stick scrupulously to wooden or plastic spoons, your pot can end up looking like chickens have been stomping on the surface.

Note: This is not a health hazard. If you swallow tiny pieces of the nonstick coating, they will pass through your body undigested.

However, when nonstick surfaces get very hot, they may

✔ Separate from the metal to which they are bound (the sides and bottom of the pot)

✔ Emit odorless fumes

If the cooking area is not properly ventilated, you may experience *polymer fume fever* — flu-like symptoms with no known long-term effect. To prevent this, keep the stove flame moderate and the windows open.

Stainless steel

Stainless steel is an alloy (a substance composed of two or more metals), mostly iron. The virtues of stainless steel are hardness and durability. The drawback is poor heat conduction. In addition, the alloy includes nickel, a metal to which many people are sensitive. If your stainless steel pot is scratched deeply enough to expose the inner layer under the shiny surface, discard it.

Plastic and paper

No, you can't use plain plastic or paper containers on a gas or electric stove. These products, which allow electromagnetic energy to pass through to the food, are meant for microwave ovens. But you can't use just any paper and plastic. You need containers made of materials labeled something like "microwave safe."

✔ Plastic containers without the "microwave safe" label may break down when exposed to electromagnetic energy, leaking plastic into your food.

✔ Paper not guaranteed "microwave safe" may contain tiny metal particles that either block microwaves or cause arcing (see the "Glass" section earlier in this chapter).

Protecting the Nutrients in Cooked Foods

Myth: All raw foods are more nutritious than cooked ones.

Fact: Some foods (such as meat, poultry, and eggs) are positively dangerous when raw (or undercooked). Other foods are less nutritious raw because they contain substances that destroy or disarm other nutrients. For example:

✔ Raw red cabbage, brussels sprouts, blueberries, and blackberries contain an enzyme that destroys thiamin (vitamin B1). Heating the food inactivates the enzyme.

✔ Raw beans, legumes, and peanuts contain enzyme inhibitors that interfere with the work of enzymes that enable your body to digest protein. Heating disarms the enzyme inhibitor.

But there's no denying that some nutrients are lost when foods are cooked. Simple strategies such as steaming food rather than boiling, or broiling rather than frying, will significantly reduce the loss of nutrients when you are cooking food.

Minerals

Virtually all minerals are unaffected by heat. A food has the same amount of calcium, phosphorus, magnesium, iron, zinc, iodine, selenium, copper, manganese, chromium, and sodium after it's cooked as it had when it was raw. The single exception to this rule is potassium, which — while not affected by heat or air — does escape out of food into the cooking liquid.

Vitamins

With the exception of vitamin K and the B vitamin niacin, which are very stable in food, many vitamins are sensitive flowers and easily destroyed when exposed to heat, air, water, or fats (cooking oils). Table 20-3 shows which nutrients are sensitive to these influences.

By the way, stainless steel is not really "stainless"

✔ When exposed to high heat, stainless steel develops a characteristic multihued "rainbow" discoloration.

✔ Starchy foods (pasta, potatoes) may darken the pot.

✔ Undissolved salt can pit the surface.

Table 20-3	What Takes Nutrients Out of Food			
Nutrient	*Heat*	*Air*	*Water*	*Fat*
Vitamin A	X			X
Vitamin D				X
Vitamin E	X	X		X
Vitamin C	X	X	X	
Thiamin	X		X	
Riboflavin			X	
Vitamin B6	X	X	X	
Folate	X	X		
Vitamin B12	X		X	
Biotin			X	
Pantothenic acid	X			
Potassium			X	

To avoid vitamin loss, keep in mind the following tips:

✔ **Vitamin A and vitamin D:** To reduce the loss of fat-soluble vitamins A and E, cook with very little oil. For example, bake or broil vitamin-A-rich liver oil-free instead of frying. Ditto for vitamin-D-rich fish.

✔ **B vitamins:** The strategies that conserve the protein in meat and poultry during cooking also work to conserve the B vitamins that leak out into cooking liquid or drippings: Use the cooking liquid in soup or sauce. *Caution:* Do not shorten cooking time or temperature in order to lessen the loss of heat-sensitive vitamin B12 from meat, fish, or poultry. These foods and their drippings must be thoroughly cooked to ensure that they are safe to eat.

Do not rinse grains (rice) before cooking unless the package advises this (some rice does need to be rinsed); washing rice once may take away as much as 25 percent of the thiamin (vitamin B1). Bake or toast cakes and breads only until the crust is light brown to preserve heat-sensitive Bs.

✔ **Vitamin C:** To reduce the loss of water-soluble, oxygen-sensitive vitamin C, cook fruits and vegetables in the least possible amount of water. For example, when you cook one cup of cabbage in 4 cups of water, the leaves lose as much as 90 percent of their vitamin C. Reverse the ratio — one cup water to 4 cups cabbage — and you hold on to more than 50 percent of the vitamin C.

Serve cooked vegetables quickly: After 24 hours in the fridge, vegetables lose one-fourth of their vitamin C; after two days, nearly half.

Root vegetables (carrots, potatoes, sweet potatoes) baked or boiled whole, in their skins, retain practically all their vitamin C.

How to Use the Info in This Chapter

Enough already. Now that you know how cooking changes food, you can move on to the recipes and techniques that help you put dinner on the table.

For more (much, much more) detail on what and how to cook, check out *Cooking For Dummies* (written by Marie Rama and Brian Miller), a compilation of the kind of no-nonsense, easy-to-follow instructions that you've come to expect from the big books with the yellow-and-black covers. If cutting fat and calories is your pleasure (or necessity), choose *Lowfat Cooking For Dummies,* written by Lynn Fisher. Both books are published by IDG Books Worldwide, Inc.

Either way, enjoy!

Chapter 21

What Happens When Food Is Frozen, Canned, Dried, or Zapped

· ·

In This Chapter

▶ How freezing protects food

▶ Who invented canned food

▶ The ancient art of drying food

▶ Using radiation to make food safe

· ·

Cold air, hot air, no air, and radioactive rays — all can be used to make food safer for longer periods of time by reducing or eliminating damage from exposure to air or organisms (microbes) that live on food.

Despite their differences, the methods described in this chapter all have one important thing in common: Used correctly, each can dramatically lengthen food's shelf life. The down side? Nothing's perfect, so you still have to monitor your food to make sure that the preservation treatment has, well, preserved it. The following pages tell you how.

Cold Comfort

Keeping food cold, sometimes very cold, slows or suspends the activity of microbes bent on digesting your food before you do.

Unlike heat, which can actually kill lots of microbes (see Chapter 20), chilling food (or freezing it) does not kill the microbes; it just puts them on the sidelines for a while. Mold spores (sort of hibernating mold organisms), for example, snuggle inside frozen food like so many comfy bears. When you thaw the food, the mold springs back into action.

For more information on storage and safety

✔ USDA Meat & Poultry Hotline

800-535-4555

10 a.m. to 4 p.m. (EST) weekdays

www.usda.gov/agency/fsis/
homepage.htm

✔ FDA

800-332-4010

10 a.m. to 4 p.m. (EST) weekdays

www.fda.gov

How long things stay safe in the refrigerator or freezer varies from food to food. Table 21-1 provides a handy guide to the limits of safe cool storage. These ranges depend on the foods being fresh to start and on the refrigerator/freezer maintaining a constant temperature. If these conditions are not met, food may spoil more quickly. Use your common sense. If food seems in any way questionable, *throw it out without tasting.*

Table 21-1	Cold Storage	
Food	*Refrigerator (40°F)*	*Freezer (0°F)*
Eggs		
Fresh, in shell	3 weeks	Don't freeze
Raw yolks, whites	2 – 4 days	1 year
Hard cooked	1 week	Doesn't freeze well
Liquid pasteurized eggs or egg substitutes, opened	3 days	Doesn't freeze well
unopened	10 days	1 year
Mayonnaise, Commercial		
Refrigerate after opening	2 months	Don't freeze
TV Dinners, Frozen Casseroles		
Keep frozen until ready to serve		3 – 4 months
Deli and Vacuum-Packed Products		
Pre-stuffed pork and lamb chops, chicken breasts stuffed with dressing	1 day	Doesn't freeze well
Store-cooked convenience meals	1 – 2 days	Doesn't freeze well

Food	Refrigerator (40°F)	Freezer (0°F)
Commercial brand vacuum-packed dinners with USDA seal	2 weeks, unopened	Doesn't freeze well
Soups and Stews		
Vegetable or meat-added	3 – 4 days	2 – 3 months
Hamburger, Ground and Stew Meats		
Hamburger and stew meats	1 – 2 days	3 – 4 months
Ground turkey, veal, pork, lamb, and mixtures of them	1 – 2 days	3 – 4 months
Hot dogs and Lunch Meats*		
Hot dogs, opened package	1 week	In freezer wrap, 1 – 2 months
unopened package	2 weeks	In freezer wrap, 1 – 2 months
Lunch meats, opened	3 – 5 days	In freezer wrap, 1 – 2 months
unopened	2 weeks	In freezer wrap, 1 – 2 months
Bacon and Sausage		
Bacon*	7 days	1 month
Sausage, raw from pork, beef, turkey	1 – 2 days	1 – 2 months
Smoked breakfast links, patties	7 days	1 – 2 months
Hard sausage — pepperoni, jerky sticks	2 – 3 weeks	1 – 2 months
Ham, Corned Beef		
Corned beef in pouch with pickling juices*	5 – 7 days	drained, wrapped, 1 month
Ham, canned, label says keep refrigerated	6 – 9 months	Don't freeze
Ham, fully cooked — whole	7 days	1 – 2 months
Ham, fully cooked — half	3 – 5 days	1 – 2 months
Ham, fully cooked — slices	3 – 4 days	1 – 2 months
Fresh Meat		
Steaks, beef	3 – 5 days	6 – 12 months
Chops, pork	3 – 5 days	4 – 6 months
Chops, lamb	3 – 5 days	6 – 9 months

(continued)

Table 21-1 *(continued)*

Food	Refrigerator (40°F)	Freezer (0°F)
Roast, beef	3 – 5 days	6 – 12 months
Roasts, lamb	3 – 5 days	6 – 9 months
Roasts, pork and veal	3 – 5 days	4 – 6 months
Variety meats — tongue, brain, kidneys, liver, heart, chitterlings	1 – 2 days	3 – 4 months
Meat Leftovers		
Cooked meat and meat dishes	3 – 4 days	2 – 3 months
Gravy and broth	1 – 2 days	2 – 3 months
Fresh Poultry		
Chicken or turkey, whole	1 – 2 days	1 year
Pieces	1 – 2 days	2 – 3 months
Giblets	1 – 2 days	3 – 4 months
Cooked Poultry, Leftover		
Fried chicken	3 – 4 days	4 months
Cooked poultry dishes	3 – 4 days	4 – 6 months
Pieces, plain	3 – 4 days	4 months
Pieces covered with broth or gravy	1 – 2 days	6 months
Chicken nuggets, patties	1 – 2 days	1 – 3 months

*Follow date on package. **Caution:** Even when food is in date and has been properly refrigerated, always boil or broil hot dogs to an internal temperature of 165°F.

Source: Food Safety and Inspection Service, "A Quick Consumer's Guide to Safe Food Handling," Home and Garden Bulletin, No. 248 (U.S. Department of Agriculture, August 1995).

How freezing affects the texture of food

When food freezes, the water inside each cell forms tiny crystals that can tear cell walls. When the food is thawed, the liquid inside the cell leaks out, leaving thawed food dryer than fresh food.

Beef that has been frozen, for example, is noticeably dryer than fresh beef. Dry cheeses, such as cheddar, turn crumbly. Bread dries, too. You can reduce the loss of moisture by thawing the food in its freezer wrap so that it has a chance to re-absorb lost moisture that is still in the package.

What's that brown spot on my burger?

Freezer burn is a harmless dry brownish spot left when moisture evaporates from the surface of frozen food.

To prevent freezer burn, wrap food securely in freezer paper or aluminum foil and put the item in a plastic bag. The more air you keep out, the fewer brown spots will develop.

You can't restore the crispness of vegetables, such as carrots, that get their crunch from stiff, high-fiber cell walls. Once ice crystals puncture the walls, the vegetable (carrots are a good example) turns mushy. The solution? Remove carrots and other crunchies, such as cabbage, before freezing the stew.

Refreezing frozen food

The official word from the U.S. Department of Agriculture is that you can re-freeze frozen food — so long as the food still has ice crystals or feels refrigerator-cold to the touch.

The personal, unofficial word from me is that I confess to feeling safer if I simply throw out partially thawed food that I'm not going to use right away. I am particularly wary of sauced frozen food, such as frozen macaroni and cheese, because it seems to me that there just have to be hidden pockets of thawed food where the bacteria are whooping it up as we speak. Call me a worrywart, if you will, but for me it's just less concerning simply to follow this rule: Partly thawed? Out the door.

Canned Food

Food is canned by heating it and sealing the container to keep out air and microbes. Like cooked food, canned food is subject to changes in appearance and nutritional content. (See the sidebar "The essence of canned food.") Heating food often changes its color and texture (see Chapter 20). It also destroys some vitamin C. But canning does effectively destroy a variety of pathogens, and it deactivates those pesky enzymes.

The essence of canned food

The technique of food canning was discovered (depending on your source) either in 1809 or 1810 by Nicholas Appert, a Frenchman who noted that if he sealed food in a container while it was heating, the food stayed edible longer than fresh food — much longer. According to

Harold McGee, author of *On Food and Cooking,* a wonderful guide to food technology, a tin of 114-year-old canned meat was once eaten without making anyone sick. To be fair, I must note that nobody cried, "Oh, wow, this is good," either.

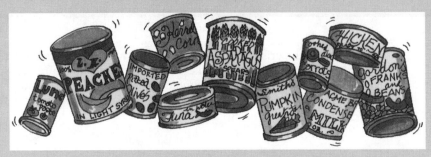

A modern variation on canning is the sealed plastic or aluminum bag known as the "retort pouch." Food sealed in the pouch is heated, but for a shorter period than that required for canning. As a result, the pouch method does a better job at preserving flavor, appearance, and heat-sensitive vitamin C.

The sealed can or pouch also protects food from deterioration caused by light or air, so the seal must remain intact. If the seal is broken, air can seep into the can or pouch, spoiling the food.

A more serious hazard associated with canned food is *botulism,* a potentially fatal form of food poisoning caused by the failure to heat the food high enough or long enough to kill all Clostridium botulinum (or C. botulinum) bacteria. *C. botulinum* is an anaerobic (an = without; aerobic = air) organism that thrives in the absence of oxygen, a condition nicely fulfilled by a sealed can. Botulinum spores not destroyed by high heat during the canning process may produce a toxin that can kill by paralyzing your heart muscles and the muscles that enable you to breathe.

To avoid canned food contaminated with botulinum organisms, do not buy, store, or use any can that is

✔ Swollen (indicating that bacteria are growing inside and producing gas)

✔ Damaged, rusted, or deeply dented along the seam (a break in the can would permit air to enter and allow the food to spoil)

Canned history

The first canned food — salmon, oysters, and lobsters — was introduced in 1819 by New Yorkers Ezra Daggett and Thomas Kennett. Four years later, Daggett and Kennett took out a patent to "preserve animal substances in tin."

The first can with a "key" opener was patented on October 2, 1866, by New York inventor J. Osterhoudt. (For the most part, "keys" —

still found on many sardine cans and canned hams — have been replaced by "pull tabs.")

The first beer in cans (from the Krueger Brewing Company, of Newark, New Jersey) went on sale on January 24, 1935, in Richmond, Virginia.

Source: Joseph Nathan Kane, *Famous First Facts* (New York: H. W. Wilson Company, 1964).

Consumer alert: Never, never, never taste any food from a swollen or damaged can "just to see if it's all right." When in doubt, throw it out.

Dried Food: No Life without Water

Drying protects food by removing the moisture that bacteria, yeasts, and molds need to live. Drying is an ancient technique, used to produce the famous dates of the desert as well as the dried meat of the American plains.

Drying food the low-tech way means putting it out in the sun and waiting for it to dry on its own. Drying food the high-tech, modern way means putting food out on racks and employing fans to quick-dry the food at low temperature under vacuum pressure.

Another form of drying is spray drying. *Spray drying* is a technique used to dry liquids, such as milk, by blowing the liquids (in very small droplets) into a heated chamber where the droplets dry into a powder that can be reconstituted (made back into a liquid) by adding water. Instant coffee is a spray-dried product. So are instant teas and all the various instant fruit beverages.

How drying affects food's nutritional value

As always, exposure to heat and/or air (oxygen) reduces a food's vitamin C content, so dried foods have less vitamin C than fresh foods.

One good example is the plum versus the prune (a dried plum):

- ✔ One fresh, medium-size plum, weighing 66 grams (a bit more than 2 ounces) without the pit, has 6 milligrams vitamin C, 10 percent of the RDA for a healthy adult.
- ✔ An equivalent amount of prunes has only 2.6 milligrams vitamin C.

But wait! Before you leap to the conclusion that fresh is always more nutritious than dried, feed these facts into your memory banks: Dried fruit has less water than fresh fruit. That means its weight reflects more solid fruit. Although drying destroys some vitamin C, removing water concentrates other nutrients, jamming more calories and heat and/or air-resistant vitamins and minerals into a smaller space.

As a result, dried food often has surprisingly more nutritional bounce to the ounce than fresh food. Once again, consider the plum and the prune:

- ✔ A medium-size, pit-free plum weighing slightly more than 2 ounces provides 35 calories, 0.1 milligram iron, and 670 IU (67 RE) vitamin A. (What's IU? What's RE? Check Chapter 4.)
- ✔ An equivalent amount of prunes has 150 calories, 1.6 milligrams iron, and 1,261 IU (126 RE) vitamin A. (People who are trying to lose weight should be aware that dried fruit, though low in fat, is high in calories.)

When dried fruit may be hazardous to your health

Many fruits contain an enzyme (polyphenoloxidase) that darkens the fruit flesh when the fruit is exposed to air. To prevent the fruits from darkening when dried, the fruits are treated with sulfur compounds known as sulfites. The sulfites — sulfur dioxide, sodium bisulfite, sodium metabisulfite — can cause potentially serious allergic reactions in sensitive individuals. For more about sulfites, see Chapter 22.

Irradiation: A Hot Topic

Irradiation is a technique that exposes food to gamma radiation, a high-energy light stronger than the X rays your doctor uses to make a picture of your insides. Gamma rays (also known as pico rays) are ionizing radiation, the kind of radiation that kills living cells. Ionizing radiation can "sterilize" food or at least prolong its shelf life by

✔ Killing microbes and insects on plants (wheat, wheat powder, spices, dry vegetable seasonings)

✔ Killing disease-causing organisms on pork (trichinella) and poultry (salmonella)

✔ Preventing potatoes and onions from sprouting during storage

✔ Slowing the rate at which some fruits ripen

Irradiation does not change the way food looks or tastes. It does not change food texture. It does not make food "radioactive." But it does alter the structure of some chemicals in foods, breaking molecules apart to form new substances called *radiolytic products* (radio = radiation; lytic = break).

About 90 percent of all compounds identified as radiolytic products (RP) are also found in raw, heated, and/or stored foods that have not been deliberately exposed to ionizing radiation. A few compounds, called *unique radiolytic products* (URP), are found only in irradiated foods.

You can get answers online to the most commonly asked questions about food irradiation at `www.sph.umich.edu/group/eih/UMSCHPS/food.htm`.

Are URPs harmful?

Many scientific organizations, including the 27,000-member Institute of Food Technologists and an international Committee on the Wholesomeness of Irradiated Foods (which includes representatives from the United Nations, the International Atomic Energy Agency, and the World Health Organization), believe that irradiation is a safe and important weapon in the fight against food poisoning caused by microbial and parasitical contamination.

The Food and Drug Administration has been approving various uses of food irradiation since 1963. In addition, irradiation is approved for more than 40 food products in more than 37 countries around the world.

Many consumers, though, remain leery of irradiation, fearful that it may expose them to radiation (it can't; there are no radioactive residues in irradiated food) or that URPs (Unique Radiolytic Products) may eventually turn out to

be harmful. For now, irradiated food seems safe, but it is fair to point out that this is still an unfolding story.

Around the world, all irradiated food is identified with this international symbol. Just in case that's not enough to get the message across, the package must also carry the words "treated by irradiation" or "treated with irradiation." The only exception is commercially produced food that contains some irradiated ingredients, such as spices. For example, a frozen pizza seasoned with irradiated oregano would not have to put the symbol on the package.

Chapter 22

Better Eating through Chemistry

● ●

In This Chapter

▶ Understanding food additives

▶ Keeping food safe with chemicals

▶ Regulating food additives

▶ Additives that cause health problems

● ●

*T*his chapter is about the natural and synthetic ingredients added to food products to make food more nutritious; enhance its appearance, flavor, and texture; and keep it fresh on the shelf longer.

Many people think that natural additives are safer than synthetic ingredients because "synthetic" seems synonymous with "chemical." Besides, synthetic additives often have names no one can pronounce, much less translate, which makes them even more forbidding.

In fact, everything in the world is made of chemicals: your body, the air you breathe, the paper on which this book is printed, and the glasses through which you read it, as well as every food you eat and every beverage you drink. The trick with additives is simply to use safe chemicals, natural or synthetic, and to use them wisely.

The Nature of Food Additives

What are food additives? Here's a really simple definition: *Food additives* are substances added to food.

The list of common food additives includes

> ✔ Nutrients
>
> ✔ Coloring agents
>
> ✔ Flavors and flavor enhancers
>
> ✔ Preservatives

Nutrients

One example of a clearly beneficial food additive is vitamin D, added to virtually all milk sold in the United States. Most bread and grain products are fortified with added B vitamins, plus iron and other essential minerals to replace what's lost when whole grains are milled into white flour for white bread. Some people say that we'd be better off simply sticking to whole grains. But adding vitamins and minerals to white flours enhances a product many people just plain like better. Another example of a nutrient used as a food additive is the calcium found in some commercially-prepared orange juices.

Some nutrients are also useful preservatives. For example, vitamin C is an antioxidant that slows food spoilage and prevents destructive chemical reactions. Manufacturers must add vitamin C (isoascorbic adic) to bacon to prevent the formation of potentially cancer-causing compounds.

Colors and flavors

Coloring and flavoring agents make food look and taste better. Like other food additives, these two may be either natural or synthetic.

Colors

Coloring agents make food look better. An example of a natural coloring agent is beta-carotene, the natural yellow pigment in many fruits and vegetables. Beta-carotene is used to make margarine (which is naturally white) look like creamy yellow butter. Other natural coloring agents are annatto (a yellow-to-pink pigment from a tropical tree), chlorophyll (the green pigment in green plants), carmine (a reddish extract of cochineal, a pigment from a female beetle), and saffron (a yellow herb) and turmeric (a yellow spice).

An example of a synthetic coloring agent is FD&C Blue No. 1, a bright blue pigment made from coal tar and used in soft drinks, gelatin, hair dyes, and face powders, among other things. As scientists have learned more about the effects of coal tar dyes, including the fact that some are carcinogenic, many have been banned from use in food but are still allowed in cosmetics because they are considered "irreplaceable."

Flavors

Every cook worth his or her spice cabinet knows about flavors and flavor enhancers, especially the most basic natural ones such as salt, sugar, vinegar, wine, and fruit juices.

Alphabet soup

When you read the label on a food, drug, or cosmetic product containing artificial colors, you may see the letters *F, D,* and *C* — as in FD&C Yellow #5. The *F* stands for food. The *D* stands for drugs. The *C* stands for cosmetics. An additive whose name includes all three letters can be used in food, drugs, and cosmetics. An additive without the *F* is restricted to use in drugs and cosmetics "for external use" (translation: You don't take them by mouth).

For example, D&C Green No. 6 is a blue-green coloring agent used in hair oils and pomades. FD&C Blue No. 2 is a bright blue coloring agent used in hair rinses, as well as mint jellies, candies, and cereals.

Artificial flavoring agents reproduce natural flavors. For example, a teaspoon of fresh lemon juice in the batter lends cheesecake a certain *je ne sais quoi* (French for "a little something special"), but artificial lemon flavoring works just as well.

You can sweeten your morning coffee with natural sugar or with the artificial sweetener saccharin. (For more about artificial sweeteners, see Chapter 19.)

Flavor enhancers are a slightly different kettle of fish. They intensify a food's natural flavor rather than adding a new one. The best known flavor enhancer is monosodium glutamate (MSG), widely used in Asian foods. MSG may trigger headaches and other symptoms in people sensitive to the seasoning.

Preservatives

Food spoils in many different ways. Milk turns sour. Bread sprouts mold. Meat and poultry rot. Vegetables lose moisture and wilt. Fats go rancid.

The first three kinds of spoilage are caused by microbes (bacteria, mold, yeasts). The last two happen when food is exposed to oxygen (air).

All preservative techniques — cooking, chilling, canning, freezing, drying — prevent spoilage either by slowing the growth of the organisms that live on food or by protecting the food from oxygen. Chemical preservatives do essentially the same thing:

- *Antimicrobials* are preservatives that protect food by slowing the growth of bacteria, molds, and yeasts.

- *Antioxidants* are preservatives that protect food by preventing food molecules from combining with oxygen (air).

Table 22-1 is a representative list of some preservative chemicals commonly found in food.

Table 22-1	Preservatives in Food
Preservative	*Found in . . .*
Ascorbic acid	Sausages, luncheon meat
Benzoic acid	Beverages (soft drinks), ice cream, baked goods
BHA (butylated hydroxyanisole)	Potato chips and other foods
BHT (butylated hydroxytoluene)	Potato chips and other foods
Calcium propionate	Breads, processed cheese
Sodium ascorbate	Luncheon meats and other foods
Sodium benzoate	Margarine, soft drinks

Source: Ruth Winter, *A Consumer's Dictionary of Cosmetic Ingredients* (New York: Crown, 1996).

Some other additives in food

Food chemists use a variety of natural and chemical additives to improve the texture of food, to keep it smooth, or to prevent mixtures from separating:

- Texturizers such as calcium chloride keep foods such as canned apples, tomatoes, or potatoes from turning mushy.

- Emulsifiers such as lecithin and polysorbate keep liquid-plus-solids such as chocolate pudding from separating into, well, liquid and solids.

- Thickeners are natural gums and starches such as apple pectin or cornstarch that add "body" to foods.

- Stabilizers such as the alginates (alginic acid) derived from seaweed make food such as ice cream feel smoother, richer, or creamier in your mouth.

Although many of these additives are derived from foods, their real benefit is aesthetic (the food looks and taste better), not nutritional.

Natural versus Synthetic

Food additives may be natural substances or synthetic substances. For example, Vitamin C is a natural chemical preservative. *Butylated hydroxianisole* (BHA) and *butylated hydroxytoluene* (BHT) are synthetic chemical preservatives. The only difference between these preservatives is that the first occurs naturally in food, while the second two are created in a laboratory.

Every natural and synthetic chemical used as an additive in food sold in the United States comes from a group of substances known as the Generally Recognized As Safe (GRAS) list.

All chemicals on the GRAS list

✔ Are FDA-approved, meaning that the agency is satisfied that the additive is safe and effective

✔ Must be used only in specifically limited amounts

✔ Must be used to satisfy a specific need in food products, such as protection against molds

✔ Must be effective, meaning that they must actually maintain freshness and safety

✔ Must be listed accurately on the label

Determining the Safety of Food Additives

The safety of any chemical approved for use as a food additive is based on whether it is

✔ Toxic

✔ Carcinogenic

✔ Allergenic

Toxins

A toxin is a poison. Some chemicals, such as cyanide, are toxic (poisonous) in very, very small doses. Others, such as sodium ascorbate (a form of vitamin C) are nontoxic even in very large doses. All chemicals on the GRAS list are considered nontoxic in the amounts permitted in food.

Carcinogens

A *carcinogen* is a substance that causes cancer. In 1958, New York Congressman James Delaney proposed, and Congress enacted into law, an amendment to the Food, Drug, and Cosmetic Act that banned from food any synthetic chemical known to cause cancer (in animals or human beings) when ingested in any amount.

Since then, the only exception to the Delaney clause has been saccharin, exempted in 1970 because while ingesting very large amounts of the artificial sweetener is known to cause bladder cancer in animals, no similar link can be found to human cancers. In addition, saccharin has clear benefits for people who cannot use sugar. However, all products containing saccharin must carry a warning statement: *Use of this product may be hazardous to your health. This product contains saccharin, which has been determined to cause cancer in laboratory animals.*

As of this writing, the Delaney clause is still in effect, even though many scientists, including cancer specialists, consider it to be outmoded because it imposes an impossible standard — zero risk — and applies only to synthetic chemicals. The Delaney clause does not apply to natural chemicals, even those known to cause cancer.

For example, nitrates and nitrites are effective preservatives used to prevent the growth of organisms in cured meat. But when they reach your stomach, nitrates and nitrites react with natural ammonia compounds called *amines* to form *nitrosamines,* substances known to cause cancer in animals, albeit at levels much higher than those used to preserve food. (Surprise! The same reaction occurs when you eat beets, celery, eggplant, lettuce, radishes, spinach, and turnip greens, foods with naturally-occurring nitrates and nitrites.)

To take the sting out of nitrates and nitrites, the FDA sensibly requires manufacturers to add an antioxidant vitamin C compound (sodium ascorbate) or an antioxidant vitamin E compound (tocopherol) to cured meats. The antioxidant vitamins prevent the formation of nitrosamines while boosting the antimicrobe power of the nitrates and nitrites.

Allergens

Allergens are substances that trigger allergic reactions. Some foods, such as peanuts, contain natural allergens that can provoke fatal allergic reactions.

The best-known example of an allergenic food additive is sulfites, a group of preservatives that

- ✔ Keep light-colored fruits and vegetables (apples, potatoes) from browning when exposed to air
- ✔ Prevent shellfish (shrimp and lobster) from developing "black spots"
- ✔ Reduce the growth of bacteria in fermenting wine and beer
- ✔ Bleach food starches
- ✔ Make dough easier to handle

Table 22-2 is a list of foods that may contain sulfites. (Also see Figure 22-1.)

Table 22-2	Where the Sulfites May Be
Food	
Beer	
Cakes, cookies, pies	
Cider (hard)	
Condiments	
Dried fruit	
Fruit juices	
Jams and jellies	
Gravy	
Maraschino cherries	
Molasses	
Potatoes (dehydrated, precut, peeled fresh)	
Shrimp	
Soup mixes	
Tea	
Vegetables (canned)	
Vegetable juices	
Wine	

Source: Ruth Papazian, "Sulfites" (FDA *Consumer,* December 1996).

Sulfites are safe for most people, but not for all. In fact, the FDA estimates that one out of every 100 people is sensitive to these chemicals; among people with asthma, the number rises to five out of every 100. For people sensitive to sulfites, even infinitesimally small amounts may trigger a serious allergic reaction, and asthmatics may develop breathing problems by simply inhaling fumes from sulfite-treated foods.

The FDA tried to ban sulfites from food but lost in a court case brought by food manufacturers who wished to use the additive. To protect sulfite-sensitive people, the FDA created rules for using the preservatives safely. The rules called for a total ban on sulfites in food at salad bars and a requirement that sulfites be listed on the label of any food or beverage product with more than ten part sulfites to every million parts food (10 ppm). These rules, plus lots of press information about the risks of sulfites, have led to a dramatic decrease in the number of sulfite reactions, down from an average of 110 cases a year from 1984 through 1994 to just six cases in 1995.

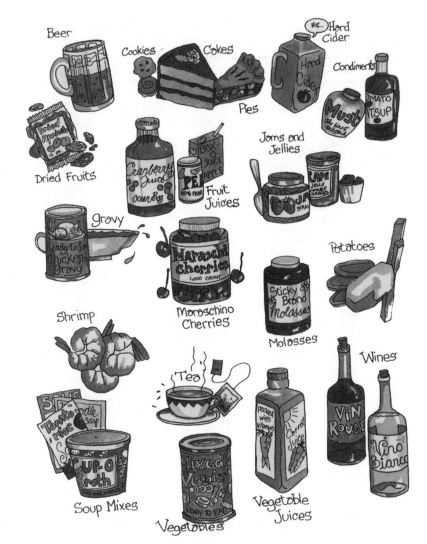

The Final Word on Additives, Straight from the Source

If you're still uneasy about the safety of food additives, you may want to read for yourself the rules governing the FDA's decision to put an additive on the GRAS list.

You can find the entire procedure spelled out on the Center for Food Safety Web page (vm.cfsan.fda.gov/~lrd/foodaddi.txt).

Part V
Food and Medicine

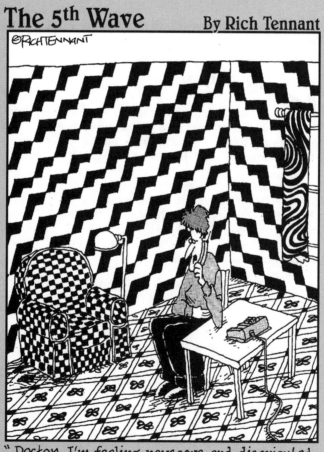

The 5th Wave   By Rich Tennant

"Doctor, I'm feeling nauseous and disoriented. Do you think I'm having a reaction to something I ate?"

In this part . . .

*H*ow come a civilization (yours) that has antibiotics, analgesics, and decongestants still serves up chicken soup for a cold, coffee for a headache, and chocolate for a broken heart? Because they work!

Food and medicine are natural partners. Sometimes they fight (the technical term is *food/drug interactions*), but more often — as you see in this part — they work together to keep your body in tip-top shape.

Chapter 23

When Food Gives You Hives

● ●

In This Chapter

▶ What a food allergy is

▶ The foods most likely to trigger allergic reactions

▶ How to tell whether you're allergic to a specific food

▶ The difference between food allergy and food intolerance

● ●

A ccording to the National Institutes of Health, true food allergies (also known as food hypersensitivity) affect about 5 million Americans, including 5 to 8 percent of all children and 2 percent of adults. Many childhood allergies seem to disappear as children grow older.

So, you may ask, why do I need a whole chapter on food allergies? Good question. Here's the answer: Food allergies that do not disappear can trigger reactions ranging from trivial (a stuffy nose the next day) to the truly dangerous (respiratory failure). So it pays to know which foods do what.

What Is a Food Allergy?

Your immune system is designed to protect your body from harmful invaders, such as bacteria. Sometimes, however, your immune system responds to substances that are normally harmless. A food allergy is just such a response — your body fighting back against specific proteins in foods. Table 23-1 lists some common allergic reactions to food.

Table 23-1	Symptoms of an Allergic Reaction to Food
Reaction	
Hives	
Itching	

(continued)

Table 23-1 *(continued)*
Reaction
Swelling of the face, tongue, lips, eyelids, hands, and feet
Rashes
Headache, migraine
Nausea and/or vomiting
Diarrhea, sometimes bloody
Sneezing, coughing
Asthma
Breathing difficulties caused by *tightening* (swelling) of tissues in the throat
Loss of consciousness (anaphylactic shock)

Two kinds of allergic reactions

Your body may respond to an allergen immediately or later on.

- ✔ Immediate reactions are more dangerous than delayed reactions because they involve a fast swelling of tissues. Immediate reactions may occur within seconds after eating, touching, or — in some cases — even smelling the offending food.

- ✔ Delayed reactions may occur as long as 24 to 48 hours after you've been exposed to the offending food, and the reaction is likely to be much more mild, perhaps a slight nasal congestion caused by swollen tissues.

How an allergic reaction occurs

When you eat a food containing a protein to which you are allergic (the allergen), your immune system releases antibodies (IgE) that recognize just that specific allergen. The antibodies circulate through your body on white blood cells (basophils) that pass into all your body tissues where they bind to immune system cells, called mast cells.

Both basophils and mast cells produce, store, and release histamine, which causes the symptoms — itching, swelling, hives — associated with allergic reactions. (That's why some allergy pills are called antihistamines.) When the antibodies carried by the basophils and mast cells come in contact with food allergens, boom! You have an allergic reaction.

Allergy lingo

allergen: Any substance that sets off an allergic reaction (see "antigen" in this sidebar)

anaphylaxis: A potentially life-threatening allergic reaction that involves many body systems

antibody: A substance in your blood that reacts to an antigen

antigen: A substance that stimulates an immune response; an allergen is an antigen

basophil: A white blood cell that carries IgE and releases histamine

ELISA: Short for *enzyme-linked immunosorbent assay,* a test used to determine the presence in your blood of antibodies, including antibodies to specific allergens

histamine: The substance released by the immune system that provides symptoms or an allergic reaction such as itching and swelling

intolerance: A nonallergic adverse reaction to food

IgE: An abbreviation for *immunoglobulin E,* the antibody that reacts to allergens

mast cell: A cell in body tissue that releases histamine

RAST: An abbreviation for *radioallergosorbent test,* a blood test used to determine whether you are allergic to certain foods

urticaria: The medical name for hives

Source: American Academy of Allergy & Immunology, International Food Information Council Foundation, "Understanding Food Allergy" (April 1995).

Who gets food allergies?

A tendency to allergies (though not the particular allergy itself) is inherited. If one of your parents has a food allergy, your risk of having the same problem is two times higher than it would be if neither of your parents were allergic to foods. If both your mother and your father have food allergies, your risk is four times higher. People with food allergies are often allergic to other things, such as dust or pollen, as well.

Are food allergies dangerous?

They can be. While most allergic reactions are unpleasant but essentially mild, about 100 people die every year in the United States from an allergic reaction to food. These people have suffered anaphylaxis *(a-na-fi-laxis),* a rare but potentially fatal condition in which many different parts of the body react to an allergen in food (or some other allergen), creating a cascade of effects beginning with sudden, severe itching and moving on to swelling of the tissue in the air passages that can lead to breathing difficulties, falling blood pressure, unconsciousness, and death.

The Foods Most Likely to Cause Allergic Reactions

Here's something to chew on: More than 90 percent of all allergic reactions to foods are caused by just eight foods (see Figure 23-1):

- ✔ Milk
- ✔ Eggs
- ✔ Peanuts
- ✔ Nuts
- ✔ Soy foods
- ✔ Wheat
- ✔ Fish
- ✔ Shellfish

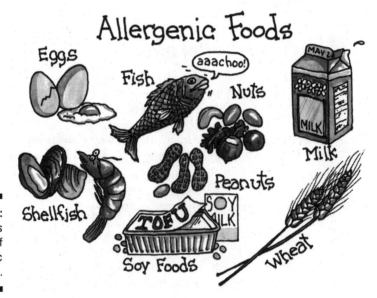

Figure 23-1: These foods can set off an allergic reaction.

The allergenic food most likely to make headlines seems to be peanuts. People allergic to peanuts may break out in hives just from touching a peanut or peanut butter and suffer a potentially fatal reaction after simply tasting chocolate made in a factory where it had touched machinery that had previously touched peanuts.

For information about potentially allergenic food additives, see Chapter 22.

Identifying Food Allergies

If you sprout hives or your skin itches or your eyelids, lips, and tongue begin to swell right after you've eaten a particular food, that's a clear sign of a food allergy. But some allergic reactions occur in milder form, many hours after you've eaten. To identify the culprit, your doctor may suggest an elimination diet.

This regimen removes from your diet foods known to cause allergic reactions in many people. Then, one at a time, the foods are added back. If you react to one, bingo! That's a clue to what triggers your immune response.

To be absolutely certain, your doctor may "challenge" your immune system by introducing foods in a form (maybe a capsule) that neither you nor he can identify as a specific food. This rules out any possibility that your reaction has been triggered by emotional stimuli — that is, seeing, tasting, or smelling the food.

Two more sophisticated tests — ELISA (enzyme-linked immunosorbent assay) and RAST (radioallergosorbent test) — can identify antibodies to specific allergens in your blood. But these two tests are rarely required.

Coping with Food Allergies

Once you know that you're allergic to a food, the best way to avoid an allergic reaction is to avoid the food. Unfortunately, the task may be harder than it sounds.

Some allergens are hidden ingredients in dishes made with other foods. For example, people allergic to peanuts have suffered serious allergic reactions after eating chili made with peanut butter. Rye bread may contain some wheat flour, which contains gluten, a protein that is a common food allergen.

Elimination diets

Because different people are sensitive to different foods, more than one elimination diet exists. The three listed here eliminate broad groups of foods known to cause allergic reactions in many people. Your doctor will pick the one that seems most useful for you.

Diet #1: No beef, pork, poultry, milk, rye, corn

Diet #2: No beef, lamb, rice, milk

Diet #3: No lamb, poultry, rye, rice, corn, milk

Source: *The Merck Manual,* 16th ed. (Rahway, N.J.: Merck Research Laboratories, 1992)

Another problem is that you may not even have to eat the food to suffer an allergic reaction. People who react to seafood — fin fish and shellfish — are known to have developed respiratory problems after simply inhaling the vapors or steam produced by cooking the fish.

If you are a person with a potentially life-threatening allergy to food (or another allergen, such as wasp venom), your doctor may suggest that you carry a syringe prefilled with *epinephrine,* a drug that counteracts the reactions. You may also wish to wear a tag that identifies you as a person with a serious allergic problem. One company that provides these tags is Medic-Alert, a 40-year-old firm located in Turloc, California. The telephone number for Medic-Alert is 1-800-633-4260.

The food industry takes food allergies so seriously that the National Restaurant Association has joined forces with the American Academy of Allergy, Asthma, and Immunology; the Food Allergy Network; and the International Food Information Council Foundation to produce the poster shown in Figure 23-2 to be hung in restaurant kitchens.

You may want to visit the following Web sites for more details on food allergies:

✔ The American Academy of Allergy, Asthma, and Immunology (www.aaaai.org)

✔ The Food Allergy Network (www.foodallergy.org)

FOOD ALLERGY
WHAT WE NEED TO KNOW

Customers allergic to some foods need our special attention. Understanding the food allergy basics on this chart will help us ensure our customers have a pleasant and safe dining experience. When a customer asks whether a certain food or ingredient is included in a menu item, you *must* answer their questions carefully and accurately. If you are unsure of the exact ingredients of a particular food, say so and refer the question to the manager on duty.

MOST COMMON ALLERGENS

The foods most likely to cause serious reactions in people with allergies are:

MILK	EGGS	FISH, SHELLFISH	WHEAT	SOY	PEANUTS	OTHER NUTS

SYMPTOMS OF ALLERGIC REACTIONS

Sometimes an allergic reaction can be so severe it may even cause death.
Call 911 and notify management if a customer experiences any of the following symptoms:

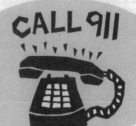

* loss of consciousness
* wheezing and hoarseness
* shortness of breath
* tightening of the throat (difficulty swallowing)

* swelling of the face, eyelids, lips, hands or feet
* hives (welts)
* itching in and around the mouth, face, scalp, hands and feet

WHAT WE NEED TO DO

We can help prevent serious allergic reactions if we:

* Carefully clean utensils, containers, and grills (to avoid cross-contamination between foods)

* When in doubt, refer customers' food allergy questions to management

FOR MORE INFORMATION

 American Academy of Allergy, Asthma and Immunology
611 East Wells Street
Milwaukee, WI 53202
1-800-822-2762

 The Food Allergy Network
10400 Eaton Place
Suite 107
Fairfax, VA 22030
1-800-929-4040
http://www.foodallergy.org/

 International Food Information Council Foundation
1100 Connecticut Avenue, N.W.
Suite 430
Washington, D.C. 20036
http://ificinfo.health.org

 National Restaurant Association
1200 Seventeenth Street, NW
Washington, DC 20036

Figure 23-2:
This food allergy poster is found in restaurant kitchens.

Other Body Reactions to Food

Allergic reactions aren't the only way your body registers a protest against certain foods.

Food intolerance is a term used to describe reactions that are common, natural, and definitely not allergic, which means that these reactions do not involve production of antibodies by the immune system. Some common food intolerance reactions are

- ✔ **A metabolic food reaction,** which is an inability to digest certain foods, such as fat or lactose (the naturally occurring sugar in milk). Metabolic food reactions can produce gas, diarrhea, or other signs of gastric revolt and are an inherited trait.

- ✔ **A physical reaction to a specific chemical** such as the laxative substance in prunes or monosodium glutamate (MSG), the flavor enhancer commonly found in Asian food. While some people are more sensitive than others to these chemicals, their reaction is a physical one, not an allergy.

- ✔ **A body response to psychological triggers.** When you are very fearful or very anxious or very excited, your body moves into hyperdrive, secreting hormones that pump up your heartbeat and respiration, speed the passage of food through your gut, and cause you to empty your bowels and bladder. The entire process, called the "fight-or-flight" reaction, prepares your body to defend itself by either fighting or running. On a more prosaic level, a strong reaction to your food may cause diarrhea. It's not an allergy; it's your hormones.

- ✔ **A change in mood and/or behavior.** Some foods, such as coffee, contain chemicals, such as caffeine, that have a real effect on mood and behavior, but that's the subject of Chapter 24. Turn the page, and it's yours.

Chapter 24

Food and Mood

• •

In This Chapter

▶ How food affects the brain

▶ Foods that increase alertness

▶ Foods that calm

▶ Meal plans that use food as an effective mood regulator

• •

Draw the curtains. Turn down the lights. Come a little closer. We're going to talk about something nutritionists never seem to write about: Food can make you feel good. I don't mean the simple warm good feelings that follow a fine meal. I mean the pick-me-up-when-I'm-low, calm-me-down-when-I'm-hyper kind of good you usually associate with serious mood-altering drugs.

Why do most nutrition books ignore this subject? Frankly, I haven't a clue. But the nice thing about writing this book is that I get the opportunity to pass along a lot of information that you may otherwise never see.

So here's a chapter on mood and food. The chapter names some of the common, naturally occurring, mood-alerting chemicals in food; explains how these chemicals work; and presents some simple strategies for increasing their effectiveness. Sit back, open a box of chocolates, pour a glass of wine, brew up the espresso — and enjoy.

How Chemicals Alter Mood

A *mood* is a feeling, an internal emotional state that can affect how you see the world. For example:

> ✔ If your team wins the World Series, your happiness may last for days, making you feel so mellow that you simply shrug off minor annoyances such as finding a ticket on your windshield because your parking meter expired while you were having lunch.

✔ If you feel sad because the project you spent six months setting up didn't work out, your disappointment can linger long enough to make your work seem temporarily unrewarding or your favorite television show unfunny.

Most of the time, your mood swings back to center fairly soon. You come down from your high or recover from your disappointment, and life resumes its normal pace — some good stuff here, some bad news there, but all in all, a relatively even field.

Occasionally, however, your mood can go haywire. Your happiness over your team's victory escalates to the point where you find yourself rushing from store to store buying things you cannot afford, or your sadness over your failure at work deepens into a gloom that steals the joy from everything else. This unpleasant state of affairs — a mood out of control — is called a mood disorder.

About one in every four human beings (women more often than men) will experience some form of mood disturbance during their lifetime. Eight or nine out of every 100 people will experience a clinical mood disorder, a mood disorder serious enough to be diagnosed as a disease.

The two most common moods are happiness and sadness. The two most common mood disorders are clinical depression (an elongated period of overly intense sadness) and clinical mania (an elongated period of overly intense elation). Clinical depression alone is called a unipolar (one-part) disorder; clinical depression plus clinical mania is a bipolar (two-part) disorder.

Today, scientists have identified naturally occurring brain chemicals that affect mood and play a role in mood disorder. Your body makes a group of substances called *neurotransmitters,* chemicals that allow brain cells to send messages back and forth. Three important neurotransmitters are

✔ Dopamine *(doe-pa-meen)*

✔ Norepinephrine *(nor-e-pee-ne-frin)*

✔ Serotonin *(se-ro-toe-nin)*

Dopamine and norepinephrine are chemicals that make you feel alert and energized. Serotonin is a chemical that can make you feel smooth and mellow.

Some forms of clinical depression and mania appear to be malfunctions of the body's ability to handle these chemicals. Drugs known as antidepressants adjust mood by making neurotransmitters more available to your brain or enabling your brain to use them more efficiently. Medications used to treat mood disorders include

✔ **Tricyclic antidepressants:** These drugs, named for their chemical structure that includes three groups of atoms shaped like rings (tri = three, cyclic = ring), relieve symptoms by increasing the availability of serotonin.

✔ **Monoamine oxidase inhibitors (also known as MAO inhibitors):** These drugs slow your body's natural destruction of dopamine and other neurotransmitters so that they remain available to your brain.

✔ **Lithium:** This drug's precise actions remain unknown, but it may increase the availability of serotonin and lower the availability of norepinephrine.

✔ **A grab-bag of chemicals unrelated to each other or to other groups of antidepressants:** Some are known to regulate the availability of serotonin; others work in ways that have not yet been identified.

How Food Affects Mood

Good morning! Time to wake up, roll out of bed, and sleepwalk into the kitchen for a cup of coffee.

Good afternoon! Time for a moderate glass of whiskey or wine to soothe away the tensions of the day.

Good grief! Your lover has left. Time for chocolate, lots of chocolate, to soothe the pain.

Good night! Time for milk and cookies to ease your way to Dreamland.

For centuries, millions of people have used these foods in these situations, secure in the knowledge that the food will work mood magic. Today, modern science knows why. Having discovered that our emotions are linked to our production or use of certain brain chemicals, nutrition scientists have been able to identify the natural chemicals in food that change the way you feel by

✔ Influencing the production of neurotransmitters

✔ Hooking onto brain cells and changing the way the cells behave

✔ Opening pathways to brain cells so that other mood-altering chemicals can come on board

The following sections describe chemicals in food most commonly known to affect mood.

Alcohol

Alcohol is the most widely used natural relaxer. Contrary to common belief, alcohol is a depressant, not a mood elevator. If you feel loosey-goosey and exuberant after one drink, it's not because the alcohol is speeding up your brain. It is because alcohol relaxes your *controls*, the brain signals that normally tell you not to put a lampshade on your head or take off your clothes in public.

For more about alcohol's effects on virtually every body organ and system, turn to Chapter 9. Here, it is enough to say that many people find that, taken with food and in moderation — defined as one drink a day for a woman, two for a man — alcohol can comfortably change one's mood from tense to mellow.

Anandamide

Anandamide is a *cannabinoid*, a chemical that hooks up to the same brain receptors that catch similar ingredients in marijuana smoke. Your brain produces some anandamide naturally, but you also get very small amounts of the chemical from (what else?) chocolate. In addition, chocolate contains two chemicals similar to anandamide, which slow the breakdown of the anandamide produced in your brain, intensifying its effects. Maybe that's why eating chocolate makes you feel very mildly mellow. Not enough to get you hauled off to the hoosegow (jail) or bring in the Feds to confiscate your candy; just enough to wipe away the tears of lost love. (Don't worry; you'd need to eat at least 25 pounds of chocolate at one time in order to get any marijuana-like effect.)

Caffeine

I don't think that I have to tell you that caffeine is a mild stimulant that

- ✔ Raises your blood pressure
- ✔ Speeds up your heartbeat
- ✔ Makes you burn calories faster
- ✔ Makes you urinate more frequently
- ✔ Causes your intestinal tract to move food more quickly through your body

Nor do I have to tell you that caffeine is a mood elevator. While it increases the level of serotonin, the calming neurotransmitter, it also hooks up at specific receptors (sites on the surface of brain cells) normally reserved for another naturally occurring tranquilizer, adenosine *(a-DEN-o-seen)*. When caffeine latches in place of adenosine, brain cells become more reactive to stimulants such as noise and light, making you talk faster and think faster. Lately, athletes who take coffee before an event have reported that it also improves performance in some endurance events.

But how people react to caffeine is a highly individual affair. Some can drink seven cups of regular (read "with caffeine") coffee a day and still stay calm all day and sleep like a baby at night. Others — me, for instance — tend to hop about on decaf. Or, as my husband often says, "What was the blur that just went through the living room?" Perhaps those who stay calm have enough brain receptors to accommodate both adenosine and caffeine, or perhaps they are more sensitive to the adenosine that manages to hook up to brain cells. Nobody really knows.

Either way, caffeine's bouncy effects may last anywhere from one to seven hours. I know that I can count on missing a night's sleep when I have real (as opposed to decaffeinated) coffee after 5 p.m. Espresso at dinner? I'll still be awake when the birds get up the next morning. Table 24-1 lists some common food sources of caffeine.

Table 24-1	Foods That Give You Caffeine
Food	*Amount of Caffeine*
5-ounce cups	
Coffee, regular, drip	80 – 150 milligrams
Coffee, regular, instant	40 – 108 milligrams
Coffee, decaffeinated	1 – 6 milligrams
Tea	20 – 110 milligrams
Tea, instant	25 – 60 milligrams
Cocoa	2 – 50 milligrams
12-ounce can	
Soft drink	30 – 72 milligrams
8-ounce container	
Chocolate milk	2 – 7 milligrams
1-ounce serving	
Milk chocolate	1 – 15 milligrams
Semisweet chocolate	5 – 35 milligrams
Bitter (baker's) chocolate	26 milligrams

Sources: George M. Briggs and Doris Howes Callaway, *Nutrition and Physical Fitness,* 11th ed. (New York: Holt, Rinehart and Winston, 1984); *Current Medical Diagnosis and Treatment,* 36th ed. (Stamford, CT: Appleton and Lange, 1997).

Tryptophan and glucose

Tryptophan is an *amino acid,* a group of chemicals commonly called the building blocks of protein (see Chapter 6). Glucose, the end product of carbohydrate metabolism, is the sugar that circulates in your blood, the basic fuel on which your body runs (see Chapter 8).

Milk and cookies, a classic calming combo, owe their power to this, the tryptophan/glucose team.

Start with the fact that the neurotransmitters dopamine, norepinephrine, and serotonin are made from the amino acids tyrosine and tryptophan, found in protein foods. Tyrosine is the most important ingredient in dopamine and norepinephrine, the alertness neurotransmitters. Tryptophan is the most important ingredient in serotonin, the calming neurotransmitter.

All amino acids ride into your brain like little trains on tiny chemical railroads. But Mother Nature — clearly a party animal! — has arranged the switches so that your brain makes way for the bouncy tyrosine train first and the soothing tryptophan train last. That's why a high-protein meal heightens your alertness.

To move the tryptophan train up the track, you need glucose. That means that you need carbohydrate foods. When you eat carbs, your pancreas releases *insulin,* a hormone that enables you to metabolize the carbs and produce glucose. The insulin also keeps tyrosine and other amino acids circulating in your blood so that tryptophan trains can travel on lots of open tracks to the brain. With more tryptophan coming in, your brain can increase its production of soothing serotonin. That's why a meal of starchy pasta (starch is composed of chains of glucose molecules, as explained in Chapter 8) makes you calm, cool, and kind of groovy.

The effects of simple sugars such as sucrose (table sugar) are more complicated. If you eat simple sugars on an empty stomach, the sugars are absorbed rapidly, triggering an equally rapid increase in the secretion of insulin, a hormone needed to digest carbohydrates. The result is a rapid decrease in the amount of sugar circulating in your blood, a condition known as "hypoglycemia" (low blood sugar) that can make you feel temporarily jumpy rather than calm. However, when eaten on a full stomach — dessert after a full meal — simple sugars are absorbed more slowly and may exert the calming effect usually linked to complex carbohydrates (starchy foods).

Some foods make you more alert (such as meat, fish, and poultry) or calm you down (such as pasta, bread, potatoes, rice, and other grains), depending on their ability to alter the amount of serotonin available to your brain. (See Figure 24-1.)

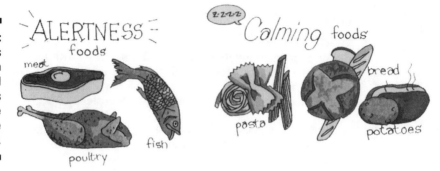

Figure 24-1: Some foods may calm you, and some foods may make you more alert.

Phenylethylalanine (PEA)

Phenylethylalanine — sometimes abbreviated PEA — is an amino acid that your body releases when you are in love, making you feel, well, good all over. A big splash occurred in the late 1980s when researchers discovered that chocolate, the food of lovers, is a fine source of PEA.

In fact, many people think that PEA has a lot to do with chocolate's reputation as the food of love and consolation. Of course, to be fair about it, chocolate also contains the mood-elevator caffeine, the muscle stimulant throbromine, and the cannabinoid anandamide (see the discussion on anandamide earlier in this chapter).

What is there to say other than, hey, can you please pass that box of chocolates down to this end of the table. . . .

Using Food to Manage Mood

No food will change your personality or alter the course of a mood disorder. But some may add a little lift or a small moment of calm to your day, increase your effectiveness at certain tasks, make you more alert, or give you a neat little push over the finish line.

The watchword is balance.

- ✔ One cup of coffee in the a.m. is a pleasant push into alertness. Seven cups of coffee a day can make your hands shake.
- ✔ One alcohol drink is generally a safe way to relax. Three may be a disaster.

- ✔ A grilled chicken breast (white meat, no skin) for breakfast — yes, breakfast — on a day when you have to be on your toes before lunch, can help make you sharp as a tack.

- ✔ Got an important lunch meeting? Order starches without fats or oils — pasta with fresh tomatoes and basil, no oil, no cheese; rice with veggies; rice with fruit. Your aim is to get the calming carbs without the high-fat food that slows thinking and makes you feel sleepy.

In this, as in other aspects of a healthy life, the point is to make sure that you use the tool (in this case, food), not the other way around.

Caution! Medicine at work

Some of the mood-altering chemicals in food interact with medicines. As you may have guessed, the two most notable examples are caffeine and alcohol.

- ✔ Caffeine makes painkillers such as aspirin and acetaminophen more effective. On the other hand, many over-the-counter (OTC) painkillers already contain caffeine. If you take the pill with a cup of java, you may increase your caffeine intake past the jitters stage.

- ✔ Alcohol is a no-no with virtually every medicine. It increases the sedative or depressant effects of some drugs, such as antihistamines and painkillers, while altering the rate at which you absorb or excrete others.

Always ask your pharmacist about food/drug interactions (you can read more about this in Chapter 25) when you fill a prescription; for OTC products, read the label. Very carefully.

Chapter 25

Food and Drug Interactions

. . . .

In This Chapter

▶ Drugs that affect appetite

▶ How some foods make some drugs less effective

▶ Which drugs should be taken with food

▶ Drugs that interact with vitamins and minerals

. . . .

*F*oods nourish your body. Medicines cure (or relieve) what ails you. You'd think the two would work together in perfect harmony to protect your body. Sometimes they do. Occasionally, however, foods and drugs square off like boxers slugging it out in the ring. (See Figure 25-1.) The drug keeps your body from absorbing or using the nutrients in food or the food (or nutrient) prevents you from getting the benefits of certain medicines.

The medical word for this state of affairs is *interaction*. This chapter describes the basic ways in which foods and drugs interact, and lays out some simple strategies that make it possible for you to get the full benefit from both.

How a Food and Drug Interaction Happens

When you eat, food moves from your mouth to your stomach to your small intestine, where the nutrients that keep you strong and healthy are absorbed into your bloodstream and distributed throughout your body.

Take medicine by mouth, and it follows pretty much the same path from your mouth to your stomach, where it is dissolved and passed along to the small intestine for absorption.

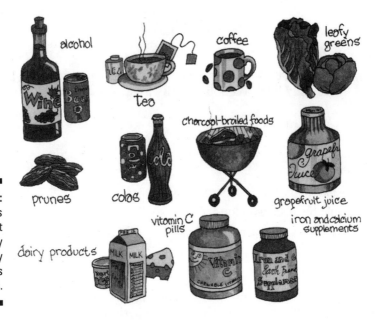

Figure 25-1:
Some foods may affect the way your body interacts with drugs.

Nothing unusual there. The problem arises when a food or drug brings the process to a screeching halt by behaving in a way that stops your body from using either the drug or the food. Many possibilities exist:

✔ Some drugs or foods change the natural acidity of your digestive tract so that you absorb nutrients less efficiently. For example, your body absorbs iron best when the inside of your stomach is acid. Taking antacids reduces stomach acidity — and iron absorption.

✔ Some drugs or foods change the rate at which food moves through your digestive tract, which means that you absorb more (or less) of a particular nutrient or drug. For example, eating prunes (a laxative food) or taking a laxative drug speeds things up so that food (and drugs) move more quickly through your body and you have less time to absorb medicine or nutrients.

✔ Some drugs and nutrients *bond* (link up with each other) to form insoluble compounds that your body cannot break apart. As a result, you get less of the drug and less of the nutrient. The best-known example: Calcium (in dairy foods) bonds to the antibiotic tetracycline so that both zip right out of your body.

✔ Some drugs and nutrients have similar chemical structures. Taking them at the same time fools your body into absorbing or using the nutrient rather than the drug. One good example is warfarin (a drug that keeps blood from clotting) and vitamin K (a nutrient that makes blood clot). Eating lots of vitamin K-rich leafy greens while taking warfarin clearly makes the drug less effective.

✔ Some foods contain chemicals that either fight or intensify the natural side effects of certain drugs. For example, the caffeine in coffee, tea, and cola drinks reduces the sedative effects of antihistamines and some antidepressant drugs, while increasing the nervousness, insomnia, and shakiness common with some diet pills and cold medications containing caffeine or a *decongestant* (an ingredient that temporarily clears a stuffy nose).

Food Fights: Drugs versus Nutrients versus Drugs

Sometimes the foods and drugs that interact are positively astounding.

Here's a prime example. Everyone knows that people with asthma may find it hard to take a deep breath around the barbecue. The culprit's all that smoke, right? Maybe not. It turns out that charcoal-broiled food speeds the body's elimination of theophylline, a widely-used asthma drug, reducing the drug's ability to protect against wheezing. Take the drug, eat the food, end up wheezing. Yipes.

Another potential troublemaker: fruit juice. Acidic beverages (colas as well as fruit juice) can send the antibiotics erythromycin, ampicillin, and penicillin down for the count. Grapefruit juice taken at the same time as the drug can alter your body's absorption of some calcium channel blockers (drugs used to treat high blood pressure), estrogen-type hormones (used at menopause), the antihistamine terfenidine, and cyclosporine (a drug used to prevent the body from rejecting a transplanted organ). The grapefruit reaction is very specific: As of this writing, orange juice is not linked to similar problems.

Water pills, more properly known as *diuretics,* make you urinate more often and more copiously, thus increasing your elimination of the mineral potassium. To make up what you lose, experts suggest adding potatoes, bananas, oranges, spinach, corn, and tomatoes to your diet. Consuming less sodium (salt) while you are using water pills makes the water pills more effective and decreases your loss of potassium.

Oral contraceptives seem to reduce the ability to absorb B vitamins, including folate. Taking lots of aspirin or other nonsteroidal anti-inflammatories such as ibuprofen can trigger a painless, slow but steady loss of small amounts of blood from the lining of your stomach that may lead to iron-deficiency anemia.

Persistent use of antacids made with aluminum compounds may lead to loss of the bone-building mineral phosphorus, which binds to aluminum and rides right out of the body. Laxatives increase the loss of minerals (calcium and others) in feces.

The anti-ulcer drugs cimetadine (Tagamet) and ranitidine (Zantac) can make you positively giddy. These drugs reduce stomach acidity, which means the body absorbs alcohol more efficiently. According to experts at the Mayo Clinic, taking ulcer medication with alcohol leads to twice the wallop, like drinking one beer and feeling the effects of two.

Of course, check with your doctor for any food and drug interaction that could affect you.

Finally, there are nutritional supplements. The vitamins and minerals in nutritional supplements are simply food reduced to its basic nutrients, so it's not surprising that drugs and supplements often interact. Table 25-1 lists some common vitamin and mineral and drug interactions.

Table 25-1	Battling Nutrients and Medications
You Absorb Less	**When You Take**
Vitamin A	Aluminum antacids Biscodyl (laxative) Cholestyramine (lower cholesterol) Fenfluramin (diet pill) Mineral oil (laxative) Neomycin (antibiotic)
Vitamin D	Biscodyl (laxative) Cholestyramine (lowers cholesterol) Mineral oil (laxative) Neomycin (antibiotic)
Vitamin K	Biscodyl (laxative) Cholestyramin (lowers cholesterol) Mineral oil (laxative) Neomycin (antibiotic)
Vitamin C	Aspirin Barbiturates (sleeping pills) Cortisone and related steroid drugs
Thiamin	Antacids (calcium) Aspirin Cortisone and related steroid drugs
Riboflavin	Birth control pills
Folate	Aspirin Cholestyramine (lowers cholesterol) Penicillin Phenobarbital, primidone, phenothiazines (antiseizure drugs) Sulfa drugs

You Absorb Less	When You Take
Vitamin B12	Cholestyramine (lowers cholesterol) Neomycin (antibiotic)
Calcium	Cortisone and related steroid drugs Diuretics ("water pills") Magnesium antacids Neomycin (antibiotic) Phosphorus laxatives Tetracycline (antibiotic)
Phosphorus	Aluminum antacids
Magnesium	Amphotericin b (antibiotic) Diuretics ("water pills") Tetracycline (antibiotic)
Iron	Aspirin and other non-steroidal anti-inflammatory drugs Calcium antacids Calcium supplements (with meals) Cholestyramine (lowers cholesterol) Neomycin (antibiotic) Penicillin (antibiotic) Tetracycline (antibiotic)
Zinc	Diuretics ("water pills")

Sources: James W. Long and James J. Rybacki, *The Essential Guide to Prescription Drugs* (New York: Harper Collins, 1995); Brian L. G. Morgan, *The Food and Drug Interaction Guide* (New York: Simon and Schuster, 1986); Eleanor Noss Whitney, Corinne Balog Cataldo, and Sharon Rady Rolfes, *Understanding Normal and Clinical Nutrition,* 4th ed. (Minneapolis/St. Paul: West Publishing, 1994).

How to Avoid Food and Drug Interactions

When you pick up an over-the-counter drug or get a new prescription, ask if there are any foods you should avoid while you are taking this drug. Read the label. Often the warnings and interactions are right there on the package. If they're not, ask your doctor or pharmacist. Go on, now — ask.

As a last resort (or a first one, if medical stuff is your thing), pick up a copy of *The Essential Guide to Prescription Drugs,* the book listed as one of the sources for the tables in this chapter. It is affordable, readable, and reliable. Go for it.

When Food Improves a Drug's Performance

Sometimes a drug works better or is less likely to cause side effects if you take it on a full stomach. For example, aspirin is less likely to upset your stomach if you take the painkiller with food, and eating stimulates the release of stomach juices that improve your ability to absorb griseofulvin, an antifungus drug.

Table 25-2 lists some drugs that may work better when your stomach is full.

Table 25-2	Drugs that Work Better on a Full Stomach
Drug	
Analgesics (painkillers)	
Acetaminophen	
Aspirin	
Codeine	
Ibuprofen	
Indomethacin	
Mefenamic acid	
Metronidazole	
Naproxen/naproxen sodium	
Antibiotics, Antivirals, Antifungals	
Ethambutol	
Griseofulvin	
Isoniazid	
Ketoconazole	
Pyrimethamine	
Antidiabetic Agents	
Glipizide	
Glyburide	
Tolazamide	
Tolbutamide	

Drug
Cholesterol-Lowering Agents
Cholestryamine
Colestipol
Lovastatin
Probucol
Ulcer Medications
Cimetadine
Ranitidine

Source: James W. Long and James J. Rybacki, *The Essential Guide to Prescription Drugs* (New York: Harper Collins, 1995).

Don't guess about drugs and food. Every time you take a pill, read the package label or check with your doctor/pharmacist to find out whether taking the medicine with food improves or reduces its ability to make you better.

With this medicine, who can eat?

Interactions aren't the only drug reactions that keep you from getting nutrients from food. Some drugs have side effects that also reduce the value of food. For example, a drug may

✔ Sharply reduce your appetite so that you simply don't eat much. The best-known example may be the amphetamine and amphetamine-like drugs such as fenfluramine used (surprise!) as "diet pills."

✔ Make food taste or smell bad or steal away your sense of taste or smell so that eating isn't pleasurable. One example is the antidepressant drug amitriptyline (Elavil), which can leave a peculiar taste in your mouth.

✔ Cause nausea, vomiting, or diarrhea so that you either cannot eat or do not retain nutrients from the food you do eat. Examples include the antibiotic erythromycin and many drugs used to treat cancer.

✔ Irritate the lining of your gut so that even if you do eat, your body has a hard time absorbing nutrients from food. One example of a drug that causes this side effect is cyclophosphamide, an antitumor medication.

The moderately good news is that new medications appear to make some drugs (including anticancer drugs) less likely to cause nausea and vomiting. The best news is that many drugs are less likely to upset your stomach or irritate your gut if you take them with food.

For example, taking aspirin and other nonprescription painkillers such as ibuprofen with food or a full glass of water may reduce their natural tendency to irritate the lining of your stomach. (See Table 25-2.)

Chapter 26

Using Food as Medicine

- -

In This Chapter

▶ Diets for special medical conditions

▶ Foods that fight cancer

▶ Using food to ease annoying but relatively minor health problems

▶ Finding your Fountain of Youth

▶ When food is not your best medicine

- -

*M*odern mainstream nutrition emphasizes using food to promote health. In other words, a good diet is one that gives you the nutrients you need to keep your body in topflight condition. It is also increasingly clear that eating right offers more benefits than simply sustaining bodily functions. A good diet may also turn out to prevent or minimize the risk of a long list of serious medical conditions including heart disease, high blood pressure, and cancer.

This chapter describes what nutritionists know right now about how to use food to prevent, alleviate, or cure what ails you.

When Food Is Medicine

Start with a definition. A food that acts like a medicine is one that increases or reduces your risk of a specific medical condition or cures or alleviates the effects of a medical condition. For example

> ✔ Eating foods such as wheat bran that are high in insoluble dietary fiber (the kind of fiber that doesn't dissolve in your gut) moves food more quickly through your intestinal tract and may reduce your risk of colon cancer. It also produces soft bulky stool that reduces your risk of constipation.

✔ Eating foods such as beans that are high in soluble dietary fiber (fiber that dissolves in your intestinal tract) seems to help your body mop up the cholesterol circulating in your bloodstream, preventing it from sticking to the walls of your arteries. This reduces your risk of heart disease.

✔ Eating very spicy foods such as chili makes the membrane lining your nose and throat "weep" a watery fluid that makes it easier to blow your nose or cough up mucus when you have a cold.

The absence of food can also be beneficial: There's no question that overweight adults who reduce to a "normal" weight (see Chapter 3 for totally reasonable weight tables) may prevent or reverse adult-onset diabetes without the use of drugs.

And don't forget mental health. As you can plainly see in Chapter 24, many common foods contain mood-altering substances such as caffeine, alcohol, and phenylethylalanine (PEA) that can change your mood, lifting you up when you're down or calming you down when you're tense.

The joy of food-as-medicine is that it's cheaper and much more pleasant than managing illness with drugs. Given the choice, who wouldn't opt to control cholesterol levels with oats or chili (all those yummy beans packed with soluble dietary fiber) than with a drug whose possible side effects include kidney failure and liver damage?

Some Diets with Absolutely, Positively Beneficial Medical Effects

Some foods and some diet plans are so obviously good for your body that no one questions their ability to keep you healthy or make you feel better if you're ill. For example, if you have ever had abdominal surgery, you know all about liquid diets — the water-gelatin-clear soup regimen your doctor prescribed right after the operation to allow you to take some nourishment by mouth without upsetting your gut.

Or if you have diabetes (an inherited inability to produce the insulin needed to process carbohydrates), you know that your ability to balance the carbohydrates, fats, and proteins in your daily diet is important to stabilizing your illness.

Other proven diet regimens include:

✔ **The soft diet.** This diet, with lots of chopped, ground, or pureed foods, is for people who have had head and neck surgery or those who, for any reason — including dentures — find it difficult to chew or swallow hard or tough food.

✔ **The sodium-restricted diet.** Sodium is hydrophilic (hydro = water; phylic = attracting). It increases the amount of water held in body tissues. A diet low in salt often lowers water retention, which can be useful in treating high blood pressure, congestive heart failure, and long-term liver disease.

By the way, not all the sodium in your diet comes from table salt. Check out Chapter 16 for a list of the sodium compounds used in food.

✔ **The low-cholesterol, low-saturated-fat diet.** The basic version, known as the Stage 1 Diet, is used as a first step in lowering a person's cholesterol level. The diet limits cholesterol consumption to no more than 300 milligrams a day and total fat intake to no more than 30 percent of your total daily calories (see Chapter 16). For a guide to the cholesterol and saturated fat of common foods, see the Appendix.

A nifty bonus to this diet is that it is a relatively painless way of losing weight.

✔ **The low-protein diet.** This diet is prescribed for people with chronic liver or kidney disease or an inherited inability to metabolize amino acids, the building blocks of proteins. The low-protein regimen reduces the amount of protein waste products in body tissues, thus reducing the possibility of tissue damage.

✔ **The high-fiber diet.** A high-fiber diet quickens the passage of food through the digestive tract. It is used to prevent constipation. If you have outpouchings (diverticuli) in the wall of your colon, a high-fiber diet may reduce the possibility of an infection. It can also alleviate the discomfort of irritable bowel syndrome (sometimes called a nervous stomach). Extra bonus: A diet high in soluble fiber also lowers cholesterol (see the preceding section "When Food Is Medicine").

✔ **The high-potassium diet.** This diet is used to counteract the loss of potassium caused by diuretics (drugs that make you urinate more frequently and more copiously, causing you to lose excess amounts of potassium in urine). Some evidence also suggests that the high-potassium diet may lower blood pressure a bit.

✔ **The high-calcium diet.** This diet, high in dairy foods (lowfat, of course) and calcium-rich vegetables such as leafy greens, protects against the age-related loss of bone density. It may also help to lower high blood pressure and reduce the incidence of colon cancer. Fish, such as canned salmon with soft edible bones, are also a good source of calcium (no, you should NEVER eat the hard bones in fresh fish!). Two surprising additions to the list of bone-builders are foods such as the soybean that are high in hormone-like chemicals called phytoestrogens (for more on these fascinating compounds see Chapter 12) and fruits rich in the mineral boron. Studies at the USDA Human Nutrition Research Center in Grand Forks, North Dakota, suggest that boron may play an important role in preventing the loss of minerals such as calcium from bone. Two apples or two or three ounces of raisins or a glass of grape juice supply 1 mg a day, the amount the USDA researchers believe may protect bones.

No one knows how much boron constitutes a toxic dose, so get your boron from food, not supplements.

Using Food to Prevent Disease

Is a good diet preventive medicine? Yes, it can be. The simplest example is the deficiency disease, a condition that occurs when you do not get sufficient amounts of a specific nutrient. For example, people deprived of vitamin C develop scurvy, the vitamin-C-deficiency disease. The identifying characteristic of a deficiency disease is that it can be cured simply by adding the missing nutrient to your diet. For example, scurvy disappears when people eat foods such as citrus fruits that are high in vitamin C. But what you really want to know is whether specific foods or specific diets can prevent illnesses other than deficiency diseases.

Using food as a general preventive is an intriguing subject. True, much anecdotal evidence ("I did this, and that happened") suggests that eating some foods and avoiding others can raise or lower your risk of some serious diseases. But anecdotes aren't science. The more important indicator is the evidence from scientific studies tracking groups of people on different diets to see how things such as eating or avoiding fat, fiber, meat, dairy foods, salt, and other foods affect their risk of specific diseases.

Sometimes, the studies show a strange effect (meat fat increases the risk of colon cancer, dairy fat doesn't). Sometimes, studies show no effect at all. And sometimes — I like this category best — they turn up results nobody expected. For example, in 1996, a study was designed to see if a diet high in selenium would reduce the risk of skin cancer. After four years, the answer was "Not so you could notice." But then researchers noticed — by accident — that people who ate lots of high-selenium foods had a lower risk of lung, breast, and prostate cancer. Naturally, researchers immediately set up another study.

Is there an anticancer diet?

Right now, the answer seems to be a definite maybe. There are many different types of cancer, and some foods may be protective against some specific cancers. For example:

 ✔ **Fruits and vegetables.** The active anti-cancer substances in fruits and vegetables include antioxidants (chemicals that prevent molecular fragments called "free radicals" from hooking up to form cancer-causing compounds); phytoestrogens (hormone-like chemicals in plants that displace natural and synthetic estrogens in our bodies); and sulfur compounds that interfere with biochemical reactions leading to the birth and growth of cancer cells. (For more about these protective substances in plant foods, see Chapter 12.)

✔ **Foods high in dietary fiber.** Human beings can't digest dietary fiber, but friendly bacteria living in your gut can. Chomping away on the fiber, the bacteria excrete fatty acids that appear to keep cells from turning cancerous. In addition, fiber helps speed food through your body, reducing the formation of carcinogenic compounds. For more than 30 years, doctors have assumed that eating lots of dietary fiber reduces the risk of colon cancer, but in 1999, data from the long-running Nurses Health Study at Boston's Brigham and Women's Hospital and Harvard's School of Public Health threw this into question.

✔ **Lowfat foods.** Dietary fat appears to increase the proliferation of various types of body cells, a situation that may lead to the out-of-control reproduction of cells known as cancer. But all fats may not be equally guilty. In several studies, fat from meat is linked to an increased risk of colon cancer, while fat from dairy foods comes up clean.

In 1996, the American Cancer Society Advisory Committee on Diet, Nutrition, and Cancer Prevention issued a set of nutrition guidelines that show how to use food to reduce the risk of cancer. These are the American Cancer Society's recommendations:

✔ **Choose most of the foods you eat from plant sources.** Eat five or more servings of fruits and vegetables every day. Eat other foods from plant sources, such as breads, cereals, grain products, rice, pasta, or beans several times a day.

✔ **Limit your intake of high-fat foods, particularly from animal sources.** Choose foods low in fat; limit consumption of meats, especially high-fat meats.

✔ **Be physically active:** Achieve and maintain a healthy weight. Be at least moderately active for 30 minutes or more on most days of the week. Stay within your healthy weight range.

✔ **Limit consumption of alcohol beverages, if you drink at all.**

Source: CA-A Cancer Journal for Clinicians, November/December 1996.

DASHing to healthy blood pressure

More than 50 million Americans have high blood pressure (a.k.a. hypertension), a major risk factor for heart disease, stroke, and heart or kidney failure.

The traditional treatment for hypertension has included drugs (some with unpleasant side effects), reduced sodium intake, weight reduction, alcohol only in moderation, and regular exercise. Now data from a National Heart, Lung and Blood Institute (NHLB) study, "Dietary Approaches to Stop Hypertension" — DASH, for short — suggest that the diet that protects your heart and reduces your risk of some forms of cancer may also help control blood pressure.

The DASH diet is rich in fruits and vegetables, plus lowfat dairy products. No surprise there. But the diet is lower in fat than the ordinary lowfat diet. The USDA/U.S. Department of Health and Human Services Dietary Guidelines for Americans (see Chapter 16) recommend that you get no more than 30 percent of your total calories from fat. DASH aims for no more than 27 percent.

The difference seems to make a difference. Your blood pressure is measured in two numbers that look something like this: 130/80. The first number is your systolic pressure, the force exerted against artery walls when your heart beats and pushes blood out into your blood vessels. The second, lower number is the diastolic pressure, the force exerted between beats.

When male and female volunteers with high blood pressure followed the DASH diet during clinical trials at medical centers in Boston, Massachusetts; Durham, North Carolina; Baltimore, Maryland; and Baton Rouge, Louisiana; their systolic blood pressure dropped an average 11.4 points, their diastolic pressure, an average 5.5 points. And unlike medication, the diet produced no unpleasant side effects — except, of course, for that occasional dream of chocolate ice cream with real whipped cream, pound cake . . . Oh well, nothing's perfect.

Can food conquer the common cold?

This section is not about chicken soup. That issue has been settled, and Dr. Mom was right. Dr. Marvin Sackler of Mt. Sinai Medical Center in Miami, Florida, published the first serious study showing that cold sufferers who got hot chicken soup felt better faster than those who got plain hot water. Nobody really knows why it works, but who cares? It works.

So let's move on to other foods that make you feel better when you have the sniffles — for example, sweet foods. Scientists do know why sweeteners — white sugar, brown sugar, honey, molasses — soothe a sore throat. All sugars are *demulcents,* substances that coat and soothe the irritated mucous membranes. Lemons aren't sweet, and they have less vitamin C than orange juice, but their popularity in the form of "hot lemonade" (tea with lemon and sugar) and sour lemon drops is unmatched. Why? Because a lemon's sharp flavor cuts through to your taste buds and makes the sugary stuff more palatable. In addition, the sour taste makes saliva flow, and that also soothes your throat.

NUTRITION SPEAK

Vegetarianism: From weird to, like, totally mainstream

Once upon a time vegetarians were regarded as really strange people. Today, vegetarianism is commonplace and, it turns out, pretty good medicine, too. Vegetarianism isn't a single diet. At least three basic variations exist:

✔ A diet for people who don't eat meat, but do eat fish and poultry or just fish. (Fairness dictates that I add that many strict vegetarians don't consider people who eat fish or poultry to be vegetarians.)

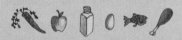

✔ A diet for people who don't eat meat, fish, or poultry, but do eat other animal products such as eggs and dairy products. Vegetarians who follow this regimen are called *ovo-lacto vegetarians* (ovo = egg, lacto = milk).

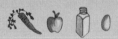

✔ A diet for people who eat absolutely no foods of animal origin. These vegetarians, who eat only plant foods, are called *vegans*.

The first two regimens — no meat, but some poultry or fish; no meat, but lots of dairy products — are completely safe from a nutritional standpoint because they contain enough different kinds of food to supply every nutrient your body needs.

A vegan diet — no meat, no poultry, no dairy foods — can be a bit dicey. It has no vitamin B12, a nutrient found only in foods from animals. Without some animal foods, it may be difficult to get enough calcium and iron. True, many plants have both minerals, but in forms your body may find hard to absorb (see Chapter 11). And unless you combine foods correctly, your proteins won't be "complete" (see Chapter 6). Of course, these "problems" are not insurmountable obstacles to good nutrition. With a little care and juggling, it is possible to get all the nutrients you need from a vegetarian diet. Juggle your foods intelligently, and you can definitely end up with a well-balanced diet that

✔ Makes losing weight without feeling deprived easy (plants are lowfat, which means low-calorie)

✔ Reduces your risk of some kinds of cancer (those wonderful antioxidant chemicals in plants)

✔ Lowers your risk of heart disease (plants have absolutely no cholesterol)

So bring on the carrots! Stir up the rice and beans!

Food and sex: What do these foods have in common?

Oysters, celery, onions, asparagus, mushrooms, truffles, chocolate, honey, caviar, bird's nest soup, and alcohol beverages. No, that's not a menu for the very, very picky. It's a partial list of foods long reputed to be *aphrodisiacs*, substances that rev up the libido and improve sexual performance. Take a second look and you will see why each is on the list.

Two (celery, asparagus) are shaped something like a male sex organ. Three (oysters, mushrooms, and truffles) are said to arouse emotion because they resemble parts of the female anatomy. (Oysters are high in zinc, the mineral that keeps the prostate gland healthy and ensures a steady production of the male hormone, testosterone. A 3-ounce serving of Pacific oysters gives you 9 milligrams of zinc, about 60 percent of the 15 milligrams a day recommended for adult men.)

Caviar (fish eggs) and bird's nest soup are symbols of fertility. Onions — like "Spanish fly" (cantharides) — contain chemicals that produce a mild burning sensation when eliminated in urine; some people, masochists to be sure, may confuse this with arousal. Honey is the quintessential sweetener: The "Song of Songs" compares it to the lips of the beloved. Alcohol beverages relax the inhibitions (but overindulgence reduces sexual performance, especially in men). As for chocolate, well, it's a veritable lover's cocktail, with stimulants (caffeine, theobromine), a marijuana-like compound called anandamide, and phenylethylalanine, a chemical produced in the bodies of people in love.

So do these foods actually make you feel sexy? Yes and no. An aphrodisiac isn't a food that sends you in search of a lover as soon as you eat it. No, it's one that makes you feel so good that you can follow through on your natural instincts. Which is as fine a description as you're likely to get of oysters, celery, onions, asparagus, mushrooms, truffles, chocolate, honey, caviar, bird's nest soup, and wine.

Hot stuff — such as peppers, horseradish (fresh-grated is definitely the most potent), and onions — contain mustard oils that irritate the membranes lining your nose and mouth and even make your eyes water. As a result, it's easier to blow your nose or cough up mucus.

Finally, there's coffee, a real boon to snifflers. When you are sick, your body piles up cytokines, chemicals that carry messages among immune system cells that fight infection. When cytokines pile up in brain tissue, you get sleepy, which may explain why you're so drowsy when you have a cold. True, rest can help to boost your immune system and fight off the cold, but once in a while you have to get up. Like to go to work.

The caffeine in even a single cup of regular coffee (or one cup of decaf if, like me, you do not ordinarily drink regular coffee) can make you more alert. It is also a mood elevator (see Chapter 24) and a vasoconstrictor (a chemical that helps shrink swollen, throbbing blood vessels). That's why it can relieve a headache. When I have a cold, one cup of espresso with tons of sugar can make life bearable. But nothing's perfect: Drinking coffee may intensify the side effects of OTC (over-the-counter) cold remedies containing deconges-tants and/or caffeine that make some people feel jittery.

Check the label warnings and directions before using coffee with your cold medicine. Vasoconstrictors reduce the diameter of certain blood vessels and may restrict proper circulation.

Is Food the Fountain of Youth?

Could be. Some foods provide nutrients that clearly lessen the natural conse-quences of growing older. For example:

- ✔ Citrus fruits are rich in vitamin C, an antioxidant vitamin that may slow the development of cataracts.

- ✔ Bran cereals give you the fiber that can rev up your intestinal tract (the contractions that move food through your gut slow a bit as you grow older, which is why older people are more likely to be constipated).

Keeping wrinkles at bay

Eating well can also protect your skin against wrinkles, the bane of the elderly — and sometimes the not-so-elderly. How soon and how much you wrinkle depends in large measure on your exposure to the sun (the more sun, the more wrinkling), plus the genes you inherit from your mother and father, but diet plays a role. Forget the fashion magazines. As you grow older, you definitely can be too thin. Eating a diet that provide enough calories to main-tain a healthful weight won't prevent all wrinkles, but theoretically it might help prevent the saggy look that sends some skinny older people off to the plastic surgeon.

Young skin also looks and feels moist. Dry skin — which seems to run in fami-lies — can occur at any age but is more common after age 40 when the glands that moisten and oil your skin secrete less moisteners. At the same time, the stratum corneum (the outer layer of your skin) gets thinner and loses its abil-ity to hold moisture. As with calories and wrinkles, a diet with sufficient amounts of fat won't totally prevent dry skin, but it does give you a measure of protection. That's one reason why virtually all sensible diet gurus, includ-ing the American Heart Association and the Dietary Guidelines, recommend some fat or oil every day.

Eating for a better brain

Finally, a word about memory. Actually, two words: varied diet. A 1983 study of 250 healthy adults, age 60 to 94, at the University of New Mexico School of Medicine in 1983, showed that the people who ate a wide range of nutritious food performed best on memory and thinking tests. According to researcher Philip J. Garry, Ph.D., Professor of Pathology at New Mexico School of Medicine, overall good food habits seemed to be more important than any one food or vitamin. Or it may just be that people with good memory are most likely to remember that they need a good diet.

Or maybe it's really the food. In 1997, another survey, this time at the University of Complutens (Madrid, Spain), showed that men and women age 60 to 90 who eat foods rich in vitamin E, vitamin C, folic acid, dietary fiber, and complex carbohydrates do better on cognitive tests. Is it the antioxidant vitamins? Does a lowfat diet protect the brain? No one knows for sure right now, but it may turn out that sticking with this same-old, same-old, lowfat, high-fiber diet as you grow older may help you to remember to stick to the lowfat, high-fiber diet — for years, and years, and years.

The Last Word on Food versus Medicine

Sometimes, people with a life-threatening illness are frightened by the side effects or the lack of certainty in standard medical treatment. In desperation, they turn down medicine and turn to diet therapy. Alas, doing this may be hazardous to their already-compromised health.

No reputable doctor denies the benefits of a healthful diet for any patient at any stage of any illness. Food not only sustains the body; it can also lift the spirit. But while food and diet may enhance the effects of many common drugs, no one has found that food or diet serves as an adequate, effective substitute for (among others) the following:

- Antibiotics and other drugs used to fight infections
- Vaccines or immunizations used to prevent communicable diseases
- Anticancer drugs

If your doctor suggests altering your diet to make your treatment more effective ("No milk when you're taking tetracycline," "More grapes with your calcium supplements," "Feeling queasy? Try a little ginger ale"), your brain will tell you, *Hey, that makes sense.* But if someone suggests chucking your doctor and tossing away your medicine in favor of food alone, heed the natural warning in your head. You know there's no free lunch and — as yet — no truly magic food, either.

Part VI
The Part of Tens

The 5th Wave · By Rich Tennant

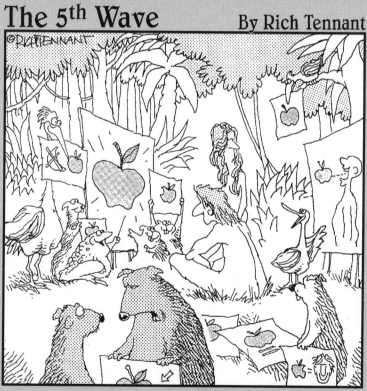

"Yes, we told them about the pectin and flavonoids, but they seem a little slow to catch on. Maybe if we just left them alone with the snake a while..."

In this part . . .

*I*f you've ever read a *...For Dummies* book, you know what to expect here — nifty lists of useful factoids that make great conversation starters and help you wind your way through the subject at hand.

In this book, that means ten great Web sites, ten superstar foods, ten ways to keep your kitchen clean and safe, and ten easy ways to cut the calories without eliminating tasty food. Who could ask for anything more?

Chapter 27

Ten Nutrition Web Sites

*H*ow did we ever manage without the Internet? Every time I open my e-mail or download an article from a journal that would have taken me hours to locate in the Bad Old Days, I feel a genuine need to toss a thank-you toward Silicon Valley.

The ten nutrition-oriented Web sites listed in this chapter give you reliable, accurate, balanced information. Point your Web browser to them to find nutritional guidelines, medical news, interactive sites, directories, and more.

And these ten sites are only a start. If IDG Books had called this section of the book The Part of Hundreds instead of The Part of Tens, I could have included a lot of super sites I don't have room for here. Like the USDA Nutrient Database at www.nal.usda.gov/fnic/cgi-bin/nut_search.pl — a site so important that I devote this book's entire Appendix to helping you use the site. Or the USDA National Agricultural Library at www.nal.usda.gov and the American Diabetes Association at www.diabetes.org and the Mayo Clinic at www.mayo.edu and Cyberdiet at www.CyberDiet.com and . . . well, you get the picture.

Cyberspace is a big world. Choosing the top sites is a hard job, but, heck, somebody has to do it. If I missed your particular favorite or you find a site you think is especially useful, don't hesitate to let me know, perhaps for inclusion in the next edition of this book. Visit my2cents.dummies.com to voice your opinion about this chapter (or any other, for that matter).

Click!

The Food and Drug Administration

`www.fda.gov`

Entering the FDA's Web site is like opening the door to the world's biggest toy store. There's so much stuff on the (virtual) shelves that you hardly know which item to grab first. Luckily, in this store, all the toys are free, and lots of links to helpful information mean you can linger here happily for days. Weeks. Years. Maybe forever.

FDA's charter includes drugs as well as food, so its home page offers information about medicines for people and pets, poisons and side effects, medical devices (think pacemaker), FDA field operations (enforcement of rules and regulations), and a place where activists can file a Freedom of Information Act (FOIA) request or report an adverse event ("I took that antibiotic and got hives!"). For foodies, though, the main event is, well, food.

On the homepage, click the Food link to visit the Center for Food Safety and Applied Nutrition page, which provides an e-mail address and a plain old-fashioned hotline through which you can comment on proposed FDA regulations. You can also find a primer on FOIA requests, plus instructions on how to access the Federal Register (Congress' record of hearings) and FDA documents on foods and cosmetics.

For more (lots more), go back to the home page and scroll down to the Information For box with links for consumers, industry, health professionals, patients, state and local officials, and women. Click Consumers to bring up a FAQ (cyber-speak for "frequently asked questions") directory.

The FAQ's categories include Food Safety (foodborne illness, food preparation, food away from home, food storage); Products (seafood, dietary supplements, fruit juice, cosmetics); Other (nutrition and weight loss); Women's Health; Food Labeling; and Miscellaneous.

The FAQ questions range from the very basic ("How do I use the %DV column on the food label") to the who-would-have-thought-to-ask ("What safety tips do you have for purchasing food through the mail?"). The answers are solid and satisfying, and you can always doodle through the site for more detail. For example, when I ordered a bunch of relishes through the mail, the jars came with no nutrition label and no expiration date. Through the FDA site, I discovered that companies with fewer than 100 full-time employees shipping fewer than 100,000 units a year don't have to have the labels. Who knew?

The Special Nutritional Adverse Event Monitoring System (AEMS)

```
vm.cfsan.fda.gov/~dms/aems.html
```

The Adverse Events Monitoring System (AEMS) was created by the FDA in 1993 along with an Office of Special Nutritionals. The AEMS Web site features reports of illness and injury associated with "special nutritionals" — dietary supplements (vitamin, minerals, herbals), infant formulas, and medical foods.

Note: Read the address carefully, and you'll see there's no "www" in front. If you forget and reflexively paste on the triple-w, you can't reach the site.

AEMS assigns an identifying number to each report — in this case an "ARMS number" — but you don't need the number to access a report. Just type the name of the product you want to research, click the button, and watch as truly terrifying charts, complete with brand name, manufacturer, ingredients, and reactions associated with using the special nutritional, appear. For example, when I typed "niacin," the dietary supplement sometimes prescribed to lower cholesterol levels, my screen filled with complaints of high blood pressure, irregular heartbeat, shortness of breath and burning sensations in various parts of the body — some of them unmentionable. Yipes!

This is not a trip for the nutritionally timid. True, FDA issues a disclaimer noting that the material in AEMS reports is almost always too scanty to prove that the adverse event is definitely linked to the nutritional product. But searching this site will probably make you stop and think every time you pop a vitamin pill.

American Dietetic Association

```
www.eatright.org
```

This site features nutrition recommendations, tips, guidelines, research, policy, and stats from the world's largest membership association of nutrition professionals, primarily registered dietitians. (For a quick run-down on who's who in nutrition science, see Chapter 1).

The ADA home page features nine links. Member Services, Classifieds, and Government Affairs are designed primarily for association members. Press Room is fun if you're addicted to press releases or enjoy browsing the ADA

Journal. Nutrition Resources has tidbits for consumers such as daily diet tips. Marketplace is an online shopping guide to ADA publications. Gateway to Related Sites is, well, self-explanatory. Find a Dietitian has a hotline for recorded nutrition messages or referral to a registered dietitian in your area (1-800-366-1655), an e-mail address (hotline@eatright.org), and — my personal favorite — an on-screen questionnaire you can fill out to find a registered dietitian, practically in your own neighborhood.

ADA's mission is to serve the public by promoting nutrition, health, and well-being. If you can bend your brain around the much-too-adorable net address (eatright? give me a break!), you'll discover this site is a true treasure trove. And golly gee, who wouldn't love having a personal dietitian to lead the way through the maze of conflicting nutritional advice?

The American Heart Association

`www.amhrt.org`

This site tells you everything you ever wanted to know about diet and heart disease. Starting at the home page, run your mouse down the left side to Family Health and then click the Nutrition link to bring up the Diet and Nutrition page. Once here, you can read AHA diet recommendations, recipes from AHA cookbooks, AHA nutrition facts, food certification program guidelines, or the AHA eating plan — a clear explanation of how to use food and diet to reduce your risk of heart disease.

Factoid fans will find Nutrition Facts total heaven. The page features a list of 33 different aspects of nutrition and heart disease, including what to do with that nasty high fat, high cholesterol chicken skin (toss it out).

The indisputable link between diet and heart disease risk, not to mention this site's user-friendly approach, makes this a must-stop on your nutritional tour of the Web.

The American Cancer Society

`www.cancer.org`

The ACS Web site is dedicated primarily to information about cancer: definitions, treatments, research, and support services. True, most of the nutrition news you find here is available elsewhere, but this site's defined focus provides easy access to other cancer-related topics.

On the ACS home page, click the Search Our Site link to bring up a form that gets you into the database on food and cancer. When the form pops up, scroll down to the Search For tab and enter a subject, such as "diet and cancer." Accept the first default setting (simple search) and use the arrow to the right of the Maximum Number of Files Retrieved box to change the number of references from the default 100 to a more manageable 10. Then click Search the Site.

Bingo! You've opened a grab-bag of ACS press releases, guidelines on diet, and the most common questions people ask about food and cancer (with answers). More targeted searches — such as "high fiber food" — yield more specific responses, such as the well-established link between a diet high in fiber and a lower risk of colon cancer.

Until now, the American Cancer Society was barely a blip on the screen of nutrition sources. Today, with a growing number of well-designed studies to demonstrate that some foods and diet regimens may reduce your risk of certain types of cancer, while others put you in harm's way, the ACS Web site offers solid reporting on this area of nutrition research.

The Food Allergy Network

`www.foodallergy.org`

The Food Allergy Network is a non-profit membership organization (membership fee: $30/year for individuals) whose participants include families, doctors, dietitians, nurses, support groups, and food manufacturers in the U.S., Canada, and Europe. The group provides education about food allergies as well as support and coping strategies for people who are allergic to specific foods.

From FAN's home page, you can link to updates, daily tips, newsletter excerpts, and all the usual service-oriented goodies. The site's best feature, an e-mail Alerts system, is free. Click the Free Alerts option, fill out the form, and e-mail it to the site. You are now connected to an early warning system with allergy-linked news and information about recalls such as a February 1997 recall of 2-ounce bags of cashews that might mistakenly contain peanuts.

This no-nonsense, highly accessible site is required reading for people with food allergies. Others, such as families and friends, can also benefit from its solid information and support services.

International Food Information Council (IFIC)

www.ificinfo.health.org

IFIC, created in 1985, is a non-profit organization dedicated to improving the relationship between the nutrition community — scientists, food manufacturers, health professionals, government officials — and the news media. (Although the Council's membership includes corporations that make and sell food products, IFIC plays no role in marketing products or promoting its members.) Its aim is to make sure that consumers get accurate information about diet and health.

The IFIC home page features ten links: About Us, What's New, Food Safety and Nutrition Information, Information for Reporters, Information for Education, Publications, Guestbook, Additional Resources, and Food Insight. The last two are probably the most useful for consumers.

Clicking the Additional Resources link takes you to a list of nutrition-related organizations, most with e-mail addresses. Clicking the Food Insight link takes you to the IFIC newsletter.

Purists may complain about IFIC positions, such as its endorsement of fat substitutes and other food additives for some people, but I like the site's intelligent approach to explaining complex and emotional issues clearly and directly so that you can make up your own mind.

American Council on Science and Health (ASCH) and The Center for Science in the Public Interest (CSPI)

www.asch.org

www.cspinet.org

The American Council on Science and Health and The Center for Science in the Public Interest are two non-profit consumer-friendly organizations that are usually on opposite sides of any nutritional issue. ASCH is cool and calm; CSPI is a hot-button advocate.

For example, CSPI believes the fat substitute Olestra is hazardous to your health; ASCH says it's useful in some foods for some people.

This kind of disagreement ensures that if you punch up the same search word or phrase on both sites, you'll find out about the pros and cons of an issue. Neat.

Both sites feature news releases, position papers, online membership enrollment, order forms for publications, and links to other sites.

Which site you prefer is pretty much a matter of personality, but you can't go wrong with either one if you're looking for highly reliable information about nutrition issues and how food and diet affect your health.

Tufts University Nutrition Navigator

`www.navigator.tufts.edu`

With so many sources of information on the Internet, you may find yourself stranded at sea in an ocean of information — maybe even some misinformation. Nutrition Navigator enables you to steer through the waves to a safe harbor.

The Nutrition Navigator is the mother of all nutrition guides, rating nearly 200 nutrition Web sites on a 25-point scale that measures content and usability. Based on their scores, sites are described as Among The Best (22–25 points), Better Than Most (17–21 points), Average (13–16 points), or Not Recommended (below 13 points).

On the home page, click the General Nutrition link to bring up the whole list of sites. Don't want to wade through the entire file? Click a specialized category such as Women or Kids to pull up a smaller list of relevant sites.

Chapter 28

Ten Superstar Foods

In This Chapter
▶ Why yogurt is good food
▶ The joy of chocolate
▶ Mood-elevators in your cup
▶ A natural remedy you should never make at home

Ever since Eve pulled that apple (really a pomegranate) off the tree of knowledge in the Garden of Eden, people have been attributing special powers to one food or another.

Perhaps the most interesting aspect of this is not whether these foods are actually cure-alls, but that so many of the foods we choose to honor contain stimulants that really do make us feel more intelligent, witty, and sexy — for a while.

This chapter is by no means a complete list of superstar foods. For example, I haven't included chicken soup, because what more can anyone say about this universal panacea? Ditto for garlic (once reputed to be a vampire slayer as effective as Buffy) and onions, both now honored as heart healthy. Winnowing down the list was hard, but somebody had to do it! So here are my nominations for the Top Ten.

Breast Milk

Human breast milk is more nutritious than cow's milk for human babies. It has a higher percentage of easily digested, high-energy fats and carbohydrates. Its proteins stimulate an infant's immune system, encouraging his or her white blood cells to produce lots of infection-fighting antibodies, including those that go after viruses linked to the infant diarrhea that accounts for 23 percent of all deaths among children younger than 5.

All in all, not a bad meal for the first few months of life.

Yogurt

Yogurt is milk with added friendly bacteria that digest milk sugar (lactose) to produce lactic acid, a natural preservative that gives yogurt its pleasant "bite." Yogurt is definitely magical for people who are "lactase deficient" (meaning they do not produce enough lactase to digest milk sugar so that they get gassy whenever they drink milk).

But there's no evidence to show that yogurt is a longevity tonic, a claim traced back to Eli Metchnikoff, a Russian Nobel prize winner (1908; physiology/medicine) who believed that people die prematurely due entirely to the action of "putrefying bacteria" in the intestines. Searching for a way to disarm the putrefiers, Metchnikoff ended up in Bulgaria, a place where lots of people lived past 50 and a significant percentage made it into their late 80s.

Historians may argue that the only way to live that long in Bulgaria was to avoid Bulgarian politics, but Metchnikoff credited the organisms used to make Bulgarian cultured milk. He was wrong. The bugs, christened L. bulgaricus, make nice yogurt but don't take up residence in the human gut. This hardly mattered to Metchnikoff, who shuffled off this mortal coil in Paris in 1916, at the relatively young age of 71. His faith in yogurt, however, continues to cycle in and out of fashion.

Apples

Apples really are a neat nutritional package. They have virtually no fat, lots of pectin (a soluble fiber known to lower cholesterol levels), and plenty of vitamin C.

They're also high in *flavonoids,* the natural chemicals in many fruits, vegetables, red wine, and tea, that appear to protect your heart. In 1993, scientists at the National Institute of Health in Bilthoven, The Netherlands, reported that men who consumed large amounts of flavonoids were 50 percent less likely to suffer a heart attack than were men who ate small amounts of flavonoids. How much is enough? One large apple a day. Wait, isn't there a saying about that? You know, "An apple a day keeps the doctor away . . . ." Hmmmmmm.

Chocolate

Westerners have been fools for chocolate ever since the Spanish conquistadors discovered it at Montezuma's Mexican court. And why not? The cocoa bean is a good source of energy, fiber, protein, carbohydrates, B vitamins, and minerals (one ounce of dark sweet chocolate has 12 percent of the iron and 33 percent of the magnesium a healthy woman needs each day).

Despite being high in saturated fats, chocolate may actually be heart-healthy. A recent study at the USDA Agricultural Research Service in Peoria, Illinois, shows that men who eat lots of *stearic acid,* the saturated fat in chocolate, reduce their risk of blood clots. And chocolate is rich in *flavonoids* (see "Apples," earlier in this chapter), the natural chemicals credited with making red wine heart-healthy. Researchers at the University of California-Davis have found that a cup of hot chocolate made with two tablespoons cocoa powder (no milk) actually has more flavonoids than a 5-ounce glass of red wine.

Finally, chocolate is a veritable happiness cocktail. It has *caffeine* (a mood elevator and central nervous system stimulant), *theobromine* (a muscle stimulant), and *phenylethylalanine* (another mood elevator). And in 1996, researchers at the Neurosciences Institute in San Diego announced that chocolate also contains *anandamide,* a chemical that stimulates the same areas of the brain that marijuana does. No, eating chocolate won't get you "high." You'd have to consume 25 pounds or more at one sitting to get the smallest marijuana-like effect. Nonetheless, I think chocolate was Montezuma's way of making up for his, ahem, "revenge."

Fish

Did your grandmother call fish "brain food"? If so, it was almost certainly because fish is rich in iodine, the mineral that makes it possible for your thyroid gland to churn out thyroid hormones vital to your ability to think and move. Once upon a time, people living far from the ocean (our best natural source of iodine) were often sluggish, sometimes even mentally retarded, due to lack of iodine. But this became rare in the U.S. after the introduction of iodized salt in the 1920s.

Fish's modern magic is its ability to reduce the risk of heart disease due to its *omega-3 fatty acids.* These fats appear to protect the heart by preventing blood clots or keeping other fats from injuring artery walls. It's clear that laboratory pigs and monkeys have cleaner arteries when their feed includes omega-3 fatty acids, and studies suggest human beings may also benefit. In the Diet and Reinfarction Trial (DART), a 2,033-man study run by the Medical Research Council Epidemiological Unit in Cardiff, Wales in the late 1980s, men who ate two servings of fatty fish a week had a lower rate of heart attack than men who either cut their fat to no more than 30 percent of their total calories or increased their dietary fiber (from grains) to 16 grams a day. And did I mention that omega-3 fatty acids also help protect bone density? Brain food, heart food, bone food — yo, bring on the salmon!

Coffee and Tea

Coffee and tea, the world's most popular beverages, share one important ingredient, that well-known pepper-upper, caffeine.

For years, there was nothing but bad news about coffee. Pancreatic cancer. Cystic breasts. High cholesterol. Heart disease. Stroke. Birth defects. But the worm — okay, the coffee bean — has turned: Later studies show no link at all between drinking coffee and an increased risk of any of these conditions. True, coffee may upset your stomach and keep you up at night, but for most people these effects are almost always linked to excess consumption. (How much is "excess consumption?" It varies from person to person, but when you hit your limit, you will definitely know. Trust me.)

But in moderation, coffee definitely qualifies for anybody's list of super foods. Its most important ingredient is caffeine, which elevates your mood and increases your ability to concentrate. It also may improve your athletic performance, can help shrink the swollen, throbbing blood vessels that make your head ache, and boosts the analgesic effect of painkillers, which is why caffeine is often included in over-the-counter analgesic products.

Like coffee, tea contains the mood elevator, caffeine. And it has theobromine, a muscle stimulant also found in chocolate. But caffeine and theobromine are on the tip of tea's wonderfulness. Drinking tea seems to lower the risk of heart disease and cancer, lower blood pressure, lower cholesterol, stabilize blood sugar levels, and, get this, prevent cavities.

Most of these effects appear to be due to antioxidants found in both the green teas popular in Asia and the "black" (dried) teas favored in the West. Antioxidants keep fragments of molecules ("free radicals") from hooking up with other fragments to make potential carcinogens.

Sure enough, in laboratory studies, chemicals derived from green tea have stopped the growth of mouse skin cancers and reduced the incidence of lung cancer in mice exposed to tobacco carcinogens. They also lower the level of LDLs ("bad cholesterol") and reduce the risk of blood clots in mice.

And cavities? Well, at least nine of the most prominent oily, floral-scented compounds that make tea smell so good can kill, wipe out, ab-so-lute-ly decimate *streptococcus mutans* (a.k.a. S. mutans), the bacteria that make the sticky gunk that enables acid-generating bacteria to glom on to your teeth and gnaw away at the surface. No sticking, no cavities. Hate tea? Then you will be pleased to know that some of these same compounds occur in coriander, sage, and thyme.

Beans

Modern science says that beans lower cholesterol levels and protect diabetics from blood sugar overload. Their effect on cholesterol appears to be due to their *gums* and *pectin,* soluble dietary fibers that mop up fats and prevent their being absorbed by your body. Oats, which are also rich in gums, particularly a gum called *beta glucans,* produce the same effect.

Beans are digested very slowly, so they produce only a gradual increase in the level of sugar circulating in your blood. As a result, when you eat beans, your body requires less insulin to control blood sugar levels than it does when you eat other high-carb foods such as pasta and potatoes. In one well-known study at the University of Kentucky, a diet rich in beans made it possible for people with Type I diabetes (their bodies produce virtually no insulin) to reduce their daily insulin intake by nearly 40 percent. Patients with Type II diabetes (their bodies produce some insulin) were able to reduce insulin intake by 98 percent.

Just about the only drawback to a diet rich in beans is gas resulting from your inability to digest dietary fiber and complex sugars (*raffinose, stachyose*). These substances are fodder for resident friendly bacteria that digest the carbs and then release carbon dioxide and (ugh) methane, a smelly gas.

One way to reduce gas production in your gut is to reduce the complex sugar content of the beans before you eat them. Here's how: Bring a pot of water to a boil. Turn off the heat. Add the beans. Let them soak for several hours. The sugars leech out into the water, which means you can discard them by draining the beans and adding fresh water to cook in. If that doesn't do the job, try two heat-and-soak sessions before cooking.

Right now, the reigning star of the bean family is the soybean, a modest beige oval packed with fiber and a prime source of phytoestrogens, the hormone-like compounds in plants that appear to reduce our risk of heart disease and some kinds of cancer. For more on phytoestrogens, see Chapter 12.

Alcohol

Alcohol beverages play so important a part in human culinary and nutrition history that they have their very own chapter earlier in this book. Simply listing alcohol's natural properties tells you right off why ancient peoples called it a "gift of the gods" or the "water of life". It is an effective antiseptic, sedative, and analgesic.

Moderate alcohol consumption relaxes muscles and mood, expands blood vessels to lower blood pressure temporarily, and appears to lower the risk of heart disease, either by reducing the stickiness of blood platelets (small particles that can clump together to form a blood clot) or by relaxing blood vessels (making them temporarily larger) or by increasing the amount of HDLs ("good cholesterol") in your blood.

While some forms of alcohol, such as red wine, have gotten more press attention with regard to these effects, the truth is that controlled studies show similar effects with all forms of alcohol beverages — wine, beer, and spirits. For more on alcohol, check out Chapter 9.

Hot Peppers

Mellow red, green, and yellow bells are a good source of vitamin A and vitamin C. Hotter black, white, and red pepper seasoning (including chili powder) can make the lining of your nose and throat "weep," thinning mucus so you can blow it out or cough it up when you have a cold. And really hot peppers, the Habaneros that can burn your hand if you handle them without wearing protective gloves, are sources of a new and effective painkiller.

The painkiller in hot peppers is *capsaicin,* the chemical that also burns. Capsaicin extracted from hot peppers is now used in over-the-counter arthritis creams. It appears to relieve pain by overstimulating nerve endings so that they can no longer transmit pain signals to your brain. Some researchers believe that capsaicin creams may also help reduce the pain of cluster headache, a type of migraine headache that comes in bunches for several days or weeks at a time.

Caution! Alert! Warning! Hot peppers are not a home remedy. NEVER attempt to self-medicate pain by applying one to your skin. Unlike the controlled dosage in an over-the-counter product, the capsaicin in these peppers — fresh or dried — is so strong it can actually blister your skin.

Tomatoes

Like sweet peppers, potatoes, and corn, tomatoes are a gift of the New World, carried home by explorers who changed the culinary history of Western Europe (imagine Italian cuisine without tomatoes!). For us, the red globular fruit once known as the "love apple" is a good source of vitamin C and folate (a B vitamin), plus a newly-important carotenoid pigment called lycopene.

Until recently, mentioning lycopene in nutrition circles drew little but yawns, because "everybody knew" that the truly valuable carotenoids were the yellow and orange pigments in deep green or yellow fruits and veggies.

But now the tomato has taken its rightful place as a nutrition star: Lycopene turns out to be an active antioxidant that reduces the risk of cancer of the prostate in human beings, and cancer of the breast and endometrium in female laboratory animals.

Tomatoes ripened to red on the vine have more lycopene than artificially-ripened tomatoes. Cooked tomato products such as catsup and tomato sauce have even more lycopene per serving.

And here's some really good news: Lycopene dissolves in fat, so it's more available to your body if you add a little fat, such as a teaspoon of olive oil, to your tomato sauce or cooked tomatoes. Can you believe it? Adding pizza and pasta with tomato sauce (lowfat cheese, please) to your diet may actually lower your risk of some kinds of cancer, including prostate cancer. And maybe heart disease, too.

In one large European study, men who ate a diet high in lycopene were at lower risk of heart attack. Don't you just love it when good-tasting food turns out to be good for you?

Chapter 29

Ten Ways to Keep Food Safe

● ●

In This Chapter

▶ The virtue of a squeaky clean kitchen

▶ How heat and cold keep food safe

▶ Why you (and your food) need soap and water

▶ When to throw food out

● ●

*E*ating healthy doesn't just mean eating healthful food. It also means handling food so as to reduce the risk of food-borne illnesses.

Every year, 21 to 81 million cases of diarrhea caused by eating microbe-
contaminated food are treated in the United States. Around the world, several
thousand people, including an estimated 9,000 Americans, fall victim to fatal
food poisoning, generally from raw or undercooked food.

The real surprise is that the numbers are so low. In 1996, when a team of
microbiologists from the University of Arizona tested various surfaces in
bathrooms and kitchens in the same houses, they found that in almost every
instance, the kitchen surfaces were dirtier. In fact — skip this if you're the
squeamish type — there were always fewer fecal bacteria on the toilet rim
than on the kitchen sink, countertops, and dish towels.

Here are some simple ways to protect yourself at home in your own kitchen.

Wash Your Hands before (And after) Touching Food

The skin on your hands, like the skin on the rest of your body, is home to millions of microbes, some friendly, some not. You can't get rid of them all, but
you can lower the population and reduce your risk of transferring microbes
from hand to food by washing your hands before touching food.

This is so basic that you'd think it would be an ingrained habit. Especially after, ahem, using the facilities. Yet many people seem seriously unconcerned about scrubbing up.

In 1996, researchers from the American Society for Microbiology and the Bayer Corporation (yes, the guys that make the aspirin), hid in stalls or pretended to comb their hair in public rest rooms in Atlanta, Chicago, New Orleans, New York, and San Francisco to check out how many people wash after using the toilet. Overall, Chicagoans come up best. Nearly 80 percent of the folks in the bathroom at Navy Pier headed for the sink before leaving. But in New York, only 60 percent of the people at Penn Station washed up, and male fans at a Braves game in Atlanta were the pits: A mere 46 percent stopped to wash. (Maybe it's a guy thing: 89 percent of the female Braves fans washed up.) Isn't it interesting to learn that when the researchers followed their on-scene survey with a telephone poll, 94 percent of those who answered the phone said they always washed after using a public rest room.

Wash All Fruits and Vegetables before You Use Them

You wouldn't want to play with people who haven't showered. Apply the same rule to fruits and veggies:

- ✔ Scrub fruits and vegetables with "hard" skins (apples, eggplants, cucumbers, and green peppers are good examples) under cool running water, dry thoroughly to prevent mold from sprouting on a damp surface, and refrigerate.

- ✔ Wash leafy greens and refrigerate them wrapped in a paper towel inside a plastic bag, or refrigerate unwashed in a plastic bag and rinse thoroughly right before use.

- ✔ Don't wash fruits and vegetables with "soft" skin (strawberries) or those that rot easily (potatoes, onions) before storing, but do rinse or scrub thoroughly before using.

In 1998, FDA sounded an alarm, warning that while washing fresh produce with running water is better than nothing, it may not be sufficient to remove all disease-causing micro-organisms that make their way onto fruits and vegetables from dirty hands or dirty soil. As a result, food scientists have been experimenting with more substantial antiseptic combinations. For example, researchers at the Virginia Polytechnic Institute in Blacksburg were able to rid apples of a deadly strain of E. coli by dunking the fruit in a non-toxic mix of vinegar and plain old hydrogen peroxide, and the Environmental Protection Agency has approved a patented chlorine-free disinfectant combo for sale to food processors (a version for home kitchens is awaiting FDA approval).

Read the Package

They may not make the best-seller list, but your food labels make good reading. Start with the date. "Sell by" tells you how long the grocer can safely sell the food. (You can usually consider the food safe for another two to three days.) "Use by" tells you how long the food remains safe to eat. "Best if used by" tells you how long the food looks and tastes best.

Many labels also offer storage advice ("do not thaw until ready to use," "keep in a cool, dry place," "refrigerate after opening") to maximize the food's nutritional value and aesthetic appeal. And occasionally there is a real surprise. For example, most people think all canned foods can be stored in a cabinet or closet. Not so. Some (canned ham is one) require refrigeration.

Handle All Raw Meat, Fish, and Poultry as though It Were Contaminated

One of every four chickens and one of every seven turkeys that reaches our kitchens comes with enough salmonella organisms to make you sick. Canpylobacter is even more common. Beef has salmonella, too, not to mention E. coli, the source of a toxin that can cause bloody diarrhea and kidney failure. As for fish? Bacteria abound.

To prevent these microbes from contaminating other foods or your kitchen surfaces

✔ Touch raw meat, fish, and poultry as little as possible.

✔ Refrigerate in the original wrap in a dish deep enough to prevent liquid spills that may contaminate your refrigerator shelf or other foods.

✔ Re-wrap meat, fish, and poultry in freezer paper or aluminum foil for long-term storage. To prevent spills, put the wrapped food in a plastic freezer bag.

✔ Wash all utensils after handling raw meat, fish, and poultry. Mop up blood and other spills with a disposable paper towel. Wipe down the counter with a solution of chlorine bleach and water, prepared as directed on the container.

✔ Finally: Wash your hands. But you knew that, right?

Cook Foods Thoroughly

Heat kills most of the disease-causing organisms on raw meat, fish, and poultry. As a general rule, cook all red meat (beef, lamb, pork, and especially ground meat) to an internal temperature of 160°F; poultry, to 180°F.

Do not rely on appearance to tell you when the meat is done. Use a meat thermometer. Stick the thermometer right into the center of the roast, burger, chop, or poultry thigh. Read the temperature. If it's high enough, wait five minutes and read it again. Now dinner's ready. (If the temperature's too low the first time you read it, remove the thermometer, wash it in hot, soapy water to remove any microbes from the still-cool center of the food, and re-test the food at 15-minute intervals.)

Keep Hot Foods Hot and Cold Foods Cold

The microbes living on food multiply most efficiently at temperatures between 40°F and 140°F, a range USDA calls "The Danger Zone." To prevent this, eat cooked food right away while it's still hot or refrigerate it right away (no cooling off on the counter first). To speed cooling in the refrigerator, take the stuffing out of poultry and store it in a separate dish, slice or divide leftovers into smaller portions, and store all hot food in shallow containers.

Keeping cold foods cold is equally important. Use a refrigerator or freezer thermometer to verify the temperature in your fridge (safe range 35–40°F) or freezer (safe range keep 0°F or lower). Keep frozen foods frozen solid. Thaw frozen foods (especially meat, fish, poultry, and mixed dishes that include eggs, cheese, or milk) in the refrigerator or in the microwave just before preparing them. Chill buffet dishes by setting the platter on a bigger platter filled with crushed ice or refill from the refrigerator rather than putting all the food out at once.

Never Eat Anything Containing Raw Eggs

Raw eggs are a haven for salmonella microbes. Even when the shell is intact, the egg inside may be contaminated. Cooking eggs (or cooking with eggs) requires the same caution you'd apply to other raw foods from animals.

Don't taste the cake batter. Cook all eggs (and egg dishes, such as custards) until the entire egg is firm, not runny. (See Table 29-1 for cooking guidelines.) And you can forget feasting on Easter eggs. What with painting, and hiding, and finding, they've been out of the fridge for more than two hours, exceeding the USDA danger zone.

Are you desperate to lick the batter bowl? Just use egg substitutes or pasteurized egg products instead of real eggs. Products such as Nabisco's Egg Beaters are pasteurized to eliminate the possibility of salmonella. (Naturally, you should follow label directions and refrigerate or freeze as directed.) Bonus: Because the egg substitutes are made solely from egg whites (the yellow comes from coloring agents), they are high protein, lowfat, and cholesterol-free. Yummy!

Table 29-1	How Long to Cook an Egg
Egg Type/Meal	*Time/Quality*
Poached	5 minutes over boiling water
Soft-cooked	7 minutes in the pot
Fried	2 to 3 minutes on each side
Scrambled	Until firm all over, no moist patches
French toast	Until crisp
Fried sandwiches	Until crisp
Custards	Firm

Zap the Sponge

I have some bad news for you: Your kitchen sponge is filthy. I know you wash it every day. I know you keep it sitting in the fresh air to dry on the sink. But it's still a true microbial zoo populated with (among others) E. coli, salmonella, pseudomonas, and staphylococcus, all thriving in the sponge's moist environment.

You could definitely improve things by using a new sponge every time you wash the dishes, but the more practical way is to heat and dry the sponge so that microbes cannot flourish. Scientists from the University of Wisconsin say that you can sterilize a dry cellulose sponge by zapping it for 30 seconds at high heat in an 800-watt microwave. Drying and sterilizing a wet sponge takes a full minute at high heat. How long this will take in your own kitchen depends on the power of your microwave oven and the thickness of your sponge. Your aim is to dry the sponge without melting it.

Isolate the Cutting Board

Once you've zapped the sponge, it's time to attack the cutting board. The conventional wisdom is that wooden boards are more likely than plastic boards to harbor microbes, but University of California at Davis microbiologist Dean Cliver says the reverse is true.

Smearing microbe-spiked chicken broth on a variety of boards, he found that plastic boards may have as much as 20 times more microbes than their wooden cousins. The absorbent wood seems to draw in and trap bacteria while the non-porous plastic keeps them pooled on top.

Cliver, who originated the zap-the-sponge technique, believes you can decontaminate wooden cutting boards in a similar fashion. (Microwaves don't work on plastic; the surface doesn't get hot enough to kill the bugs.) But others warn that microwaves can set wooden boards afire.

One alternative is the old fashioned soap-and-hot-water bath, followed by a bleach solution. Here's another possibility: Get two cutting boards. Use one exclusively for raw meat, fish, and poultry; the other for fruits and vegetables, bread, cheese, whatever. Wash them both, but don't mix foods, so you don't transfer bugs from raw food to cooked food. Holy leaping salmonella, what a revolutionary move!

When in Doubt, Throw It Out

You open the can, and the salmon smells funny. You tear off the wrapper, and there's a spot of green mold on the cheese. You fold out the spout, and the orange juice fizzes when you pour it.

Should you take a taste to see if it's okay? Not on your life. Some spoiled foods tell you loud and clear they've gone South. The smells of sour milk and rotten eggs come quickly to mind. Others, such as that fizzy (fermented) orange juice, give a more gentle but no less certain hint.

Potentially carcinogenic molds have no unusual flavor or odor, and food harboring potentially fatal botulinum or E. coli organisms may look, smell, and even taste just fine. Lacking sophisticated laboratory equipment, you simply cannot be sure what's lurking in the slightly "off" luncheon meat or canned green beans.

Here's the better way: Where food safety is concerned, "When in doubt, throw it out."

Chapter 30

Ten Easy Ways to Cut Calories

· ·

In This Chapter

▶ The value of lowfat foods

▶ Cutting down, not cutting out

▶ Substitutes that work

▶ A special tip for chopped meat

· ·

*L*osing weight is simple math. If you cut 3,500 calories out of your diet in the course of a week without reducing your daily activity, you can say good-bye to one whole pound of fat.

Yes, I know reading that sentence is easier than actually doing it, so I am ready to give you two tricks to make the job easier. First, cut your calories in small increments, 50 here, 100 there, rather than one big lump. Second, instead of giving up foods you really love (and feeling deprived), switch to lowfat versions.

This chapter tells you how to accomplish both. I've included some brand-name products just so that you can compare different versions made by the same company.

Switch to Lowfat or No-Fat Dairy Products

Milk and milk products are the best source for the calcium that keeps bones strong. But these same products may also be high in cholesterol, saturated fat, and calories. You can reduce all three by choosing a low- or no-fat milk product.

For example, a cup of whole milk has 150 calories; a cup of skim milk, only 85. One slice of regular Kraft American cheese has 60 calories; one slice of Kraft Free American cheese, only 30. A sandwich made with three slices of cheese is 90 calories lighter if the cheese is "free."

Substitute Sugar Substitutes

Coffee has no calories, but there are 15 big ones in every teaspoon of sugar. Multiply that by four (one teaspoon in four cups of coffee), and your naturally no-cal beverage can add 60 calories a day to your diet. Sixty calories a day times seven days a week. Yipes! 420 calories. That's about as much as you would get from four or five pieces of unbuttered toast or 5 medium apples. So is this a good time to mention that one packet of sugar substitute has absolutely zero calories? I thought so.

Serve Stew Instead of Steak

No matter how you slice it, red meat is red meat, cholesterol, saturated fats, and all. But if you stew your beef or lamb or pork, rather than broiling or roasting it, you can skim off a lot of high-calorie fat. Just make the stew, and then stick it in the fridge for a couple of hours until a layer of fat hardens on top. Spoon it off: Every tablespoon of pure fat subtracts 100 calories from dinner.

Choose Lowfat Desserts

Who says you have to suffer to cut calories? Not me. One half cup of Häagen-Dazs chocolate ice cream has 270 calories. One half cup of Häagen-Dazs no-fat chocolate sorbet has 140 calories. Believe me: Switching from the first to the second is no problem. If you're a true chocoholic, you'll send me valentines for this suggestion.

Peel the Poultry

Most of the fat in poultry is in the skin. A fried chicken breast with skin has 217 calories; without the skin, 160. Half a roasted duck (with skin) has a whopping 1,287 calories; without skin, it's 444. Even if you have a fried chicken breast every night for a week, you can save 399 calories by taking the skin off before you cook the bird. Share seven half ducks with a friend and you each save 2,950 calories a week. Wow. That's practically a pound right there.

Don't Oil the Salad

True, salad can be a lowfat, low-calorie meal. Even if you throw in some breast of chicken and a couple of no-fat croutons or cheese cubes, it's still mostly crunch.

But the dressing can do you in. For example, two tablespoons of Wishbone Italian Dressing or one tablespoon of Hellmann's regular "real mayonnaise" have 100 calories. What to do? Ah, c'mon, you know the answer: Switch.

Two tablespoons of Wishbone Fat Free Italian dressing adds just 15 — count 'em, 15! — calories. One tablespoon of Hellmann's Light, 50 calories; one tablespoon of Hellmann's Lowfat, a mere 25. Have salad once a day for a week, and you can save 595 calories with fat-free versus regular salad dressing, 525 calories with lowfat mayonnaise versus regular. Neat.

Don't oil your pots and pans, either. Bake with parchment paper instead of greasing the pan. Sauté with natural juices in non-stick pans. Every tablespoon of fat you don't use means 100 calories cut from the "cost" of the dish.

Make One-Slice Sandwiches

One slice of bread in your daily luncheon sandwich has anywhere from 65 to 100 calories, depending on the brand. Eliminate one slice — serve your sandwich open, and you can save up to 700 calories a week.

Eliminate the High-Fat Ingredient

A bacon, lettuce, and tomato sandwich usually comes with three strips of bacon, each one worth 100 calories. Leave off one strip and save 100 calories. Leave off two, save 200 calories. Leave off three, save 300 calories — and enjoy your lettuce and tomato sandwich with lowfat mayonnaise.

Other ways to eliminate fat calories:

- Make spaghetti sauce without olive oil (100 calories a tablespoon).
- Make split pea soup without ham (55 to 90 calories an ounce).
- Make cream sauces with skim milk instead of cream (470 calories per cup for the cream; 85 to 90 calories for the skim milk).

Don't Butter the Veggies

This one's a no-brainer. Season your vegetables with herbs instead of greasing them, and you save 100 calories for every unused tablespoon of butter, margarine, or oil.

Wash the Chopped Meat

Yes, you read that right. Heat a teapot of water. Put the chopped meat in a pan and cook it until it browns. Pour off the fat, turn the meat into a strainer, and pour a cup of hot water over it. Repeat two times. Every tablespoon of fat that melts or drains from the meat saves you 100 calories, plus cholesterol and saturated fat. Use the de-fatted meat in spaghetti sauce. (Check out Figure 30-1 for the visual presentation!)

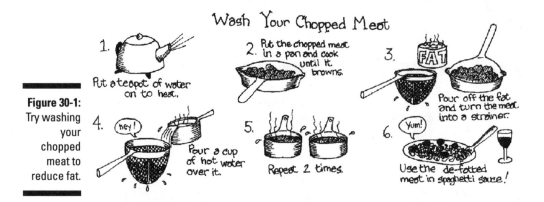

Figure 30-1: Try washing your chopped meat to reduce fat.

Appendix
The Nutrients in Food

*T*he chart on the following pages is an adaptation of the USDA Nutrient Database prepared by the Human Nutrition Information Service. It lists the nutrient values for specific, real-life servings of hundreds of different foods and beverages. Each entry on the chart is identified with an NDB (Nutrition Data Base) number and gives you a snap-shot of a specific food serving ("raw apple with skin") that shows how much the serving weighs (in grams) and lists the amount of

- Water (as a percentage of the serving's weight)
- Food energy (calories)
- Protein
- Carbohydrates
- Dietary fiber
- Calcium
- Phosphorus
- Iron
- Sodium
- Potassium
- Magnesium

- Vitamin A
- Thiamin (vitamin B1)
- Riboflavin (vitamin B2)
- Niacin
- Vitamin B6
- Folate
- Vitamin B12
- Vitamin C
- Fat
- Saturated, monounsaturated, and polyunsaturated fat
- Cholesterol

The Foods on This Chart

The actual Human Nutrition Information Service chart has more than 5,000 (!) entries, including baby food and fast food. The *Nutrition For Dummies* chart is considerably shorter, of course. (I tell you how to access the *big* chart in a minute.)

What you find here are absolutely basic foods. For example, a raw apple with skin rather than a baked apple or apple pie. Why the distinction? Because it is relatively easy to figure out how many calories and what nutrients you get from a plain raw apple, but when you bake the apple or put it into a pie, you begin to add ingredients in amounts that may vary from one dish to another.

For fresh foods (that raw apple, again), the values in this chart apply to the part of the food you actually eat — corn without the cob, meat without bones, the apple without pits and core. The values for cooked foods, such as vegetables or toast, do not include extra ingredients, such as butter or salt.

Sometimes you will find two sets of values for the same portion of cooked meat or poultry — one for a simple combination of fat and lean parts, a second for lean meat (meat from which the fat has been removed before or after cooking) or poultry without skin.

For the most part, no brand-name foods appear on this list. The recipes used to determine the nutrient values of breads or pastas or jellies and jams are based on standard recipes. The bread or pasta or jelly or jam you buy may not conform precisely to these recipes.

But not to worry. The wonderful new food labels (see Chapter 17) tell you everything you need to know about these foods. Think of this as your government's gift to healthy eating!

Accessing the Whole She-bang

Are you consumed with a mad desire to access the entire online Human Nutrition Food chart? Are you computer literate? Then the task is easy as pie — apple, no sugar, plain crust — well, you get the picture.

Your goal is to get to the USDA Nutrient Database on the Web, a site that allows you to search for foods either by NDB number or (more likely) by name. Here's how.

1. **Go directly to the search page for the USDA Nutrient Database at** `www.nal.usda.gov/fnic/cgi-bin/nut_search.pl`

   If you don't have the NDB number and just plan to look for a food by name, be prepared to make some choices. For example, say that you are curious about the banana you've decided to wolf down as a late afternoon snack and decided to search for "banana" on the USDA Nutrient Database site (see Figure A-1).

2. Search for your food by entering the name or the NBD number and then pressing Enter.

A search for "banana" turns up (can you believe this?) 38 items — including, of course, the plain, raw one that you're looking for. But, hey, you may change your mind in mid-bite and go for another version.

3. Click the link to the food item that you want (see Figure A-2).

You now get a choice of serving sizes and/or weights to choose from.

Search the USDA Nutrient Database for Standard Reference

This interface allows simple searches. Enter one keyword which best describes your food item or the NDB No. If you don't get a match, check your spelling or try a related term. If you get too many items, try a more specific keyword. If you enter two or more keywords, the program will search for items which contain all of the keywords. They do not have to be adjacent or in the same order you entered them.

You can search this index. Type the keyword(s) you want to search for:

banana

Figure A-1: Begin your nutrition journey here.

- Babyfood, cereal, rice, with applesauce and bananas, strained
- Babyfood, cereal, rice, with bananas, dry
- Babyfood, fruit, bananas with tapioca, junior
- Babyfood, cereal, mixed, with bananas, prepared with whole milk
- Babyfood, cereal, oatmeal, with bananas, prepared with whole milk
- Babyfood, cereal, rice, with bananas, prepared with whole milk
- Cereals, CREAM OF WHEAT, mix'n eat, apple, banana and maple flavored, dry
- Cereals, CREAM OF WHEAT, mix'n eat, apple, banana and maple flavored, prepared
- Bananas, raw
- Bananas, dehydrated, or banana powder
- Fruit salad, (pineapple and papaya and banana and guava), tropical, canned, heavy syrup, solids and liquids
- Bread banana, prepared from recipe, made with margarine
- Bread, banana, prepared from recipe, made with vegetable shortening
- Pie, banana cream, prepared from mix, no-bake type
- Pie, banana cream, prepared from recipe
- Desserts, puddings, banana, dry mix, instant, prepared with 2% milk
- Desserts, puddings, banana, dry mix, regular, prepared with 2% milk
- Desserts, puddings, banana, ready-to-eat
- Desserts, puddings, banana, dry mix, instant
- Desserts, puddings, banana, dry mix, instant, prepared with whole milk
- Desserts, puddings, banana, dry mix, regular
- Desserts, puddings, banana, dry mix, regular, prepared with whole milk

Figure A-2: Here are some of your choices for the "banana" search.

4. Pick a serving size (or several) and click the Report button.

For example, as you can see from Figure A-3, I chose 1 cup (mashed), 1 small, and 1 large banana.

Here comes your customized report, which includes even more details than you can find on the *Nutrition For Dummies* chart. For example, did you know that 1 cup of raw mashed bananas has 0.108 grams of lysine? Wow! (Hey, wait: What's lysine? Hint: The answer's in Chapter 6.) A list of some of the stuff found in the database is shown in Figure A-4.

Select weights to be reported. If you select 100 grams, number of samples(N) and standard error (SE) will also be reported. You may select up to 5 weights or 100 grams and up to 3 weights.

☐ 100 grams
☑ 1 cup, mashed = 225.0 g
☐ 1 cup, sliced = 150.0 g
☑ 1 small (6" to 6-7/8" long) = 101.0 g
☐ 1 extra small (less than 6" long) = 81.0 g
☐ 1 medium (7" to 7-7/8" long) = 118.0 g
☐ 1 extra large (9" or longer) = 152.0 g
☑ 1 large (8" to 8-7/8" long) = 136.0 g

[report]   [clear]

Figure A-3: Make your choice and ask for a report.

NDB No: 09040

Nutrient	Units	1 cup, mashed = 225.0 g	1 small (6" to 6-7/8" long) = 101.0 g	1 large (8" to 8-7/8" long) = 136.0 g
Proximates				
Moisture	g	167.085	75.003	100.994
Energy	kcal	207.000	92.920	125.120
Energy	kj	864.000	387.840	522.240
Protein	g	2.317	1.040	1.401
Lipids	g	1.080	0.485	0.653
Carbohydrates, by difference	g	52.718	23.664	31.865
Fiber, total dietary	g	5.400	2.424	3.264
Ash	g	1.800	0.808	1.088
Minerals				
Calcium, Ca	mg	13.500	6.060	8.160
Iron, Fe	mg	0.698	0.313	0.422

Figure A-4: Part of your banana nutrition report.

Eating by the Numbers

The *Nutrition For Dummies* chart and the Human Nutrition Information Service database listings can give you the real facts about what's in the food on your plate. After you know why you need the various nutrients — protein, fat, carbs, vitamins, and minerals — the charts give you the information you need to make healthy food choices that also satisfy your palate.

NDB #	Description & Serving	Grams	Water	Calories	Protein	Carbohydrates	Fiber	Calcium	Phosphorus	Iron	Sodium	Potassium	Magnesium
			gm	kcal	gm	gm	gm	mg	mg	mg	mg	mg	mg
Beans (legumes) and bean products													
16015	Black beans, cooked, boiled, wo/salt 1 cup	172	113.07	227.04	15.24	40.78	14.96	46.44	240.8	3.61	1.72	610.6	120.4
16058	Chickpeas (garbanzo beans, bengal gm), seeds, canned 1 cup	240	167.26	285.6	11.88	54.29	10.56	76.8	216	3.24	717.6	412.8	69.6
16028	Kidney beans, all types, cooked, boiled, wo/salt 1 cup	177	118.48	224.79	15.35	40.37	11.33	49.56	251.34	5.2	3.54	713.31	79.65
16070	Lentils, cooked, boiled, wo/salt 1 cup	198	137.89	229.68	17.86	39.88	15.64	37.62	356.4	6.59	3.96	730.62	71.28
16072	Lima beans, lrg, cooked, boiled, wo/salt 1 cup	188	131.21	216.2	14.66	39.27	13.16	31.96	208.68	4.49	3.76	955.04	80.84
16038	Navy beans, cooked, boiled, wo/salt 1 cup	182	114.99	258.44	15.83	47.88	11.65	127.4	285.74	4.51	1.82	669.76	107.38
16086	Peas, split, cooked, boiled, wo/salt 1 cup	196	136.2	231.28	16.35	41.38	16.27	27.44	194.04	2.53	3.92	709.52	70.56
16090	Peanuts, all types, dry-roasted, w/salt 1 oz	28.35	0.44	165.85	6.71	6.1	2.27	15.31	101.49	0.64	230.49	186.54	49.9
16098	Peanut butter, smooth style, w/salt 2 tablespoons	32	0.39	189.76	8.07	6.17	1.89	12.16	118.08	0.59	149.44	214.08	50.88
16109	Soybeans, cooked, boiled, wo/salt 1 cup	172	107.59	297.56	28.62	17.06	10.32	175.44	421.4	8.84	1.72	885.8	147.92
Dairy products													
Butter													
01145	Butter, without salt 1 tablespoon	14.2	2.55	101.81	0.12	0.01	0	3.34	3.24	0.02	1.56	3.69	0.28
Cheese													
01007	Camembert 1 wedge	38	19.68	113.83	7.52	0.18	0	147.29	131.7	0.13	319.85	70.9	7.59
01009	Cheddar 1 cup, diced	132	48.51	531.4	32.87	1.69	0	952.12	675.97	0.9	819.06	129.89	36.67
01012	Cottage cheese, creamed, lrg curd 1 cup (not packed, large curd)	210	165.82	217.03	26.23	5.63	0	126	276.78	0.29	850.08	177.03	11.05
01014	Cottage cheese, uncrmd, dry, lrg or sml curd 1 cup (not packed)	145	115.67	122.66	25.04	2.68	0	45.97	150.8	0.33	18.56	46.98	5.71
01015	Cottage cheese, 2% fat 1 cup (not packed)	226	179.24	202.68	31.05	8.2	0	154.81	340.13	0.36	917.56	217.41	13.56
01016	Cottage cheese, 1% fat 1 cup (not packed)	226	186.4	163.62	28	6.15	0	137.63	302.39	0.32	917.56	193.23	12.07
01017	Cream cheese 1 tablespoon	14.5	7.79	50.61	1.09	0.39	0	11.59	15.14	0.17	42.85	17.31	0.93
01186	Cream cheese, fat free 100 grams	100	75.53	96	14.41	5.8	0	185	434	0.18	545	163	14
01026	Mozzarella, whole milk 1 oz	28.35	15.35	79.77	5.51	0.63	0	146.57	105.09	0.05	105.77	19.02	5.27
01028	Mozzarella, part skim milk 1 oz	28.35	15.25	72.08	6.88	0.79	0	183.06	131.26	0.06	132.11	23.73	6.58

NDB #	Zinc	Copper	Vitamin A	Thiamin	Riboflavin	Niacin	Vitamin B6	Folate	Vitamin B12	Vitamin C	Fat	Fat. Saturated	Fat. Monounsaturated	Fat. Polyunsaturated	Cholesterol
	mg	mg	IU	mg	mg	mg	mg	mcg	mcg	mg	gm	gm	gm	gm	mg
Beans (legumes) and bean products															
16015	1.93	0.36	10.32	0.42	0.1	0.87	0.12	255.94	0	0	0.93	0.24	0.08	0.4	0
16058	2.54	0.42	57.6	0.07	0.08	0.33	1.14	160.32	0	9.12	2.74	0.28	0.62	1.22	0
16028	1.89	0.43	0	0.28	0.1	1.02	0.21	229.39	0	2.12	0.89	0.13	0.07	0.49	0
16070	2.51	0.5	15.84	0.33	0.14	2.1	0.35	357.98	0	2.97	0.75	0.1	0.13	0.35	0
16072	1.79	0.44	0	0.3	0.1	0.79	0.3	156.23	0	0	0.71	0.17	0.06	0.32	0
16038	1.93	0.54	3.64	0.37	0.11	0.97	0.3	254.62	0	1.64	1.04	0.27	0.09	0.45	0
16086	1.96	0.35	13.72	0.37	0.11	1.74	0.09	127.2	0	0.78	0.76	0.11	0.16	0.32	0
16090	0.94	0.19	0	0.12	0.03	3.83	0.07	41.19	0	0	14.08	1.95	6.99	4.45	0
16098	0.93	0.04	0	0.03	0.03	4.29	0.15	23.68	0	0	16.33	3.31	7.77	4.41	0
16109	1.98	0.7	15.48	0.27	0.49	0.69	0.4	92.54	0	2.92	15.43	2.23	3.41	8.71	0
Dairy products															
Butter															
01145	0.01	0	434.24	0	0	0.01	0	0.4	0.02	0	11.52	7.17	3.33	0.43	31.08
Cheese															
01007	0.9	0.01	350.74	0.01	0.19	0.24	0.09	23.63	0.49	0	9.21	5.8	2.67	0.28	27.36
01009	4.11	0.04	1397.88	0.04	0.5	0.11	0.1	24.02	1.09	0	43.74	27.84	12.4	1.24	138.47
01012	0.78	0.06	342.3	0.04	0.34	0.26	0.14	25.62	1.31	0	9.47	5.99	2.7	0.29	31.29
01014	0.68	0.04	43.5	0.04	0.21	0.22	0.12	21.46	1.2	0	0.61	0.4	0.16	0.02	9.72
01015	0.95	0.06	158.2	0.05	0.42	0.33	0.17	29.61	1.61	0	4.36	2.76	1.24	0.13	18.98
01016	0.86	0.06	83.62	0.05	0.37	0.29	0.15	28.02	1.43	0	2.31	1.46	0.66	0.07	9.94
01017	0.08	0	206.92	0	0.03	0.01	0.01	1.91	0.06	0	5.06	3.19	1.43	0.18	15.91
01186	0.88	0.05	930	0.05	0.17	0.16	0.05	37	0.55	0	1.36	0.9	0.33	0.06	8
01026	0.63	0.01	224.53	0	0.07	0.02	0.02	1.98	0.19	0	6.12	3.73	1.86	0.22	22.23
01028	0.78	0.01	165.56	0.01	0.09	0.03	0.02	2.49	0.23	0	4.51	2.87	1.28	0.13	16.39

NDB #	Description & Serving	Grams	Water	Calories	Protein	Carbohydrates	Fiber	Calcium	Phosphorus	Iron	Sodium	Potassium	Magnesium
			gm	kcal	gm	gm	gm	mg	mg	mg	mg	mg	mg
01032	Parmesan, grated 1 tablespoon	5	0.88	22.79	2.08	0.19	0	68.79	40.36	0.05	93.08	5.36	2.54
01036	Ricotta, whole milk 1/2 cup	124	88.91	215.68	13.96	3.77	0	256.68	196.04	0.47	104.28	129.7	14.01
01037	Ricotta, part skim milk 1 cup	246	183.05	339.62	28.02	12.64	0	669.12	449.2	1.08	306.76	307.5	36.33
01040	Swiss 1 cup, diced	132	49.12	496.01	37.53	4.46	0	1268.39	798.07	0.22	343.2	146.12	47.4
Eggs													
01123	Egg, whole, raw, fresh 1 extra large	58	43.69	86.42	7.24	0.71	0	28.42	103.24	0.84	73.08	70.18	5.8
01124	Egg, white, raw, fresh 1 large egg white	33.4	29.33	16.7	3.51	0.34	0	2	4.34	0.01	54.78	47.76	3.67
01125	Egg, yolk, raw, fresh 1 large egg yolk	16.6	8.1	59.43	2.78	0.3	0	22.74	81.01	0.59	7.14	15.6	1.49
Milk and cream													
Milk													
01077	Milk, whole, 3.3% fat 1 cup	244	214.7	149.92	8.03	11.37	0	291.34	227.9	0.12	119.56	369.66	32.79
01079	Milk, lofat, 2% fat, w/ vit A 1 cup	244	217.67	121.2	8.13	11.71	0	296.7	232.04	0.12	121.76	376.74	33.35
01082	Milk, lofat, 1% fat, w/ vit A 1 cup	244	219.8	102.15	8.03	11.66	0	300.12	234.73	0.12	123.22	380.88	33.72
01085	Milk, skim, w/ vit A 1 cup	245	222.46	85.53	8.35	11.88	0	302.33	247.21	0.1	126.18	405.72	27.83
Cream													
01049	Cream, half and half 1 tablespoon	15	12.09	19.55	0.44	0.65	0	15.74	14.28	0.01	6.11	19.44	1.53
01052	Cream, light whipping 1 cup, fluid (yields 2 cups whipped)	239	151.77	698.88	5.19	7.07	0	165.87	146.03	0.07	81.98	231.35	17.28
01053	Cream, heavy whipping 1 tablespoon	15	10.28	36.56	0.37	0.52	0	13.53	10.59	0.01	5.55	17.18	1.26
01056	Cream, sour, cultured 1 cup	230	163.19	492.79	7.27	9.82	0	267.72	195.27	0.14	122.59	331.2	25.83
Ice cream, ice milk													
19270	Ice cream, chocolate 1/2 cup (4 fl oz)	66	36.76	142.56	2.51	18.61	0.79	71.94	70.62	0.61	50.16	164.34	19.14
19271	Ice cream, strawberry 1/2 cup (4 fl oz)	66	39.6	126.72	2.11	18.22	0.2	79.2	66	0.14	39.6	124.08	9.24
19095	Ice cream, vanilla 1/2 cup (4 fl oz)	66	40.26	132.66	2.31	15.58	0	84.48	69.3	0.06	52.8	131.34	9.24
19088	Ice milk, vanilla 1/2 cup (4 fl oz)	66	45.01	91.74	2.51	14.98	0	91.74	71.94	0.07	56.1	139.26	9.9
Yogurt													
01116	Yogurt, plain, whole milk 1 cup (8 fl oz)	245	215.36	150.48	8.5	11.42	0	295.72	232.51	0.12	113.68	378.77	28.37

NDB #	Zinc	Copper	Vitamin A	Thiamin	Riboflavin	Niacin	Vitamin B6	Folate	Vitamin B12	Vitamin C	Fat	Fat: Saturated	Fat: Monounsaturated	Fat: Polyunsaturated	Cholesterol
	mg	mg	IU	mg	mg	mg	mg	mcg	mcg	mg	gm	gm	gm	gm	mg
01032	0.16	0	35.05	0	0.02	0.02	0.01	0.4	0.07	0	1.5	0.95	0.44	0.03	3.94
01036	1.44	0.03	607.6	0.02	0.24	0.13	0.05	15.13	0.42	0	16.1	10.29	4.5	0.48	62.74
01037	3.3	0.08	1062.72	0.05	0.46	0.19	0.05	32.23	0.72	0	19.46	12.12	5.69	0.64	75.77
01040	5.15	0.04	1115.4	0.03	0.48	0.12	0.11	8.45	2.21	0	36.23	23.47	9.6	1.28	121.04
Eggs															
01123	0.64	0.01	368.3	0.04	0.29	0.04	0.08	27.26	0.58	0	5.81	1.8	2.21	0.79	246.5
01124	0	0	0	0	0.15	0.03	0	1	0.07	0	0	0	0	0	0
01125	0.52	0	322.87	0.03	0.11	0	0.07	24.24	0.52	0	5.12	1.59	1.95	0.7	212.65
Milk and cream															
Milk															
01077	0.93	0.02	307.44	0.09	0.4	0.2	0.1	12.2	0.87	2.29	8.15	5.07	2.35	0.3	33.18
01079	0.95	0.02	500.2	0.1	0.4	0.21	0.1	12.44	0.89	2.32	4.68	2.92	1.35	0.17	18.3
01082	0.95	0.02	500.2	0.1	0.41	0.21	0.1	12.44	0.9	2.37	2.59	1.61	0.75	0.1	9.76
01085	0.98	0.03	499.8	0.09	0.34	0.22	0.1	12.74	0.93	2.4	0.44	0.29	0.12	0.02	4.41
Cream															
01049	0.08	0	65.1	0.01	0.02	0.01	0.01	0.38	0.05	0.13	1.73	1.07	0.5	0.06	5.54
01052	0.6	0.02	2693.53	0.06	0.3	0.1	0.07	8.84	0.47	1.46	73.87	46.22	21.73	2.11	265.29
01053	0.04	0	141.3	0	0.02	0.01	0	0.35	0.03	0.11	3.75	2.33	1.08	0.14	13.13
01056	0.62	0.04	1817	0.08	0.34	0.15	0.04	24.84	0.69	1.98	48.21	30.01	13.92	1.79	102.12
Ice cream, ice milk															
19270	0.38	0.09	274.56	0.03	0.13	0.15	0.04	10.56	0.19	0.46	7.26	4.49	2.12	0.27	22.44
19271	0.22	0.02	211.2	0.03	0.17	0.11	0.03	7.92	0.2	5.08	5.54	3.43	0	0	19.14
19095	0.46	0.02	269.94	0.03	0.16	0.08	0.03	3.3	0.26	0.4	7.26	4.48	2.09	0.27	29.04
19088	0.29	0.01	108.9	0.04	0.17	0.06	0.04	3.96	0.44	0.53	2.84	1.74	0.81	0.11	9.24
Yogurt															
01116	1.45	0.02	301.35	0.07	0.35	0.18	0.08	18.13	0.91	1.3	7.96	5.14	2.19	0.23	31.12

NDB #	Description & Serving	Grams	Water	Calories	Protein	Carbohydrates	Fiber	Calcium	Phosphorus	Iron	Sodium	Potassium	Magnesium
			gm	kcal	gm	gm	gm	mg	mg	mg	mg	mg	mg
01117	Yogurt, plain, lowfat 1 cup (8 fl oz)	245	208.42	155.05	12.86	17.25	0	447.37	351.58	0.2	171.99	572.81	42.75
01118	Yogurt, plain, skim milk 1 cup (8 fl oz)	245	208.81	136.64	14.04	18.82	0	487.8	383.43	0.22	187.43	624.51	46.8

Fats and oils

Fats

NDB #	Description & Serving	Grams	Water	Calories	Protein	Carbohydrates	Fiber	Calcium	Phosphorus	Iron	Sodium	Potassium	Magnesium
04071	Margarine, reg, hard, corn (hydr) 1 teaspoon	4.7	0.74	33.78	0.04	0.04	0	1.41	1.08	0	44.34	1.99	0.12
04092	Margarine, soft, corn (hydr & reg) 1 teaspoon	4.7	0.76	33.67	0.04	0.02	0	1.25	0.95	0	50.7	1.77	0.11
04585	Margarine blend, 60% corn oil & 40% butter 1 tablespoon	14.2	2.24	101.96	0.12	0.09	0	3.98	3.27	0.01	127.37	5.11	0.28

Oils

NDB #	Description & Serving	Grams	Water	Calories	Protein	Carbohydrates	Fiber	Calcium	Phosphorus	Iron	Sodium	Potassium	Magnesium
04582	Canola oil 1 tablespoon	14	0	123.76	0	0	0	0	0	0	0	0	0
04518	Corn, salad or cooking oil 1 tablespoon	13.6	0	120.22	0	0	0	0	0	0	0	0	0
04053	Olive, salad or cooking oil 1 tablespoon	13.5	0	119.34	0	0	0	0.02	0.16	0.05	0.01	0	0
04042	Peanut, salad or cooking oil 1 tablespoon	13.5	0	119.34	0	0	0	0.01	0	0	0.01	0	0.01

Fruits and fruit juices

NDB #	Description & Serving	Grams	Water	Calories	Protein	Carbohydrates	Fiber	Calcium	Phosphorus	Iron	Sodium	Potassium	Magnesium
09003	Apples, raw, with skin 1 cup, quartered or chopped	125	104.91	73.75	0.24	19.06	3.38	8.75	8.75	0.23	0	143.75	6.25
09021	Apricots, raw 1 cup, halves	155	133.84	74.4	2.17	17.24	3.72	21.7	29.45	0.84	1.55	458.8	12.4
09032	Apricots, dried, sulfured, uncooked 1 half	3.5	1.09	8.33	0.13	2.16	0.32	1.58	4.1	0.16	0.35	48.23	1.65
09038	Avocados, raw, California 1 fruit, without skin and seeds	173	125.53	306.21	3.65	11.95	8.48	19.03	72.66	2.04	20.76	1096.82	70.93
09039	Avocados, raw, Florida 1 fruit, without skin and seeds	304	242.38	340.48	4.83	27.09	16.11	33.44	118.56	1.61	15.2	1483.52	103.36
09040	Bananas, raw 1 cup, sliced	150	111.39	138	1.55	35.15	3.6	9	30	0.47	1.5	594	43.5
09050	Blueberries, raw 1 pint, as purchased, yields	402	340.13	225.12	2.69	56.8	10.85	24.12	40.2	0.68	24.12	357.78	20.1
09087	Dates, domestic, nat & dry 1 cup, pitted, chopped	178	40.05	489.5	3.51	130.85	13.35	56.96	71.2	2.05	5.34	1160.56	62.3
09094	Figs, dried, uncooked 1 fig	19	5.4	48.45	0.58	12.42	1.77	27.36	12.92	0.42	2.09	135.28	11.21
09111	Grapefruit, raw, pink & red & white, all areas 1 cup sections with juice	230	209.05	73.6	1.45	18.58	2.53	27.6	18.4	0.21	0	319.7	18.4
09131	Grapes, American type (slip skin), raw 1 cup	92	74.8	57.96	0.58	15.78	0.92	12.88	9.2	0.27	1.84	175.72	4.6
09132	Grapes, European type (adherent skin), raw 1 cup, seedless	160	128.9	113.6	1.06	28.43	1.6	17.6	20.8	0.42	3.2	296	9.6
09148	Kiwi fruit, (Chinese gooseberries), fresh, raw 1 large fruit, without skin	91	75.58	55.51	0.9	13.54	3.09	23.66	36.4	0.37	4.55	302.12	27.3

NDB #	Zinc	Copper	Vitamin A	Thiamin	Riboflavin	Niacin	Vitamin B6	Folate	Vitamin B12	Vitamin C	Fat	Fat: Saturated	Fat: Monounsaturated	Fat: Polyunsaturated	Cholesterol
	mg	mg	IU	mg	mg	mg	mg	mcg	mcg	mg	gm	gm	gm	gm	mg
01117	2.18	0.03	161.7	0.11	0.52	0.28	0.12	27.44	1.38	1.96	3.8	2.45	1.04	0.11	14.95
01118	2.38	0.04	17.15	0.12	0.57	0.3	0.13	29.89	1.5	2.13	0.44	0.28	0.12	0.01	4.41

Fats and oils

Fats

NDB #	Zinc	Copper	Vitamin A	Thiamin	Riboflavin	Niacin	Vitamin B6	Folate	Vitamin B12	Vitamin C	Fat	Fat: Saturated	Fat: Monounsaturated	Fat: Polyunsaturated	Cholesterol
04071	0	0	167.84	0	0	0	0	0.06	0	0.01	3.78	0.62	2.15	0.85	0
04092	0	0	167.84	0	0	0	0	0.05	0	0.01	3.78	0.66	1.49	1.47	0
04585	0	0	507.08	0	0	0	0	0.28	0.01	0.01	11.46	4.04	4.65	2.26	12.5

Oils

NDB #	Zinc	Copper	Vitamin A	Thiamin	Riboflavin	Niacin	Vitamin B6	Folate	Vitamin B12	Vitamin C	Fat	Fat: Saturated	Fat: Monounsaturated	Fat: Polyunsaturated	Cholesterol
04582	0	0	0	0	0	0	0	0	0	0	14	0.99	8.25	4.14	0
04518	0	0	0	0	0	0	0	0	0	0	13.6	1.73	3.29	7.98	0
04053	0.01	0	0	0	0	0	0	0	0	0	13.5	1.82	9.95	1.13	0
04042	0	0	0	0	0	0	0	0	0	0	13.5	2.28	6.24	4.32	0

Fruits and fruit juices

NDB #	Zinc	Copper	Vitamin A	Thiamin	Riboflavin	Niacin	Vitamin B6	Folate	Vitamin B12	Vitamin C	Fat	Fat: Saturated	Fat: Monounsaturated	Fat: Polyunsaturated	Cholesterol
09003	0.05	0.05	66.25	0.02	0.02	0.1	0.06	3.5	0	7.13	0.45	0.07	0.02	0.13	0
09021	0.4	0.14	4048.6	0.05	0.06	0.93	0.08	13.33	0	15.5	0.6	0.04	0.26	0.12	0
09032	0.03	0.02	253.4	0	0.01	0.1	0.01	0.36	0	0.08	0.02	0	0.01	0	0
09038	0.73	0.46	1058.76	0.19	0.21	3.32	0.48	113.32	0	13.67	29.98	4.48	19.4	3.53	0
09039	1.28	0.76	1860.48	0.33	0.37	5.84	0.85	162.03	0	24.02	26.96	5.34	14.8	4.5	0
09040	0.24	0.16	121.5	0.07	0.15	0.81	0.87	28.65	0	13.65	0.72	0.28	0.06	0.13	0
09050	0.44	0.25	402	0.19	0.2	1.44	0.14	25.73	0	52.26	1.53	0.13	0.22	0.67	0
09087	0.52	0.51	89	0.16	0.18	3.92	0.34	22.43	0	0	0.8	0.34	0.27	0.06	0
09094	0.1	0.06	25.27	0.01	0.02	0.13	0.04	1.43	0	0.15	0.22	0.04	0.05	0.11	0
09111	0.16	0.11	285.2	0.08	0.05	0.58	0.1	23.46	0	79.12	0.23	0.03	0.03	0.06	0
09131	0.04	0.04	92	0.08	0.05	0.28	0.1	3.59	0	3.68	0.32	0.1	0.01	0.09	0
09132	0.08	0.14	116.8	0.15	0.09	0.48	0.18	6.24	0	17.28	0.93	0.3	0.04	0.27	0
09148	0.15	0.14	159.25	0.02	0.05	0.46	0.08	34.58	0	89.18	0.4	0.03	0.04	0.22	0

NDB #	Description & Serving	Grams	Water	Calories	Protein	Carbohydrates	Fiber	Calcium	Phosphorus	Iron	Sodium	Potassium	Magnesium
			gm	*kcal*	*gm*	*gm*	*gm*	*mg*	*mg*	*mg*	*mg*	*mg*	*mg*
09176	**Mangos, raw** 1 fruit, without refuse	207	169.14	134.55	1.06	35.19	3.73	20.7	22.77	0.27	4.14	322.92	18.63
09181	**Melons, cantaloupe, raw** 1 cup, balls	177	158.91	61.95	1.56	14.8	1.42	19.47	30.09	0.37	15.93	546.93	19.47
09184	**Melons, honeydew, raw** 1 cup, diced (approx 20 pieces per cup)	170	152.42	59.5	0.78	15.61	1.02	10.2	17	0.12	17	460.7	11.9
09193	**Olives, ripe, canned (small-extra lrg)** 1 large	4.4	3.52	5.06	0.04	0.28	0.14	3.87	0.13	0.15	38.37	0.35	0.18
09201	**Oranges, raw, California, Valencias** 1 fruit (2-5/8" dia, sphere)	121	104.47	59.29	1.26	14.39	3.03	48.4	20.57	0.11	0	216.59	12.1
09202	**Oranges, raw, California, navels** 1 fruit (2-7/8" dia)	140	121.53	64.4	1.44	16.28	3.36	56	26.6	0.17	1.4	249.2	14
09203	**Oranges, raw, Florida** 1 fruit (2-5/8" dia, sphere)	141	122.87	64.86	0.99	16.27	3.38	60.63	16.92	0.13	0	238.29	14.1
09206	**Orange juice, raw** 1 cup	248	218.98	111.6	1.74	25.79	0.5	27.28	42.16	0.5	2.48	496	27.28
09218	**Tangerines (mandarin oranges), raw** 1 large (2-1/2" dia)	98	85.85	43.12	0.62	10.97	2.25	13.72	9.8	0.1	0.98	153.86	11.76
09226	**Papayas, raw** 1 cup, cubes	140	124.36	54.6	0.85	13.73	2.52	33.6	7	0.14	4.2	359.8	14
09236	**Peaches, raw** 1 large (2-3/4" dia) (approx 2 1/2 per lb)	157	137.63	67.51	1.1	17.43	3.14	7.85	18.84	0.17	0	309.29	10.99
09252	**Pears, raw** 1 medium (approx 2 1/2 per lb)	166	139.12	97.94	0.65	25.08	3.98	18.26	18.26	0.42	0	207.5	9.96
09266	**Pineapple, raw** 1 cup, diced	155	134.08	75.95	0.6	19.2	1.86	10.85	10.85	0.57	1.55	175.15	21.7
09279	**Plums, raw** 1 fruit (2-1/8" dia)	66	56.23	36.3	0.52	8.59	0.99	2.64	6.6	0.07	0	113.52	4.62
09291	**Prunes, dried, uncooked** 1 prune	8.4	2.72	20.08	0.22	5.27	0.6	4.28	6.64	0.21	0.34	62.58	3.78
09298	**Raisins, seedless** 1 cup, packed	165	25.44	495	5.31	130.56	6.6	80.85	160.05	3.43	19.8	1239.15	54.45
09302	**Raspberries, raw** 1 cup	123	106.48	60.27	1.12	14.23	8.36	27.06	14.76	0.7	0	186.96	22.14
09316	**Strawberries, raw** 1 cup, halves	152	139.19	45.6	0.93	10.67	3.5	21.28	28.88	0.58	1.52	252.32	15.2
09326	**Watermelon, raw** 1 cup, balls	154	140.93	49.28	0.95	11.06	0.77	12.32	13.86	0.26	3.08	178.64	16.94

Grain products

Breads

NDB #	Description & Serving	Grams	Water	Calories	Protein	Carbohydrates	Fiber	Calcium	Phosphorus	Iron	Sodium	Potassium	Magnesium
18001	**Bagels, plain, enriched, w/ca prop (incl onion, poppy, sesame)** 1 bagel (3" dia)	57	18.58	156.75	5.99	30.44	1.31	42.18	54.72	2.03	304.38	57.57	16.53
18080	**Breadsticks, plain** 1 small stick (approx 4-1/4" long)	5	0.31	20.6	0.6	3.42	0.15	1.1	6.05	0.21	32.85	6.2	1.6

NDB #	Zinc	Copper	Vitamin A	Thiamin	Riboflavin	Niacin	Vitamin B6	Folate	Vitamin B12	Vitamin C	Fat	Fat: Saturated	Fat: Monounsaturated	Fat: Polyunsaturated	Cholesterol
	mg	mg	IU	mg	mg	mg	mg	mcg	mcg	mg	gm	gm	gm	gm	mg
09176	0.08	0.23	8060.58	0.12	0.12	1.21	0.28	28.98	0	57.34	0.56	0.14	0.21	0.11	0
09181	0.28	0.07	5706.48	0.06	0.04	1.02	0.2	30.09	0	74.69	0.5	0.13	0.01	0.19	0
09184	0.12	0.07	68	0.13	0.03	1.02	0.1	10.2	0	42.16	0.17	0.04	0	0.07	0
09193	0.01	0.01	17.73	0	0	0	0	0	0	0.04	0.47	0.06	0.35	0.04	0
09201	0.07	0.04	278.3	0.11	0.05	0.33	0.08	46.71	0	58.69	0.36	0.04	0.07	0.07	0
09202	0.08	0.08	256.2	0.12	0.06	0.41	0.1	47.18	0	80.22	0.13	0.02	0.02	0.03	0
09203	0.11	0.05	282	0.14	0.06	0.56	0.07	24.39	0	63.45	0.3	0.04	0.05	0.06	0
09206	0.12	0.11	496	0.22	0.07	0.99	0.1	75.14	0	124	0.5	0.06	0.09	0.1	0
09218	0.24	0.03	901.6	0.1	0.02	0.16	0.07	19.99	0	30.18	0.19	0.02	0.03	0.04	0
09226	0.1	0.02	397.6	0.04	0.04	0.47	0.03	53.2	0	86.52	0.2	0.06	0.05	0.04	0
09236	0.22	0.11	839.95	0.03	0.06	1.55	0.03	5.34	0	10.36	0.14	0.02	0.05	0.07	0
09252	0.2	0.18	33.2	0.03	0.07	0.17	0.03	12.12	0	6.64	0.66	0.04	0.14	0.16	0
09266	0.12	0.17	35.65	0.14	0.06	0.65	0.13	16.43	0	23.87	0.67	0.05	0.07	0.23	0
09279	0.07	0.03	213.18	0.03	0.06	0.33	0.05	1.45	0	6.27	0.41	0.03	0.27	0.09	0
09291	0.04	0.04	166.91	0.01	0.01	0.16	0.02	0.31	0	0.28	0.04	0	0.03	0.01	0
09298	0.45	0.51	13.2	0.26	0.15	1.35	0.41	5.45	0	5.45	0.76	0.25	0.03	0.22	0
09302	0.57	0.09	159.9	0.04	0.11	1.11	0.07	31.98	0	30.75	0.68	0.02	0.07	0.38	0
09316	0.2	0.07	41.04	0.03	0.1	0.35	0.09	26.9	0	86.18	0.56	0.03	0.08	0.28	0
09326	0.11	0.05	563.64	0.12	0.03	0.31	0.22	3.39	0	14.78	0.66	0.07	0.16	0.22	0

Grain products

Breads

NDB #	Zinc	Copper	Vitamin A	Thiamin	Riboflavin	Niacin	Vitamin B6	Folate	Vitamin B12	Vitamin C	Fat	Fat: Saturated	Fat: Monounsaturated	Fat: Polyunsaturated	Cholesterol
18001	0.5	0.09	0	0.31	0.18	2.6	0.03	12.54	0	0	0.91	0.13	0.07	0.4	0
18080	0.04	0.01	0	0.03	0.03	0.26	0	1.5	0	0	0.48	0.07	0.19	0.18	0

NDB #	Description & Serving	Grams	Water	Calories	Protein	Carbohydrates	Fiber	Calcium	Phosphorus	Iron	Sodium	Potassium	Magnesium
			gm	kcal	gm	gm	gm	mg	mg	mg	mg	mg	mg
18347	Dinner rolls, wheat 1 roll (1 oz)	28.35	10.49	77.4	2.44	13.04	1.07	49.9	33.45	1.01	96.39	37.71	11.91
18258	English muffins, plain, enriched, w/ca prop (incl sourdough) 1 muffin	57	24	133.95	4.39	26.22	1.54	99.18	75.81	1.43	264.48	74.67	11.97
18029	French or vienna bread (incl sourdough) 1 large slice (5" x 2-1/2" x 1")	35	12.01	95.9	3.08	18.17	1.05	26.25	36.75	0.89	213.15	39.55	9.45
18350	Hamburger or hot dog, plain rolls 1 roll	43	14.62	122.98	3.66	21.63	1.16	59.77	37.84	1.36	240.8	60.63	8.6
18353	Hard (incl kaiser) rolls 1 roll (3-1/2" dia)	57	17.67	167.01	5.64	30.04	1.31	54.15	57	1.87	310.08	61.56	15.39
18033	Italian bread 1 large slice (4-1/2" x 3-1/4" x 3/4")	30	10.71	81.3	2.64	15	0.81	23.4	30.9	0.88	175.2	33	8.1
18041	Pita, white, enriched bread 1 large pita (6-1/2" dia)	60	19.26	165	5.46	33.42	1.32	51.6	58.2	1.57	321.6	72	15.6
18042	Pita, whole-wheat bread 1 large pita (6-1/2" dia)	64	19.58	170.24	6.27	35.2	4.74	9.6	115.2	1.85	340.48	108.8	44.16
18044	Pumpernickel bread 1 regular slice	26	9.85	65	2.26	12.35	1.69	17.68	46.28	0.75	174.46	54.08	14.04
18047	Raisin, enriched bread 1 large slice	32	10.75	87.68	2.53	16.74	1.38	21.12	34.88	0.93	124.8	72.64	8.32
18060	Rye bread 1 slice	32	11.94	82.88	2.72	15.46	1.86	23.36	40	0.91	211.2	53.12	12.8
18064	Wheat (incl wheat berry) bread 1 slice	25	9.28	65	2.28	11.8	1.08	26.25	37.5	0.83	132.5	50.25	11.5
18069	White bread, commly prep (incl soft bread crumbs) 1 cup, crumbs	45	16.52	120.15	3.69	22.28	1.04	48.6	42.3	1.36	242.1	53.55	10.8
18360	Taco shells, baked 1 large (6-1/2" dia)	21	1.26	98.28	1.51	13.1	1.58	33.6	52.08	0.53	77.07	37.59	22.05
18363	Tortillas, rtb or -fry, corn 1 medium tortilla (approx 6" dia)	26	11.47	57.72	1.48	12.12	1.35	45.5	81.64	0.36	41.86	40.04	16.9
18364	Tortillas, rtb or -fry, flour 1 medium tortilla (approx 6" dia)	32	8.58	104	2.78	17.79	1.06	40	39.68	1.06	152.96	41.92	8.32
Flours and meals													
20011	Buckwheat flour, whole-groat 1 cup	120	13.38	402	15.14	84.71	12	49.2	404.4	4.87	13.2	692.4	301.2
20022	Cornmeal, degermed, enriched, yellow 1 cup	138	15.99	505.08	11.7	107.2	10.21	6.9	115.92	5.7	4.14	223.56	55.2
20020	Cornmeal, whole-grain, yellow 1 cup	122	12.52	441.64	9.91	93.81	8.91	7.32	294.02	4.21	42.7	350.14	154.94
20061	Rice flour, white 1 cup	158	18.79	578.28	9.4	126.61	3.79	15.8	154.84	0.55	0	120.08	55.3
20063	Rye flour, dark 1 cup	128	14.17	414.72	17.96	87.99	28.93	71.68	808.96	8.26	1.28	934.4	317.44
20076	Wheat flour, durum 1 cup	192	21	650.88	26.27	136.57	0	65.28	975.36	6.76	3.84	827.52	276.48
20080	Wheat flour, whole-grain 1 cup	120	12.32	406.8	16.44	87.08	14.64	40.8	415.2	4.66	6	486	165.6

NDB #	Zinc	Copper	Vitamin A	Thiamin	Riboflavin	Niacin	Vitamin B6	Folate	Vitamin B12	Vitamin C	Fat	Fat: Saturated	Fat: Monounsaturated	Fat: Polyunsaturated	Cholesterol
	mg	mg	IU	mg	mg	mg	mg	mcg	mcg	mg	gm	gm	gm	gm	mg
18347	0.29	0.04	0	0.12	0.08	1.15	0.02	4.25	0	0	1.79	0.43	0.92	0.3	0
18258	0.4	0.07	0	0.25	0.16	2.21	0.02	21.09	0.02	0.06	1.03	0.15	0.17	0.51	0
18029	0.3	0.07	0	0.18	0.12	1.66	0.02	10.85	0	0	1.05	0.22	0.43	0.24	0
18350	0.27	0.05	0	0.21	0.13	1.69	0.02	11.61	0.01	0	2.19	0.51	1.07	0.39	0
18353	0.54	0.09	0	0.27	0.19	2.42	0.03	8.55	0	0	2.45	0.35	0.65	0.98	0
18033	0.26	0.06	0	0.14	0.09	1.31	0.01	9	0	0	1.05	0.26	0.24	0.42	0
18041	0.5	0.1	0	0.36	0.2	2.78	0.02	14.4	0	0	0.72	0.1	0.06	0.32	0
18042	0.97	0.18	0	0.22	0.05	1.82	0.15	22.4	0	0	1.66	0.26	0.22	0.68	0
18044	0.38	0.07	0	0.09	0.08	0.8	0.03	8.84	0	0	0.81	0.11	0.24	0.32	0
18047	0.23	0.06	0.64	0.11	0.13	1.11	0.02	10.88	0	0.16	1.41	0.35	0.73	0.22	0
18060	0.36	0.06	1.28	0.14	0.11	1.22	0.02	16.32	0	0.06	1.06	0.2	0.42	0.26	0
18064	0.26	0.05	0	0.1	0.07	1.03	0.02	10.25	0	0	1.03	0.22	0.43	0.23	0
18069	0.28	0.06	0	0.21	0.15	1.79	0.03	15.3	0.01	0	1.62	0.36	0.73	0.33	0.45
18360	0.29	0.03	73.5	0.05	0.01	0.28	0.08	1.26	0	0	4.75	0.7	1.99	1.81	0
18363	0.24	0.04	62.92	0.03	0.02	0.39	0.06	3.9	0	0	0.65	0.09	0.17	0.29	0
18364	0.23	0.09	0	0.17	0.09	1.14	0.02	3.84	0	0	2.27	0.35	0.92	0.89	0
Flours and meals															
20011	3.74	0.62	0	0.5	0.23	7.38	0.7	64.8	0	0	3.72	0.81	1.14	1.14	0
20022	0.99	0.11	569.94	0.99	0.56	6.95	0.35	66.24	0	0	2.28	0.31	0.57	0.98	0
20020	2.22	0.24	572.18	0.47	0.25	4.43	0.37	30.99	0	0	4.38	0.62	1.16	2	0
20061	1.26	0.21	0	0.22	0.03	4.09	0.69	6.32	0	0	2.24	0.61	0.7	0.6	0
20063	7.19	0.96	0	0.4	0.32	5.47	0.57	76.8	0	0	3.44	0.4	0.42	1.54	0
20076	7.99	1.06	0	0.8	0.23	12.94	0.8	83.14	0	0	4.74	0.87	0.66	1.88	0
20080	3.52	0.46	0	0.54	0.26	7.64	0.41	52.8	0	0	2.24	0.39	0.28	0.93	0

NDB #	Description & Serving	Grams	Water	Calories	Protein	Carbohydrates	Fiber	Calcium	Phosphorus	Iron	Sodium	Potassium	Magnesium
			gm	kcal	gm	gm	gm	mg	mg	mg	mg	mg	mg
20081	Wheat flour, white, all-purpose, enriched, bleached												
	1 cup	125	14.9	455	12.91	95.39	3.38	18.75	135	5.8	2.5	133.75	27.5
20581	Wheat flour, white, all-purpose, enriched, unbleached												
	1 cup	125	14.9	455	12.91	95.39	3.38	18.75	135	5.8	2.5	133.75	27.5
	Grains and cereals												
20006	Barley, pearled, cooked												
	1 cup	157	108.02	193.11	3.55	44.31	5.97	17.27	84.78	2.09	4.71	146.01	34.54
20013	Bulgur, cooked												
	1 cup	182	141.52	151.06	5.61	33.82	8.19	18.2	72.8	1.75	9.1	123.76	58.24
20029	Couscous, cooked												
	1 cup, cooked	157	113.93	175.84	5.95	36.46	2.2	12.56	34.54	0.6	7.85	91.06	12.56
20034	Oat bran, cooked												
	1 cup	219	183.96	87.6	7.03	25.05	5.69	21.9	260.61	1.93	2.19	201.48	87.6
08121	Oats, reg & quick & instant, wo/fort, cooked w/water, wo/salt (oats)												
	1 cup	234	199.6	145.08	6.08	25.27	3.98	18.72	177.84	1.59	2.34	131.04	56.16
08123	Oats, instant, fort, plain, prep w/water (oats)												
	1 cup, cooked	234	200.07	138.06	5.85	23.87	3.98	215.28	175.5	8.33	376.74	131.04	56.16
20037	Rice, brown, long-grain, cooked												
	1 cup	195	142.53	216.45	5.03	44.77	3.51	19.5	161.85	0.82	9.75	83.85	83.85
20041	Rice, brown, medium-grain, cooked												
	1 cup	195	142.27	218.4	4.52	45.84	3.51	19.5	150.15	1.03	1.95	154.05	85.8
20345	Rice, white, long-grain, reg, cooked, enriched, w/salt												
	1 cup	158	108.14	205.4	4.25	44.51	0.63	15.8	67.94	1.9	603.56	55.3	18.96
20055	Rice, white, glutinous, cooked												
	1 cup, cooked	174	133.34	168.78	3.51	36.7	1.74	3.48	13.92	0.24	8.7	17.4	8.7
20066	Semolina, enriched												
	1 cup	167	21.16	601.2	21.18	121.63	6.51	28.39	227.12	7.28	1.67	310.62	78.49
20067	Sorghum												
	1 cup	192	17.66	650.88	21.7	143.29	0	53.76	551.04	8.45	11.52	672	0
08084	Wheat germ, toasted, plain												
	1 cup	113	6.33	431.66	32.88	56.05	14.58	50.85	1294.98	10.27	4.52	1070.11	361.6
20089	Wild rice, cooked												
	1 cup	164	121.25	165.64	6.54	35	2.95	4.92	134.48	0.98	4.92	165.64	52.48
Pasta													
20100	Macaroni, cooked, enriched												
	1 cup elbow shaped	140	92.39	197.4	6.68	39.68	1.82	9.8	75.6	1.96	1.4	43.4	25.2
20108	Macaroni, whole-wheat, cooked												
	1 cup elbow shaped	140	94.01	173.6	7.46	37.16	3.92	21	124.6	1.48	4.2	61.6	42
20110	Noodles, egg, cooked, enriched												
	1 cup	160	109.92	212.8	7.6	39.74	1.76	19.2	110.4	2.54	11.2	44.8	30.4
20113	Noodles, chinese, chow mein												
	1 cup	45	0.33	237.15	3.77	25.89	1.76	9	72.45	2.13	197.55	54	23.4
20115	Noodles, japanese, soba, cooked												
	1 cup	114	83.23	112.86	5.77	24.44	0	4.56	28.5	0.55	68.4	39.9	10.26

NDB #	Zinc	Copper	Vitamin A	Thiamin	Riboflavin	Niacin	Vitamin B6	Folate	Vitamin B12	Vitamin C	Fat	Fat: Saturated	Fat: Monounsaturated	Fat: Polyunsaturated	Cholesterol
	mg	mg	IU	mg	mg	mg	mg	mcg	mcg	mg	gm	gm	gm	gm	mg
20081	0.88	0.18	0	0.98	0.62	7.38	0.06	32.5	0	0	1.23	0.19	0.11	0.52	0
20581	0.88	0.18	0	0.98	0.62	7.38	0.06	32.5	0	0	1.23	0.19	0.11	0.52	0

Grains and cereals

NDB #	Zinc	Copper	Vitamin A	Thiamin	Riboflavin	Niacin	Vitamin B6	Folate	Vitamin B12	Vitamin C	Fat	Fat: Saturated	Fat: Monounsaturated	Fat: Polyunsaturated	Cholesterol
20006	1.29	0.16	10.99	0.13	0.1	3.24	0.18	25.12	0	0	0.69	0.15	0.09	0.34	0
20013	1.04	0.14	0	0.1	0.05	1.82	0.15	32.76	0	0	0.44	0.08	0.06	0.18	0
20029	1.37	0.22	0	0.33	0.14	5.19	0.27	79.2	0	0	0.84	0.15	0.12	0.34	0
20034	1.16	0.14	0	0.35	0.07	0.32	0.05	13.14	0	0	1.88	0.36	0.64	0.74	0
08121	1.15	0.13	37.44	0.26	0.05	0.3	0.05	9.36	0	0	2.34	0.42	0.75	0.87	0
08123	1.15	0.13	1996.02	0.7	0.37	7.23	0.98	198.9	0	0	2.34	0.42	0.75	0.87	0
20037	1.23	0.2	0	0.19	0.05	2.98	0.28	7.8	0	0	1.76	0.35	0.64	0.63	0
20041	1.21	0.16	0	0.2	0.02	2.59	0.29	7.8	0	0	1.62	0.32	0.59	0.58	0
20345	0.77	0.11	0	0.26	0.02	2.33	0.15	4.74	0	0	0.44	0.12	0.14	0.12	0
20055	0.71	0.09	0	0.03	0.02	0.5	0.05	1.74	0	0	0.33	0.07	0.12	0.12	0
20066	1.75	0.32	0	1.35	0.95	10	0.17	120.24	0	0	1.75	0.25	0.21	0.72	0
20067	0	0	0	0.46	0.27	5.62	0	0	0	0	6.34	0.88	1.91	2.63	0
08084	18.84	0.7	0	1.89	0.93	6.32	1.11	397.76	0	6.78	12.09	2.07	1.7	7.48	0
20089	2.2	0.2	0	0.09	0.14	2.11	0.22	42.64	0	0	0.56	0.08	0.08	0.35	0

Pasta

NDB #	Zinc	Copper	Vitamin A	Thiamin	Riboflavin	Niacin	Vitamin B6	Folate	Vitamin B12	Vitamin C	Fat	Fat: Saturated	Fat: Monounsaturated	Fat: Polyunsaturated	Cholesterol
20100	0.74	0.14	0	0.29	0.14	2.34	0.05	9.8	0	0	0.94	0.13	0.11	0.38	0
20108	1.13	0.23	0	0.15	0.06	0.99	0.11	7	0	0	0.76	0.14	0.11	0.3	0
20110	0.99	0.14	32	0.3	0.13	2.38	0.06	11.2	0.14	0	2.35	0.5	0.69	0.65	52.8
20113	0.63	0.08	38.25	0.26	0.19	2.68	0.05	9.9	0	0	13.84	1.97	3.46	7.8	0
20115	0.14	0.01	0	0.11	0.03	0.58	0.05	7.98	0	0	0.11	0.02	0.03	0.04	0

NDB #	Description & Serving	Grams	Water	Calories	Protein	Carbohydrates	Fiber	Calcium	Phosphorus	Iron	Sodium	Potassium	Magnesium
		gm	gm	kcal	gm	gm	gm	mg	mg	mg	mg	mg	mg
20121	Spaghetti, cooked, enriched, wo/ salt 1 cup	140	92.39	197.4	6.68	39.68	2.38	9.8	75.6	1.96	1.4	43.4	25.2
20125	Spaghetti, whole-wheat, cooked 1 cup	140	94.01	173.6	7.46	37.16	6.3	21	124.6	1.48	4.2	61.6	42

Meat

Beef

NDB #	Description & Serving	Grams	Water	Calories	Protein	Carbohydrates	Fiber	Calcium	Phosphorus	Iron	Sodium	Potassium	Magnesium
13034	Chuck, arm pot rst, lean & fat, 1/4" fat, braised 3 oz	85	40.79	282.2	23.32	0	0	8.5	187	2.64	51	209.1	16.15
13073	Rib, whole (ribs 6-12), lean & fat, 1/4" fat, roasted 3 oz	85	40.37	304.3	19.13	0	0	9.35	148.75	1.99	53.55	255.85	17
13184	Eye of round, lean, 1/4" fat, roasted 3 oz	85	55.25	142.8	24.64	0	0	4.25	192.1	1.66	52.7	335.75	22.95
13238	Tenderloin, lean & fat, 1/4" fat, broiled 3 oz	85	45.08	247.35	21.47	0	0	6.8	178.5	2.68	50.15	312.8	22.1
13298	Ground, extra lean, broiled, med 3 oz	85	48.67	217.6	21.59	0	0	5.95	136.85	2	59.5	266.05	17.85
13327	Liver, pan-fried 3 oz	85	47.33	184.45	22.71	6.67	0	9.35	391.85	5.34	90.1	309.4	19.55

Lamb

NDB #	Description & Serving	Grams	Water	Calories	Protein	Carbohydrates	Fiber	Calcium	Phosphorus	Iron	Sodium	Potassium	Magnesium
17014	Dom, leg, whole (shk & sirl), lean, 1/4" fat, choice, roasted 3 oz	85	54.31	162.35	24.06	0	0	6.8	175.1	1.8	57.8	287.3	22.1
17025	Dom, loin, lean & fat, 1/4" fat, choice, roasted 3 oz	85	44.63	262.65	19.17	0	0	15.3	153	1.8	54.4	209.1	19.55

Veal

NDB #	Description & Serving	Grams	Water	Calories	Protein	Carbohydrates	Fiber	Calcium	Phosphorus	Iron	Sodium	Potassium	Magnesium
17103	Leg, lean, roasted 3 oz	85	56.96	127.5	23.86	0	0	5.1	200.6	0.77	57.8	334.05	23.8
17109	Loin, lean, roasted 3 oz	85	54.9	148.75	22.37	0	0	17.85	188.7	0.72	81.6	289	22.1
17115	Rib, lean, roasted 3 oz	85	54.94	150.45	21.9	0	0	10.2	175.95	0.82	82.45	264.35	20.4

Pork

NDB #	Description & Serving	Grams	Water	Calories	Protein	Carbohydrates	Fiber	Calcium	Phosphorus	Iron	Sodium	Potassium	Magnesium
10011	Frsh, (ham), whole, lean, roasted 3 oz	85	51.56	179.35	25	0	0	5.95	238.85	0.95	54.4	317.05	21.25
10027	Frsh, loin, whole, lean, roasted 3 oz	85	51.87	177.65	24.33	0	0	15.3	211.65	0.93	49.3	361.25	23.8
10050	Frsh, center rib (chops), bone-in, lean, broiled 3 oz	85	48.41	186.15	26.15	0	0	26.35	208.25	0.7	55.25	357	23.8
10124	Cured, bacon, broiled, pan-fried or roasted 3 medium slices packed 20/lb raw, after cooking	19	2.46	109.44	5.79	0.11	0	2.28	63.84	0.31	303.24	92.34	4.56
10131	Cured, canadian-style bacon, grilled 2 slices (6 per 6-oz pkg.)	46.5	28.69	86.03	11.27	0.63	0	4.65	137.64	0.38	718.89	181.35	9.77
10153	Cured, ham, whole, lean, roasted 3 oz	85	55.91	133.45	21.29	0	0	5.95	192.95	0.8	1127.95	268.6	18.7

Poultry: Chicken (broilers or fryers)

NDB #	Description & Serving	Grams	Water	Calories	Protein	Carbohydrates	Fiber	Calcium	Phosphorus	Iron	Sodium	Potassium	Magnesium
05031	Light meat, meat & skin, fried, flour 1/2 chicken, bone removed	130	71.06	319.8	39.59	2.37	0.13	20.8	276.9	1.57	100.1	310.7	35.1

NDB #	Zinc	Copper	Vitamin A	Thiamin	Riboflavin	Niacin	Vitamin B6	Folate	Vitamin B12	Vitamin C	Fat	Fat: Saturated	Fat: Monounsaturated	Fat: Polyunsaturated	Cholesterol
	mg	mg	IU	mg	mg	mg	mg	mcg	mcg	mg	gm	gm	gm	gm	mg
20121	0.74	0.14	0	0.29	0.14	2.34	0.05	9.8	0	0	0.94	0.13	0.11	0.38	0
20125	1.13	0.23	0	0.15	0.06	0.99	0.11	7	0	0	0.76	0.14	0.11	0.3	0

Meat

Beef

NDB #	Zinc	Copper	Vitamin A	Thiamin	Riboflavin	Niacin	Vitamin B6	Folate	Vitamin B12	Vitamin C	Fat	Fat: Saturated	Fat: Monounsaturated	Fat: Polyunsaturated	Cholesterol
13034	5.81	0.11	0	0.06	0.2	2.7	0.24	7.65	2.51	0	20.24	7.97	8.68	0.77	84.15
13073	4.55	0.07	0	0.06	0.14	2.9	0.2	5.95	2.16	0	24.66	9.95	10.6	0.88	71.4
13184	4.03	0.09	0	0.08	0.14	3.19	0.32	5.95	1.84	0	4.17	1.51	1.77	0.14	58.65
13238	4.15	0.13	0	0.09	0.22	2.99	0.33	5.1	2.05	0	17.22	6.76	7.06	0.65	73.1
13298	4.63	0.06	0	0.05	0.23	4.22	0.23	7.65	1.84	0	13.88	5.46	6.08	0.52	71.4
13327	4.63	3.8	30689.25	0.18	3.52	12.27	1.22	187	95.03	19.55	6.8	2.27	1.38	1.45	409.7

Lamb

NDB #	Zinc	Copper	Vitamin A	Thiamin	Riboflavin	Niacin	Vitamin B6	Folate	Vitamin B12	Vitamin C	Fat	Fat: Saturated	Fat: Monounsaturated	Fat: Polyunsaturated	Cholesterol
17014	4.2	0.1	0	0.09	0.25	5.39	0.14	19.55	2.24	0	6.58	2.35	2.88	0.43	75.65
17025	2.9	0.1	0	0.09	0.2	6.04	0.09	16.15	1.88	0	20.05	8.7	8.23	1.59	80.75

Veal

NDB #	Zinc	Copper	Vitamin A	Thiamin	Riboflavin	Niacin	Vitamin B6	Folate	Vitamin B12	Vitamin C	Fat	Fat: Saturated	Fat: Monounsaturated	Fat: Polyunsaturated	Cholesterol
17103	2.62	0.11	0	0.05	0.28	8.57	0.26	13.6	1	0	2.88	1.04	1.01	0.25	87.55
17109	2.75	0.1	0	0.05	0.26	8.04	0.31	13.6	1.11	0	5.9	2.19	2.12	0.48	90.1
17115	3.82	0.09	0	0.05	0.25	6.38	0.23	11.9	1.34	0	6.32	1.77	2.26	0.57	97.75

Pork

NDB #	Zinc	Copper	Vitamin A	Thiamin	Riboflavin	Niacin	Vitamin B6	Folate	Vitamin B12	Vitamin C	Fat	Fat: Saturated	Fat: Monounsaturated	Fat: Polyunsaturated	Cholesterol
10011	2.77	0.09	7.65	0.59	0.3	4.19	0.38	10.2	0.61	0.34	8.02	2.81	3.78	0.72	79.9
10027	2.15	0.05	6.8	0.86	0.28	5.01	0.47	5.95	0.62	0.51	8.19	2.98	3.67	0.65	68.85
10050	2.02	0.06	5.1	0.95	0.28	5.24	0.4	2.55	0.65	0.26	8.28	2.94	3.78	0.53	68.85
10124	0.62	0.03	0	0.13	0.05	1.39	0.05	0.95	0.33	0	9.36	3.31	4.5	1.1	16.15
10131	0.79	0.03	0	0.38	0.09	3.22	0.21	1.86	0.36	0	3.92	1.32	1.88	0.38	26.97
10153	2.18	0.07	0	0.58	0.22	4.27	0.4	3.4	0.6	0	4.68	1.56	2.15	0.54	46.75

Poultry: Chicken (broilers or fryers)

NDB #	Zinc	Copper	Vitamin A	Thiamin	Riboflavin	Niacin	Vitamin B6	Folate	Vitamin B12	Vitamin C	Fat	Fat: Saturated	Fat: Monounsaturated	Fat: Polyunsaturated	Cholesterol
05031	1.64	0.08	88.4	0.1	0.17	15.65	0.7	5.2	0.43	0	15.72	4.32	6.24	3.5	113.1

NDB #	Description & Serving	Grams	Water	Calories	Protein	Carbohydrates	Fiber	Calcium	Phosphorus	Iron	Sodium	Potassium	Magnesium
			gm	kcal	gm	gm	gm	mg	mg	mg	mg	mg	mg
05032	Light meat, meat & skin, roasted 1/2 chicken, bone removed	132	79.87	293.04	38.31	0	0	19.8	264	1.5	99	299.64	33
05037	Dark meat, meat & skin, roasted 1/2 chicken, bone removed	167	97.91	422.51	43.37	0	0	25.05	280.56	2.27	145.29	367.4	36.74
05028	Chicken, liver, all classes, simmered 1 cup, chopped or diced	140	95.63	219.8	34.1	1.23	0	19.6	436.8	11.86	71.4	196	29.4
Poultry: Duck													
05140	Duck, domesticated, meat & skin, roasted 1 cup, chopped or diced	140	72.58	471.8	26.59	0	0	15.4	218.4	3.78	82.6	285.6	22.4
Poultry: Turkey													
05192	Turkey, breast, meat & skin, roasted 1/2 breast, bone removed	864	546.22	1632.96	248.05	0	0	181.44	1814.4	12.1	544.32	2488.32	233.28
05194	Turkey, leg, meat & skin, roasted 1 leg, bone removed	546	334.1	1135.68	152.17	0	0	174.72	1086.54	12.56	420.42	1528.8	125.58
Nuts, seeds, and related products													
12063	Almonds, dry roasted, unblanched, wo/salt 1 cup whole kernels	138	4.14	810.06	22.54	33.35	18.91	389.16	756.24	5.24	15.18	1062.6	419.52
12085	Cashew nuts, dry roasted, wo/salt 1 cup, halves and whole	137	2.33	786.38	20.97	44.79	4.11	61.65	671.3	8.22	21.92	774.05	356.2
12131	Macadamia nuts, dried 1 oz (11 whole kernels)	28.35	0.82	199.02	2.35	3.89	2.64	19.85	38.56	0.68	1.42	104.33	32.89
12133	Macadamia nuts, oil roasted, wo/salt 1 cup, whole or halves	134	2.24	962.12	9.73	17.29	12.46	60.3	268	2.41	9.38	440.86	156.78
12143	Pecans, dry roasted, wo/salt 1 oz	28.35	0.31	186.83	2.26	6.33	2.64	9.92	86.18	0.62	0.28	104.9	37.71
12152	Pistachio nuts, dry roasted, wo/salt 1 cup	128	2.68	775.68	19.11	35.24	13.82	89.6	609.28	4.06	7.68	1241.6	166.4
12537	Sunflower seed kernels, dry roasted, w/salt 1 cup	128	1.54	744.96	24.74	30.81	11.52	89.6	1478.4	4.86	998.4	1088	165.12
12023	Sesame seeds, whole, dried 1 tablespoon	9	0.42	51.57	1.6	2.11	1.06	87.75	56.61	1.31	0.99	42.12	31.59
12036	Sunflower seed kernels, dried 1 cup, with hulls, edible yield	46	2.47	262.2	10.48	8.63	4.83	53.36	324.3	3.11	1.38	316.94	162.84
12154	Walnuts, black, dried 1 cup, chopped	125	5.45	758.75	30.44	15.13	6.25	72.5	580	3.84	1.25	655	252.5
Seafood													
Fish													
15189	Bluefish, cooked, dry heat 3 oz	85	53.24	135.15	21.84	0	0	7.65	247.35	0.53	65.45	405.45	35.7
15235	Catfish, channel, farmed, cooked, dry heat 3 oz	85	60.84	129.2	15.91	0	0	7.65	208.25	0.7	68	272.85	22.1
15016	Cod, Atlantic, cooked, dry heat 3 oz	85	64.53	89.25	19.41	0	0	11.9	117.3	0.42	66.3	207.4	35.7
15029	Flatfish (flounder & sole sp), cooked, dry heat 3 oz	85	62.19	99.45	20.54	0	0	15.3	245.65	0.29	89.25	292.4	49.3
15032	Grouper, mxd sp, cooked, dry heat 3 oz	85	62.36	100.3	21.11	0	0	17.85	121.55	0.97	45.05	403.75	31.45

NDB #	Zinc	Copper	Vitamin A	Thiamin	Riboflavin	Niacin	Vitamin B6	Folate	Vitamin B12	Vitamin C	Fat	Fat: Saturated	Fat: Monounsaturated	Fat: Polyunsaturated	Cholesterol
	mg	mg	IU	mg	mg	mg	mg	mcg	mcg	mg	gm	gm	gm	gm	mg
05032	1.62	0.07	145.2	0.08	0.16	14.7	0.69	3.96	0.42	0	14.32	4.03	5.62	3.05	110.88
05037	4.16	0.13	335.67	0.11	0.35	10.62	0.52	11.69	0.48	0	26.35	7.3	10.34	5.83	151.97
05028	6.08	0.52	22925	0.21	2.45	6.23	0.81	1078	27.15	22.12	7.63	2.58	1.88	1.26	883.4

Poultry: Duck

NDB #	Zinc	Copper	Vitamin A	Thiamin	Riboflavin	Niacin	Vitamin B6	Folate	Vitamin B12	Vitamin C	Fat	Fat: Saturated	Fat: Monounsaturated	Fat: Polyunsaturated	Cholesterol
05140	2.6	0.32	294	0.24	0.38	6.76	0.25	8.4	0.42	0	39.69	13.54	18.06	5.11	117.6

Poultry: Turkey

NDB #	Zinc	Copper	Vitamin A	Thiamin	Riboflavin	Niacin	Vitamin B6	Folate	Vitamin B12	Vitamin C	Fat	Fat: Saturated	Fat: Monounsaturated	Fat: Polyunsaturated	Cholesterol
05192	17.54	0.41	0	0.49	1.13	54.99	4.15	51.84	3.11	0	64.02	18.14	21.17	15.55	639.36
05194	23.31	0.84	0	0.33	1.32	19.44	1.8	49.14	1.97	0	53.62	16.71	15.67	14.85	464.1

Nuts, seeds, and related products

NDB #	Zinc	Copper	Vitamin A	Thiamin	Riboflavin	Niacin	Vitamin B6	Folate	Vitamin B12	Vitamin C	Fat	Fat: Saturated	Fat: Monounsaturated	Fat: Polyunsaturated	Cholesterol
12063	6.76	1.69	0	0.18	0.83	3.89	0.1	88.04	0	0.97	71.21	6.75	46.24	14.94	0
12085	7.67	3.04	0	0.27	0.27	1.92	0.35	94.8	0	0	63.5	12.55	37.42	10.74	0
12131	0.48	0.08	0	0.1	0.03	0.61	0.06	4.45	0	0	20.9	3.13	16.49	0.36	0
12133	1.47	0.4	12.06	0.29	0.15	2.71	0.27	21.31	0	0	102.54	15.35	80.91	1.77	0
12143	1.61	0.35	37.71	0.09	0.03	0.26	0.06	11.54	0	0.57	18.31	1.47	11.42	4.53	0
12152	1.74	1.55	304.64	0.54	0.31	1.8	0.33	75.65	0	9.34	67.61	8.56	45.64	10.22	0
12537	6.77	2.34	0	0.14	0.31	9.01	1.03	303.87	0	1.79	63.74	6.68	12.17	42.09	0
12023	0.7	0.37	0.81	0.07	0.02	0.41	0.07	8.7	0	0	4.47	0.63	1.69	1.96	0
12036	2.33	0.81	23	1.05	0.12	2.07	0.35	104.6	0	0.64	22.8	2.39	4.35	15.06	0
12154	4.28	1.28	370	0.27	0.14	0.86	0.69	81.88	0	4	70.73	4.54	15.91	46.87	0

Seafood

Fish

NDB #	Zinc	Copper	Vitamin A	Thiamin	Riboflavin	Niacin	Vitamin B6	Folate	Vitamin B12	Vitamin C	Fat	Fat: Saturated	Fat: Monounsaturated	Fat: Polyunsaturated	Cholesterol
15189	0.88	0.06	390.15	0.06	0.08	6.16	0.39	1.7	5.29	0	4.62	1	1.95	1.15	64.6
15235	0.89	0.1	42.5	0.36	0.06	2.14	0.14	5.95	2.38	0.68	6.82	1.52	3.53	1.18	54.4
15016	0.49	0.03	39.1	0.07	0.07	2.14	0.24	6.89	0.89	0.85	0.73	0.14	0.11	0.25	46.75
15029	0.54	0.02	32.3	0.07	0.1	1.85	0.2	7.82	2.13	0	1.3	0.31	0.2	0.55	57.8
15032	0.43	0.04	140.25	0.07	0.01	0.32	0.3	8.67	0.59	0	1.11	0.25	0.23	0.34	39.95

NDB #	Description & Serving	Grams	Water	Calories	Protein	Carbohydrates	Fiber	Calcium	Phosphorus	Iron	Sodium	Potassium	Magnesium
		gm	gm	kcal	gm	gm	gm	mg	mg	mg	mg	mg	mg
15041	**Herring, Atlantic, pickled** 1 oz, boneless	28.35	15.65	74.28	4.02	2.73	0	21.83	25.23	0.35	246.65	19.56	2.27
15069	**Pompano, Florida, cooked, dry heat** 3 oz	85	53.52	179.35	20.14	0	0	36.55	289.85	0.57	64.6	540.6	26.35
15209	**Salmon, Atlantic, wild, cooked, dry heat** 3 oz	85	50.68	154.7	21.62	0	0	12.75	217.6	0.88	47.6	533.8	31.45
15212	**Salmon, pink, cooked, dry heat** 3 oz	85	59.23	126.65	21.73	0	0	14.45	250.75	0.84	73.1	351.9	28.05
15086	**Salmon, sockeye, cooked, dry heat** 3 oz	85	52.56	183.6	23.21	0	0	5.95	234.6	0.47	56.1	318.75	26.35
15088	**Sardine, Atlantic, canned in oil, drained sol w/bone** 1 oz	28.35	16.9	58.97	6.98	0	0	108.3	138.92	0.83	143.17	112.55	11.06
15102	**Snapper, mxd sp, cooked, dry heat** 3 oz	85	59.8	108.8	22.36	0	0	34	170.85	0.2	48.45	443.7	31.45
15111	**Swordfish, cooked, dry heat** 3 oz	85	58.44	131.75	21.58	0	0	5.1	286.45	0.88	97.75	313.65	28.9
15116	**Trout, rainbow, wild, cooked, dry heat** 3 oz	85	59.93	127.5	19.48	0	0	73.1	228.65	0.32	47.6	380.8	26.35
15118	**Tuna, fresh, bluefin, cooked, dry heat** 3 oz	85	50.23	156.4	25.42	0	0	8.5	277.1	1.11	42.5	274.55	54.4
15221	**Tuna, yellowfin, fresh, cooked, dry heat** 3 oz	85	53.39	118.15	25.47	0	0	17.85	208.25	0.8	39.95	483.65	54.4
	Shellfish												
15159	**Clam, mxd sp, cooked, moist heat** 20 small clams	190	120.92	281.2	48.55	9.75	0	174.8	642.2	53.12	212.8	1193.2	34.2
15137	**Crab, Alaska king, cooked, moist heat** 1 leg	134	103.92	129.98	25.93	0	0	79.06	375.2	1.02	1436.48	351.08	84.42
15148	**Lobster, northern, cooked, moist heat** 3 oz	85	64.63	83.3	17.43	1.09	0	51.85	157.25	0.33	323	299.2	29.75
15165	**Mussel, blue, cooked, moist heat** 3 oz	85	51.98	146.2	20.23	6.28	0	28.05	242.25	5.71	313.65	227.8	31.45
15167	**Oyster, eastern, wild, raw** 6 medium	84	71.53	57.12	5.92	3.28	0	37.8	113.4	5.59	177.24	131.04	39.48
15171	**Oyster, Pacific, raw** 3 oz	85	69.75	68.85	8.03	4.21	0	6.8	137.7	4.34	90.1	142.8	18.7
15173	**Scallop, mxd sp, cooked, breaded & fried** 2 large scallops	31	18.12	66.65	5.6	3.14	0	13.02	73.16	0.25	143.84	103.23	18.29
15151	**Shrimp, mxd sp, cooked, moist heat** 4 large	22	17	21.78	4.6	0	0	8.58	30.14	0.68	49.28	40.04	7.48
	Vegetables and vegetable juices												
11008	**Artichokes (globe or French), cooked, boiled, drained, wo/salt** 1 medium artichoke	120	100.76	60	4.18	13.42	6.48	54	103.2	1.55	114	424.8	72
11011	**Asparagus, raw** 1 small spear (5" long or less)	12	11.09	2.76	0.27	0.54	0.25	2.52	6.72	0.1	0.24	32.76	2.16
11053	**Beans, snap, green, cooked, boiled, drained, wo/salt** 1 cup	125	111.53	43.75	2.36	9.86	4	57.5	48.75	1.6	3.75	373.75	31.25
11081	**Beets, cooked, boiled, drained** 1/2 cup slices	85	74	37.4	1.43	8.47	1.7	13.6	32.3	0.67	65.45	259.25	19.55

NDB #	Zinc	Copper	Vitamin A	Thiamin	Riboflavin	Niacin	Vitamin B6	Folate	Vitamin B12	Vitamin C	Fat	Fat. Saturated	Fat. Monounsaturated	Fat. Polyunsaturated	Cholesterol
	mg	mg	IU	mg	mg	mg	mg	mcg	mcg	mg	gm	gm	gm	gm	mg
15041	0.15	0.03	244.09	0.01	0.04	0.94	0.05	0.68	1.21	0	5.1	0.68	3.39	0.48	3.69
15069	0.59	0.07	102	0.58	0.13	3.23	0.2	14.71	1.02	0	10.32	3.82	2.82	1.24	54.4
15209	0.7	0.27	37.4	0.23	0.41	8.57	0.8	24.65	2.59	0	6.91	1.07	2.29	2.77	60.35
15212	0.6	0.08	115.6	0.17	0.06	7.25	0.2	4.25	2.94	0	3.76	0.61	1.02	1.47	56.95
15086	0.43	0.06	177.65	0.18	0.15	5.67	0.19	4.25	4.93	0	9.32	1.63	4.5	2.05	73.95
15088	0.37	0.05	63.5	0.02	0.06	1.49	0.05	3.35	2.53	0	3.25	0.43	1.1	1.46	40.26
15102	0.37	0.04	97.75	0.05	0	0.29	0.39	4.93	2.98	1.36	1.46	0.31	0.27	0.5	39.95
15111	1.25	0.14	116.45	0.04	0.1	10.02	0.32	1.96	1.72	0.94	4.37	1.2	1.68	1	42.5
15116	0.43	0.05	42.5	0.13	0.08	4.9	0.29	16.15	5.36	1.7	4.95	1.38	1.48	1.56	58.65
15118	0.65	0.09	2142	0.24	0.26	8.96	0.45	1.87	9.25	0	5.34	1.37	1.75	1.57	41.65
15221	0.57	0.07	57.8	0.43	0.05	10.15	0.88	1.7	0.51	0.85	1.04	0.26	0.17	0.31	49.3
Shellfish															
15159	5.19	1.31	1083	0.29	0.81	6.37	0.21	54.72	187.89	41.99	3.71	0.36	0.33	1.05	127.3
15137	10.21	1.58	38.86	0.07	0.07	1.8	0.24	68.34	15.41	10.18	2.06	0.18	0.25	0.72	71.02
15148	2.48	1.65	73.95	0.01	0.06	0.91	0.07	9.44	2.64	0	0.5	0.09	0.14	0.08	61.2
15165	2.27	0.13	258.4	0.26	0.36	2.55	0.09	64.26	20.4	11.56	3.81	0.72	0.86	1.03	47.6
15167	76.28	3.74	84	0.08	0.08	1.16	0.05	8.4	16.35	3.11	2.07	0.65	0.26	0.81	44.52
15171	14.13	1.34	229.5	0.06	0.2	1.71	0.04	8.5	13.6	6.8	1.96	0.43	0.3	0.76	42.5
15173	0.33	0.02	23.25	0.01	0.03	0.47	0.04	5.64	0.41	0.71	3.39	0.83	1.39	0.89	18.91
15151	0.34	0.04	48.18	0.01	0.01	0.57	0.03	0.77	0.33	0.48	0.24	0.06	0.04	0.1	42.9
Vegetables and vegetable juices															
11008	0.59	0.28	212.4	0.08	0.08	1.2	0.13	61.2	0	12	0.19	0.04	0.01	0.08	0
11011	0.06	0.02	69.96	0.02	0.02	0.14	0.02	15.36	0	1.58	0.02	0.01	0	0.01	0
11053	0.45	0.13	832.5	0.09	0.12	0.77	0.07	41.63	0	12.13	0.35	0.08	0.01	0.18	0
11081	0.3	0.06	29.75	0.02	0.03	0.28	0.06	68	0	3.06	0.15	0.02	0.03	0.05	0

NDB #	Description & Serving	Grams	Water	Calories	Protein	Carbohydrates	Fiber	Calcium	Phosphorus	Iron	Sodium	Potassium	Magnesium
		gm	gm	kcal	gm	gm	gm	mg	mg	mg	mg	mg	mg
11090	**Broccoli, raw** 1 cup, flowerets	71	64.39	19.88	2.12	3.72	2.13	34.08	46.86	0.62	19.17	230.75	17.75
11099	**Brussels sprouts, cooked, boiled, drained, wo/salt** 1/2 cup	78	68.11	30.42	1.99	6.76	2.03	28.08	43.68	0.94	16.38	247.26	15.6
11109	**Cabbage, raw** 1 cup, shredded	70	64.51	17.5	1.01	3.8	1.61	32.9	16.1	0.41	12.6	172.2	10.5
11113	**Cabbage, red, cooked, boiled, drained, wo/salt** 1/2 cup shredded	75	70.2	15.75	0.79	3.48	1.5	27.75	21.75	0.26	6	105	8.25
11115	**Cabbage, savoy, cooked, boiled, drained, wo/salt** 1 cup, shredded	145	133.4	34.8	2.61	7.84	4.06	43.5	47.85	0.55	34.8	266.8	34.8
11124	**Carrots, raw** 1 cup, grated	110	96.57	47.3	1.13	11.15	3.3	29.7	48.4	0.55	38.5	355.3	16.5
11960	**Carrots, baby, raw** 1 medium	10	8.98	3.8	0.08	0.82	0.18	2.3	3.8	0.08	3.5	27.9	1.2
11135	**Cauliflower, raw** 1 cup	100	91.91	25	1.98	5.2	2.5	22	44	0.44	30	303	15
11143	**Celery, raw** 1 cup, diced	120	113.57	19.2	0.9	4.38	2.04	48	30	0.48	104.4	344.4	13.2
11162	**Collards, cooked, boiled, drained, wo/salt** 1 cup, chopped	190	174.53	51.3	2.57	11.65	5.32	43.7	15.2	0.3	30.4	248.9	13.3
11168	**Corn, swt, yellow, cooked, boiled, drained, wo/salt** 1 baby ear	8	5.57	8.64	0.27	2.01	0.22	0.16	8.24	0.05	1.36	19.92	2.56
11205	**Cucumber, with peel, raw** 1/2 cup slices	52	49.93	6.76	0.36	1.44	0.42	7.28	10.4	0.14	1.04	74.88	5.72
11210	**Eggplant, cooked, boiled, drained, wo/salt** 1 cup (1" cubes)	99	90.85	27.72	0.82	6.57	2.48	5.94	21.78	0.35	2.97	245.52	12.87
11213	**Endive, raw** 1/2 cup, chopped	25	23.45	4.25	0.31	0.84	0.78	13	7	0.21	5.5	78.5	3.75
11234	**Kale, cooked, boiled, drained, wo/salt** 1 cup, chopped	130	118.56	41.6	2.47	7.32	2.6	93.6	36.4	1.17	29.9	296.4	23.4
11242	**Kohlrabi, cooked, boiled, drained, wo/salt** 1 cup, sliced	165	149	47.85	2.97	11.04	1.82	41.25	74.25	0.66	34.65	561	31.35
11247	**Leeks (bulb & lower leaf-portion), cooked, boiled, drained, wo/salt** 1/4 cup chopped or diced	26	23.61	8.06	0.21	1.98	0.26	7.8	4.42	0.29	2.6	22.62	3.64
11250	**Lettuce, butterhead (incl Boston & bibb types), raw** 1 cup, shredded or chopped	55	52.57	7.15	0.71	1.28	0.55	17.6	12.65	0.17	2.75	141.35	7.15
11251	**Lettuce, cos or romaine, raw** 1/2 cup shredded	28	26.57	4.48	0.45	0.66	0.48	10.08	12.6	0.31	2.24	81.2	1.68
11252	**Lettuce, iceberg (incl crisphead types), raw** 1 cup, shredded or chopped	55	52.74	6.6	0.56	1.15	0.77	10.45	11	0.28	4.95	86.9	4.95
11253	**Lettuce, looseleaf, raw** 1/2 cup shredded	28	26.32	5.04	0.36	0.98	0.53	19.04	7	0.39	2.52	73.92	3.08
11260	**Mushrooms, raw** 1 cup, whole	96	88.14	24	2.01	4.46	1.15	4.8	99.84	1.19	3.84	355.2	9.6
11950	**Mushrooms, enoki, raw** 1 large	5	4.47	1.7	0.12	0.35	0.13	0.05	5.65	0.04	0.15	19.05	0.8
11268	**Mushrooms, shiitake, dried** 1 mushroom	3.6	0.34	10.66	0.34	2.71	0.41	0.4	10.58	0.06	0.47	55.22	4.75

NDB #	Zinc	Copper	Vitamin A	Thiamin	Riboflavin	Niacin	Vitamin B6	Folate	Vitamin B12	Vitamin C	Fat	Fat, Saturated	Fat, Monounsaturated	Fat, Polyunsaturated	Cholesterol
	mg	mg	IU	mg	mg	mg	mg	mcg	mcg	mg	gm	gm	gm	gm	mg
11090	0.28	0.03	1094.82	0.05	0.08	0.45	0.11	50.41	0	66.17	0.25	0.04	0.02	0.12	0
11099	0.26	0.06	560.82	0.08	0.06	0.47	0.14	46.8	0	48.36	0.4	0.08	0.03	0.2	0
11109	0.13	0.02	93.1	0.04	0.03	0.21	0.07	30.1	0	22.54	0.19	0.02	0.01	0.09	0
11113	0.11	0.05	20.25	0.03	0.02	0.15	0.11	9.45	0	25.8	0.15	0.02	0.01	0.07	0
11115	0.33	0.08	1289.05	0.07	0.03	0.03	0.22	67.14	0	24.65	0.13	0.02	0.01	0.06	0
11124	0.22	0.05	30941.9	0.11	0.06	1.02	0.16	15.4	0	10.23	0.21	0.03	0.01	0.08	0
11960	0.02	0	197.2	0	0.01	0.09	0.01	3.3	0	0.84	0.05	0.01	0	0.03	0
11135	0.28	0.04	19	0.06	0.06	0.53	0.22	57	0	46.4	0.21	0.03	0.01	0.1	0
11143	0.16	0.04	160.8	0.06	0.05	0.39	0.1	33.6	0	8.4	0.17	0.04	0.03	0.08	0
11162	0.21	0.06	5181.3	0.04	0.1	0.55	0.1	11.4	0	22.99	0.36	0.05	0.03	0.17	0
11168	0.04	0	17.36	0.02	0.01	0.13	0	3.71	0	0.5	0.1	0.02	0.03	0.05	0
11205	0.1	0.02	111.8	0.01	0.01	0.11	0.02	6.76	0	2.76	0.07	0.02	0	0.03	0
11210	0.15	0.11	63.36	0.08	0.02	0.59	0.09	14.26	0	1.29	0.23	0.04	0.02	0.09	0
11213	0.2	0.02	512.5	0.02	0.02	0.1	0.01	35.5	0	1.63	0.05	0.01	0	0.02	0
11234	0.31	0.2	9620	0.07	0.09	0.65	0.18	17.29	0	53.3	0.52	0.07	0.04	0.25	0
11242	0.51	0.22	57.75	0.07	0.03	0.64	0.25	19.97	0	89.1	0.18	0.02	0.01	0.09	0
11247	0.02	0.02	11.96	0.01	0.01	0.05	0.03	6.32	0	1.09	0.05	0.01	0	0.03	0
11250	0.09	0.01	533.5	0.03	0.03	0.17	0.03	40.32	0	4.4	0.12	0.02	0	0.06	0
11251	0.07	0.01	728	0.03	0.03	0.14	0.01	38	0	6.72	0.06	0.01	0	0.03	0
11252	0.12	0.02	181.5	0.03	0.02	0.1	0.02	30.8	0	2.15	0.1	0.01	0	0.06	0
11253	0.08	0.01	532	0.01	0.02	0.11	0.02	13.94	0	5.04	0.08	0.01	0	0.04	0
11260	0.7	0.47	0	0.1	0.43	3.95	0.09	20.26	0	3.36	0.4	0.05	0.01	0.16	0
11950	0.03	0	0.35	0	0.01	0.18	0	1.5	0	0.6	0.02	0	0	0.01	0
11268	0.28	0.19	0	0.01	0.05	0.51	0.03	5.88	0	0.13	0.04	0.01	0.01	0.01	0

NDB #	Description & Serving	Grams	Water	Calories	Protein	Carbohydrates	Fiber	Calcium	Phosphorus	Iron	Sodium	Potassium	Magnesium
		gm	gm	kcal	gm	gm	gm	mg	mg	mg	mg	mg	mg
11269	Mushrooms, shiitake, cooked, wo/salt 1 cup (pieces)	145	121.05	79.75	2.26	20.71	3.05	4.35	42.05	0.64	5.8	169.65	20.3
11282	Onions, raw 1 cup, chopped	160	143.49	60.8	1.86	13.81	2.88	32	52.8	0.35	4.8	251.2	16
11283	Onions, cooked, boiled, drained, wo/salt 1 cup	210	184.51	92.4	2.86	21.32	2.94	46.2	73.5	0.5	6.3	348.6	23.1
11291	Onions, spring (incl tops & bulb), raw 1 tablespoon, chopped	6	5.39	1.92	0.11	0.44	0.16	4.32	2.22	0.09	0.96	16.56	1.2
11297	Parsley, raw 1 cup	60	52.63	21.6	1.78	3.8	1.98	82.8	34.8	3.72	33.6	332.4	30
11305	Peas, green, cooked, boiled, drained, wo/salt 1 cup	160	124.59	134.4	8.58	25.02	8.8	43.2	187.2	2.46	4.8	433.6	62.4
11333	Peppers, sweet, green, raw 1 cup, chopped	149	137.36	40.23	1.33	9.58	2.68	13.41	28.31	0.69	2.98	263.73	14.9
11951	Peppers, sweet, yellow, raw 10 strips	52	47.85	14.04	0.52	3.29	0.47	5.72	12.48	0.24	1.04	110.24	6.24
11363	Potatoes, baked, flesh, wo/salt 1 potato (2-1/3" x 4-3/4")	156	117.66	145.08	3.06	33.63	2.34	7.8	78	0.55	7.8	609.96	39
11364	Potatoes, baked, skin, wo/salt 1 potato skin	58	27.44	114.84	2.49	26.72	4.58	19.72	58.58	4.08	12.18	332.34	24.94
11365	Potatoes, boiled, cooked in skin, flesh, wo/salt 1 potato (2-1/2" dia, sphere)	136	104.69	118.32	2.54	27.38	2.45	6.8	59.84	0.42	5.44	515.44	29.92
11429	Radishes, raw 1 cup, slices	116	110.01	19.72	0.7	4.16	1.86	24.36	20.88	0.34	27.84	269.12	10.44
11458	Spinach, cooked, boiled, drained, wo/salt 1 cup	180	164.18	41.4	5.35	6.75	4.32	244.8	100.8	6.43	126	838.8	156.6
11480	Squash, summer, zucchini, incl skin, frz, cooked, boiled, drained, wo/salt 1 cup	223	211.27	37.91	2.56	7.94	2.9	37.91	55.75	1.07	4.46	432.62	28.99
11483	Squash, winter, acorn, cooked, baked, wo/salt 1 cup, cubes	205	169.95	114.8	2.3	29.89	9.02	90.2	92.25	1.91	8.2	895.85	88.15
11486	Squash, winter, butternut, cooked, baked, wo/salt 1 cup, cubes	205	179.99	82	1.85	21.5	0	84.05	55.35	1.23	8.2	582.2	59.45
11490	Squash, winter, hubbard, cooked, baked, wo/salt 1 cup, cubes	205	174.46	102.5	5.08	22.16	0	34.85	47.15	0.96	16.4	733.9	45.1
11496	Succotash (corn & limas), cooked, boiled, drained, wo/salt 1 cup	192	131.27	220.8	9.73	46.81	8.64	32.64	224.64	2.92	32.64	787.2	101.76
11508	Sweet potato, cooked, baked in skin, wo/salt 1 large	180	131.13	185.4	3.1	43.69	5.4	50.4	99	0.81	18	626.4	36
11529	Tomatoes, red, ripe, raw, year-round average 1 cup, chopped or sliced	180	168.77	37.8	1.53	8.35	1.98	9	43.2	0.81	16.2	399.6	19.8
11530	Tomatoes, red, ripe, cooked, boiled, wo/salt 2 medium	246	226.71	66.42	2.63	14.34	2.46	14.76	76.26	1.38	27.06	686.34	34.44

NDB #	Zinc	Copper	Vitamin A	Thiamin	Riboflavin	Niacin	Vitamin B6	Folate	Vitamin B12	Vitamin C	Fat	Fat: Saturated	Fat: Monounsaturated	Fat: Polyunsaturated	Cholesterol
	mg	mg	IU	mg	mg	mg	mg	mcg	mcg	mg	gm	gm	gm	gm	mg
11269	1.93	1.3	0	0.05	0.25	2.18	0.23	30.31	0	0.44	0.32	0.08	0.1	0.04	0
11282	0.3	0.1	0	0.07	0.03	0.24	0.19	30.4	0	10.24	0.26	0.04	0.04	0.1	0
11283	0.44	0.14	0	0.09	0.05	0.35	0.27	31.5	0	10.92	0.4	0.07	0.06	0.15	0
11291	0.02	0	23.1	0	0	0.03	0	3.84	0	1.13	0.01	0	0	0	0
11297	0.64	0.09	3120	0.05	0.06	0.79	0.05	91.2	0	79.8	0.47	0.08	0.18	0.07	0
11305	1.9	0.28	955.2	0.41	0.24	3.23	0.35	101.28	0	22.72	0.35	0.06	0.03	0.16	0
11333	0.18	0.1	941.68	0.1	0.04	0.76	0.37	32.78	0	133.06	0.28	0.04	0.02	0.15	0
11951	0.09	0.06	123.76	0.01	0.01	0.46	0.09	13.52	0	95.42	0.11	0	0	0	0
11363	0.45	0.34	0	0.16	0.03	2.18	0.47	14.2	0	19.97	0.16	0.04	0	0.07	0
11364	0.28	0.47	0	0.07	0.06	1.78	0.36	12.53	0	7.83	0.06	0.02	0	0.02	0
11365	0.41	0.26	0	0.14	0.03	1.96	0.41	13.6	0	17.68	0.14	0.04	0	0.06	0
11429	0.35	0.05	9.28	0.01	0.05	0.35	0.08	31.32	0	26.45	0.63	0.03	0.02	0.05	0
11458	1.37	0.31	14742	0.17	0.42	0.88	0.44	262.44	0	17.64	0.47	0.08	0.01	0.19	0
11480	0.45	0.1	963.36	0.09	0.09	0.86	0.1	17.39	0	8.25	0.29	0.06	0.02	0.12	0
11483	0.35	0.18	877.4	0.34	0.03	1.81	0.4	38.34	0	22.14	0.29	0.06	0.02	0.12	0
11486	0.27	0.13	14352.05	0.15	0.03	1.99	0.25	39.36	0	30.96	0.18	0.04	0.01	0.08	0
11490	0.31	0.09	12371.75	0.15	0.1	1.14	0.35	33.21	0	19.48	1.27	0.26	0.09	0.53	0
11496	1.21	0.34	564.48	0.32	0.18	2.55	0.22	62.98	0	15.74	1.54	0.28	0.3	0.73	0
11508	0.52	0.37	39279.6	0.13	0.23	1.09	0.43	40.68	0	44.28	0.2	0.04	0.01	0.09	0
11529	0.16	0.13	1121.4	0.11	0.09	1.13	0.14	27	0	34.38	0.59	0.08	0.09	0.24	0
11530	0.27	0.23	1827.78	0.17	0.14	1.84	0.23	31.98	0	56.09	1.01	0.14	0.15	0.42	0

Index

• *C* •

• *B* •

• G •

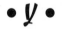

• Z •

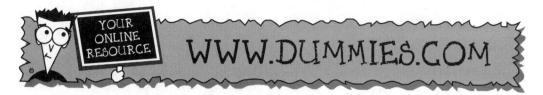

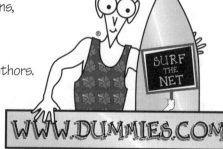

IDG BOOKS WORLDWIDE
BOOK REGISTRATION

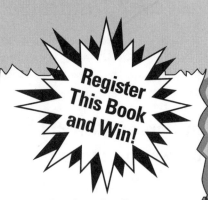

We want to hear from you!

Visit **http://my2cents.dummies.com** to register this book and tell us how you liked it!

✔ Get entered in our monthly prize giveaway.

✔ Give us feedback about this book — tell us what you like best, what you like least, or maybe what you'd like to ask the author and us to change!

✔ Let us know any other ...*For Dummies*® topics that interest you.

Your feedback helps us determine what books to publish, tells us what coverage to add as we revise our books, and lets us know whether we're meeting your needs as a ...*For Dummies* reader. You're our most valuable resource, and what you have to say is important to us!

Not on the Web yet? It's easy to get started with *Dummies 101*®: *The Internet For Windows*® *98* or *The Internet For Dummies*®, 6th Edition, at local retailers everywhere.

Or let us know what you think by sending us a letter at the following address:

...*For Dummies* Book Registration
Dummies Press
10475 Crosspoint Blvd.
Indianapolis, IN 46256

™

**BESTSELLING
BOOK SERIES**